Exacerbations of Asthma

Exacerbations of Asthma

Editors

Sebastian L Johnston MBBS PhD FRCP
Professor of Respiratory Medicine
National Heart and Lung Institute
Imperial College London, London, UK

Paul M O'Byrne MB FRCPI FRCP (C) FRCPE
Firestone Institute for Respiratory Health
Hamilton, ON, Canada

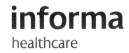

informa
healthcare

First published in 2007 by Informa Healthcare, Telephone House, 69-77 Paul Street, London EC2A 4LQ, UK.

Simultaneously published in the USA by Informa Healthcare, 52 Vanderbilt Avenue, 7th Floor, New York, NY 10017, USA.

Informa Healthcare is a trading division of Informa UK Ltd. Registered Office: 37–41 Mortimer Street, London W1T 3JH, UK. Registered in England and Wales number 1072954.

A CIP record for this book is available from the British Library.

Library of Congress Cataloging-in-Publication Data available on application

ISBN-13: 9781842143186

Orders may be sent to: Informa Healthcare, Sheepen Place, Colchester, Essex CO3 3LP, UK
Telephone: +44 (0)20 7017 5540
Email: CSDhealthcarebooks@informa.com
Website: http://informahealthcarebooks.com/

For corporate sales please contact: CorporateBooksIHC@informa.com
For foreign rights please contact: RightsIHC@informa.com
For reprint permissions please contact: PermissionsIHC@informa.com

Contents

Contributors

Simon Bourne MBBS MRCP
Queen Alexandra Hospital, Portsmouth, UK

William W Busse MD
Department of Medicine, University of
Wisconsin School of Medicine and Public
Health, Madison, WI, USA

Anoop J Chauhan MB ChB FRCP PhD
St Mary's Hospital, Portsmouth, UK

Marco Contoli
Department of Clinical and Experimental
Medicine, Research Centre on Asthma and
COPD, University of Ferrara, Ferrara, Italy

Azzeddine Dakhama PhD
Department of Pediatrics, National Jewish
Medical and Research Center, Denver, CO, USA

Donna E Davies
Brooke Laboratories, University of
Southampton, Southampton, UK

Jeffrey M Drazen MD
Harvard Medical School, Boston, MA, USA

M Patricia Fabian MS
Department of Environmental Health, Harvard
School of Public Health, Boston, MA, USA

John V Fahy MD
Pulmonary Division, Department of
Medicine/Cardiovascular Research Institute,
University of California, San Francisco,
CA, USA

Erwin W Gelfand MD
Department of Pediatrics, National
Jewish Medical and Research Center,
Denver, CO, USA

James E Gern MD
University of Wisconsin-Madison, Madison,
WI, USA

Peter G Gibson MBBS FRACP
Hunter Medical Research Institute,
John Hunter Hospital, New Lambton,
Australia

Brian DW Harrison MA MB BChir FRCP
Department of Respiratory Medicine,
Norfolk and Norwich University Hospital,
and Honorary Professor in School
of Medicine at the University of
East Anglia, Norwich, UK

Stephen T Holgate MD MRCP FRCPath
Brooke Laboratories, University of
Southampton, Southampton, UK

Anh L Innes MD
Department of Medicine/Cardiovascular
Research Institute, University of California,
San Francisco, CA, USA

Neil W Johnston MSc
Firestone Institute for Respiratory Health
and Department of Medicine, Faculty of
Health Sciences, McMaster University,
Hamilton, ON, Canada

Sebastian L Johnston MBBS PhD FRCP
National Heart and Lung Institute, Imperial
College London, London, UK

Vasile Laza-Stanca MD
Department of Respiratory Medicine,
National Heart and Lung Institute,
Imperial College London, London, UK

Todd A Lee PharmD PhD
Midwest Center for Health Services
and Policy Research, Hines VA Hospital,
Hines, IL, USA

Robert F Lemanske Jr MD
Division of Pediatric Allergy, Immunology,
and Rheumatology, University of Wisconsin
School of Medicine and Public Health,
Madison, WI, USA

James J McDevitt PhD MHS CIH
Department of Environmental Health, Harvard
School of Public Health, Boston, MA, USA

Simon Message MB BSc MRCP
Department of Respiratory Medicine,
National Heart and Lung Institute,
Imperial College London, London, UK

Donald K Milton MD DrPH
Department of Work Environment,
School of Health and Environment,
University of Massachusetts, Lowell and
Department of Environmental Health,
Harvard School of Public Health,
Boston, MA, USA

Paul M O'Byrne MB FRCPI FRCP(C) FRCPE
Firestone Institute for Respiratory Health,
Hamilton, ON, Canada

Alberto Papi
Department of Clinical and Experimental
Medicine, Research Centre on Asthma and
COPD, University of Ferrara, Ferrara, Italy

Giovanni Piedimonte MD
Department of Pediatrics, West Virginia
University School of Medicine and WVU
Children's Hospital, Morgantown, WV, USA

Heather Powell MMedSci (Clin Epi)
Respiratory and Sleep Medicine, John Hunter
Hospital, Newcastle, Australia

Helen K Reddel MBBS PhD FRACP
Woolcock Institute of Medical Research,
Camperdown, Australia

Malcolm R Sears MB ChB
Firestone Institute for Respiratory Health, and
Department of Medicine, Faculty of Health
Sciences, McMaster University, Hamilton,
ON, Canada

Malcolm G Semple PhD BMBCh MRCPCH PGCMedEd
School of Reproductive and Developmental
Medicine, University of Liverpool,
Liverpool, UK

Jane R Smith PGDip BSC
School of Medicine, University of East Anglia,
Norwich, UK

Rosalind L Smyth MA MBBS MD FRCPCH FMedSci
School of Reproductive and
Developmental Medicine,
University of Liverpool, Liverpool, UK

Luminita A Stanciu MD PhD
Department of Respiratory Medicine, National
Heart and Lung Institute, Imperial College
London, London, UK

William W Storms MD
University of Colorado Health Sciences
Center, Denver, CO, USA

Anne E Tattersfield MD FRCP FmedSci
Division of Respiratory Medicine, Nottingham
University Hospital, Nottingham, UK

Sara J Uekert MD
Department of Medicine, University of
Wisconsin Medical School, Madison, WI, USA

Stephen D Vincent MBBS
Woolcock Institute of Medical Research,
Camperdown, Australia

Peter AB Wark
Brooke Laboratories, University of
Southampton, Southampton, UK

Preface

Asthma is the most common chronic respiratory condition, now affecting approximately 1 in 5 adults and children in westernized countries. Currently available treatments such as inhaled steroids and long-acting β-agonists are very successful at treating the great majority of these, but leave one aspect of the disease poorly treated, namely acute exacerbations. Unfortunately, despite use of the best available current therapies, the majority of acute exacerbations continue to occur. This strongly suggests that available therapies fail to address the pathogenesis of acute exacerbations adequately.

Acute exacerbations are also, unfortunately, the major cause of morbidity, mortality and health-care costs associated with asthma. The importance of exacerbations is clearly recognized by their being the primary outcome variable in the majority of clinical trials, investigating current and new therapies in the treatment of asthma.

In the past 10 years or so, we have fortunately begun to understand a great deal more about the risk factors and causes of acute exacerbations, though of course, much remains to be learned. We can be fairly certain that the great majority of exacerbations are precipitated by virus infections, often in concert with high exposure to an allergen that the patient is sensitized to. Recent evidence also suggests that atypical bacterial infections may contribute. Given this increased focus on the importance of exacerbations and our improving understanding, we feel the time has come for a major thrust in asthma research to further address the causes and pathogenesis of these distressing events so that we can develop and study new therapies that better address the causes and mechanisms of exacerbations.

We therefore feel it is timely to bring together world experts on asthma exacerbations to summarize our current state of knowledge and provide guidance on directions that future research should take. For this reason we are proud to present this volume entitled *Exacerbations of Asthma* in which we consider the epidemiology and pathophysiology in exacerbations, describe the *in vitro* and *in vivo* experimental models available to study mechanisms of exacerbations and consider treatment and prevention strategies, including of course, delivery of care. We hope very much that you find the contents stimulating and that this volume will provoke further efforts to research the etiology and pathogenesis and will lead to the development of new treatments to prevent and treat acute attacks of asthma more effectively.

Sebastian L Johnston
Paul M O'Byrne

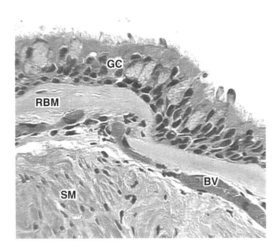

Color Plate I Airway pathology in asthma is depicted in this photomicrograph of a section from an endobronchial biopsy taken during bronchoscopy from a subject with mild chronic asthma. Goblet cell (GC) hyperplasia, reticular basement membrane (RBM) fibrosis, smooth muscle (SM) hypertrophy and blood vessel (BV) engorgement are shown. (Hematoxylin and eosin stain)

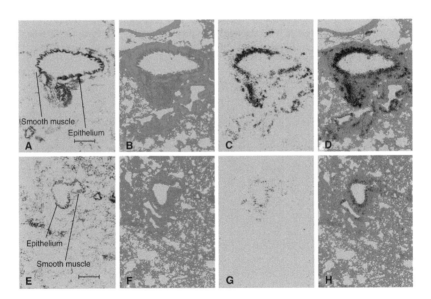

Color Plate II Autoradiographic mapping of substance P (SP) binding sites in the lungs of respiratory syncytial virus (RSV)-infected (A-B-C-D) and pathogen-free (E-F-G-H) rats 5 days after inoculation. The illustration shows, from left to right: schematic diagrams (A and E), hematoxylin/eosin (H&E) preparations (B and F), autoradiographic images (C and G) and autoradiography digitally superimposed on H&E (D and H). Specific SP binding was detected over the bronchial mucosa and the wall of adjacent pulmonary vessels and was consistently and markedly increased in infected airways. No significant binding was detected over the airway smooth muscle and the alveolar tissue. Internal scale, 0.5 mm. Reproduced with permission from reference 95, Chapter 9

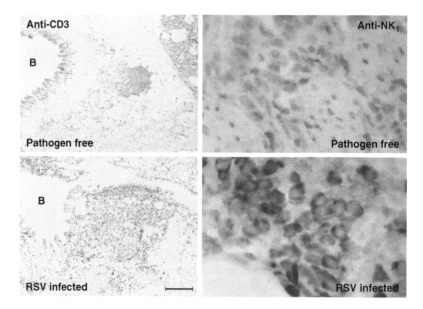

Color Plate III   Lung sections from rats sacrificed 5 days after the intratracheal inoculation of virus-free medium (upper panels) or respiratory syncytial virus (RSV) (lower panels). Immunoperoxidase staining was performed using antibodies specific for the all-T antigen CD3 (left panels) and the high-affinity substance P receptor NK_1 (right panels). The dark-brown reaction reveals predominance of T cells in the hypertrophic bronchus-associated lymphoid tissue of RSV-infected airways with strong overexpression of the NK_1 receptor on discrete lymphocyte subpopulations. Internal scale, 40 µm. Reproduced with permission from reference 102, Chapter 9

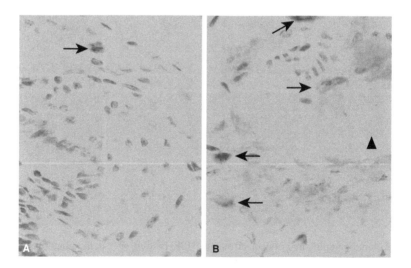

Color Plate IV   Mast cells–nerve interactions. Lung sections from weanling rats sacrificed 5 days after the intranasal inoculation of virus-free medium (A) or respiratory syncytial virus (RSV) suspension (B). Mast cells (arrows) were identified by immunohistochemistry using a monoclonal antibody specific for tryptase. An average seven-fold increase in mast cell density was found in the lung sections from RSV-infected rats compared to pathogen-free controls. These mast cells were always clustered in close proximity to nerve fibers (arrowhead)

PART I

Epidemiology

CHAPTER 1

Asthma exacerbations: the size of the problem

Anne E Tattersfield

Asthma is characterized by airway inflammation and a reduction in airway caliber, both of which fluctuate over time. Bronchoconstriction can be precipitated by a wide range of stimuli, both organic and physical; it may be transient with a rapid return to previous lung function, or it may persist and be labeled an exacerbation. Exacerbations are a cardinal feature of asthma, reflecting one end of the spectrum of the fluctuations that are an inherent part of the disease.

Acute exacerbations of asthma are frightening and distressing for patients and for their relatives. They may necessitate a visit to a nurse, doctor or emergency department or require admission to hospital. Exacerbations cause loss of schooling and work, and disruption to families and family life. Families live with the knowledge that, although most exacerbations resolve satisfactorily, the outcome is occasionally fatal. Knowing whether and when to call for help is therefore an additional concern for patients and relatives.

THE NATURE OF EXACERBATIONS

Exacerbations of asthma come in various forms. They can be mild and self-limiting or severe and life-threatening, and they may develop gradually or rapidly.

A retrospective review of the nature of the 425 exacerbations in the FACET (Formoterol And Corticosteroids Establishing Therapy) study[1] showed that the nadir in terms of the lowest peak flow value was preceded by an initial gradual fall in peak flow over a few days followed by a more rapid fall over 1 to 2 days (Figure 1.1). The fall in peak flow was accompanied by an increase in symptoms and in use of β-agonists as relief medication. The relatively rapid deterioration over 24–48 hours leaves limited time for interventions that are designed to abort an exacerbation to be effective.

This description, based on the FACET study,[2] looks at the pattern of an average exacerbation as seen in patients considered to be suitable for a long-term intervention study. The study excluded patients with very brittle asthma or those with very mild asthma, and hence is not necessarily representative of exacerbations as seen amongst patients with the full spectrum of asthma severity.

Most exacerbations develop relatively gradually, as seen in the FACET study.[1] Even most fatal or life-threatening exacerbations appear to have been preceded by more gradual deterioration in asthma control, which was unrecognized or ignored.[3-6] Nevertheless, some severe exacerbations have a rapid onset[3-6] and, although less common, they are of great concern since the outcome is more likely to be fatal. Exacerbations that develop rapidly show some differences in terms of their natural history and pathology when compared with exacerbations with a rather more gradual onset. A rapidly developing

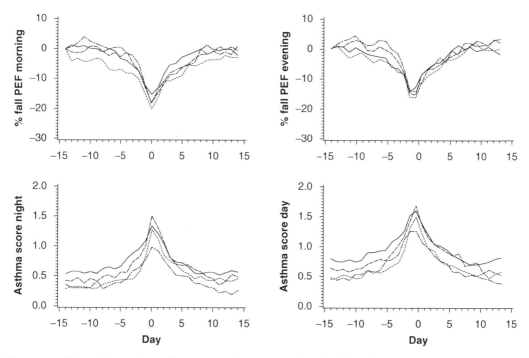

Figure 1.1 Change in morning and evening peak expiratory flow (PEF) (% change from day −14) and daytime and nocturnal symptoms over the 14 days before and after an exacerbation in relation to treatment in the FACET study. Budesonide 200 μg daily, solid line; budesonide 200 μg daily + formoterol (12 μg) twice daily, dotted line; budesonide 800 μg daily, dashed line; budesonide 800 μg daily + formoterol (12 μg) twice daily, dashed/dot line. From reference 1. See text (page 6) for definition of a severe exacerbation

or sudden-onset exacerbation is more likely to have been precipitated by allergen, exercise or psychological stress rather than infection,[6] and although they can be life-threatening they also respond more promptly to treatment.[6] Studies in patients who have died from rapidly developing asthma show more neutrophils and fewer eosinophils in the lungs, when compared with the lungs of patients in whom the onset of the exacerbation was more gradual.[7]

Death from asthma is fortunately relatively rare and tends to present in one of two ways. It occurs in a proportion of patients, usually middle-aged or elderly, with severe chronic asthma who have responded poorly to maximum recommended treatment including oral corticosteroids. Such deaths can be regarded as an inevitable consequence of having severe asthma, given current treatments available. Death can also occur following an acute exacerbation in patients who are reasonably well at other times, sometimes with normal lung function and few or no symptoms between attacks, and this can occur in young patients. Such deaths are considered to be preventable, and several studies have looked in detail at the factors associated with death or near fatal attacks of asthma to try to determine the cause. Factors identified include previous life-threatening attacks, social and psychological problems and failure to take medication as prescribed, including poor compliance with preventive medication and undue reliance on β-agonists.[8–10] Increased fluctuations in diurnal peak flow recordings often precede a fatal attack or ventilatory arrest.[11] Some of these fatal attacks follow rapidly developing exacerbations ('sudden-onset fatal asthma') but in others it is clear that the patient has been deteriorating for some days prior to the respiratory arrest (the so-called 'slow onset, late arrival' attacks).[12] Information about the events preceding a fatal attack are often limited, so the proportion that follow sudden acute exacerbations is unknown.

Most deaths occur outside hospital, making it difficult to determine the precise sequence of events prior to death and the relative contribution of asphyxia, hypoxia and/or an arrhythmia. Autopsies inevitably show changes of acute asthma but cannot determine the nature of the terminal event. The characteristics of ten patients with asthma who had a respiratory arrest within 20 minutes of arriving at hospital showed evidence of asphyxia, with a marked respiratory acidosis (mean pH 7.01), hypokalemia and a mean arterial carbon dioxide tension of 13 kPa.[13] The patients in this study may not be typical of patients who die from an acute exacerbation of asthma, in that they lived long enough to reach hospital, unlike the majority of patients who die at home following an exacerbation.

ASSESSING MORBIDITY FROM EXACERBATIONS OF ASTHMA

It is clear from the number of hospital admissions and doctor visits for asthma attacks that exacerbations of asthma are a large problem. Estimating the size of the problems attributable to acute exacerbations is difficult, however, and must take the following factors into account.

(1) Acute exacerbations are easy to describe but difficult to define. A reasonable description might be 'an acute deterioration in asthma control compared to the patient's usual control'. Asthma is a fluctuating disease and an exacerbation is one end of the spectrum of deteriorating asthma; any cut-off between what might be described as mildly deteriorating asthma or the patient's usual daily variation in asthma control and

an exacerbation has to be arbitrary. Definitions are not required in clinical practice and patients will adjust their treatment or ask for help according to changes in their symptoms and previous experience, aided sometimes by changes in lung function.

When exacerbations are being assessed in clinical trials of asthma, a more rigorous definition is required but none is perfect. Definitions based on change in daily peak flow fluctuations, for example, are problematic and cannot be relied upon to identify exacerbations.[14] A 20% fall in peak flow may be less representative of a true exacerbation (i.e. deterioration from usual asthma control) in someone whose diurnal variation in peak flow is usually around 15%, than in someone whose peak flow is relatively stable. Basing the definition of an acute exacerbation on the need for an increase in treatment is a pragmatic solution that fits with clinical practice. The need for an increase in inhaled treatment or a requirement for oral prednisolone would be generally judged to relate to mild and severe exacerbations, respectively.

(2) The size of the problem will vary according to age and sex. It will also vary according to location, because of the large variation in asthma prevalence between countries. This chapter focuses mainly on westernized countries where the prevalence of asthma is high and where more data are available.

(3) The size of the problem attributable to exacerbations of asthma can be measured in different ways. It needs to be considered in terms of mortality and morbidity, and for some patients there may also be adverse effects from medication. The problem can also be assessed in terms of the financial costs to the patient and their family, which might include the costs of medication to treat or prevent exacerbations and sometimes to prevent adverse effects, as with bisphosphonates in patients taking higher doses of corticosteroids. Finally, there are

the financial costs to the health service and to society at large.

Bearing these various caveats in mind, this chapter attempts to gauge the impact of exacerbations of asthma by pulling together a range of different measures that reflect the frequency and severity of exacerbations and their impact on patients and health resources.

FREQUENCY AND SEVERITY OF ASTHMA EXACERBATIONS AS MEASURED IN PROSPECTIVE STUDIES

Exacerbations can be measured under relatively controlled conditions in clinical trials. They were an infrequent primary endpoint, however, until the past decade, despite their importance to patients and to health services. They tended to be included under adverse effects, and were often not clearly defined. This changed following publication of the FACET study in 1997, and several recent studies have made exacerbations a primary outcome measure.

Since the definition of an exacerbation varies between studies for reasons outlined above, the frequency will vary inversely with the severity of the exacerbations as defined; exacerbations that depend on the need for oral corticosteroids, for example, will occur less often than those that do not require such an intervention. Although this is not an exact science, an analysis of the frequency and severity of exacerbations in the literature provides some insight into the size of the problem.

The first major study to identify exacerbations as a primary outcome was the FACET study.[2] The study had four parallel limbs and was designed to compare high- and low-dose budesonide with and without formoterol or placebo. The strength of the study was that it included over 800 patients, and patients were followed for a year. Exacerbations were the primary endpoint and were assessed as being severe or mild. Severe

exacerbations were defined by the need for oral corticosteroids or a fall in peak expiratory flow of 30% below baseline values on 2 days. In the event, 73% of severe exacerbations were diagnosed by the perceived need for oral corticosteroids rather than a fall in peak flow rate. Mild exacerbations were defined as occurring when, on 2 successive days, peak flow values were 20% below baseline, terbutaline use had increased by three puffs or more or patients woke at night because of asthma. The mean frequency of severe exacerbations in the four limbs of the study ranged from 0.34 to 0.91 per patient per year depending on whether patients were randomized to high- or low-dose budesonide or to formoterol or placebo. The frequency of mild exacerbation days was much higher, as expected, ranging from 13.4 to 35.4 per person per year in the four limbs.

The frequency of exacerbations has been measured as a primary or secondary endpoint in other recent therapeutic trials in patients with asthma. Table 1.1 provides details from some of the larger studies in which it is possible to measure an annual rate of exacerbations, by extrapolation to a yearly rate when necessary.[2,15–22] The studies were selected as having at least 150 subjects and follow-up of at least 3 months, since frequency measurements will be more reliable in longer-term studies. As can be seen (Table 1.1) the frequency of exacerbations varies considerably, from 0.12 to 1.3 per patient per year (excluding mild exacerbations in the FACET study, since the definition here was considerably less stringent than that used in any of the other studies). The lowest figures for exacerbation frequency were seen in the START study, by Pauwels et al.,[22] reflecting the fact that the subjects had mild asthma and only the need for a course of oral corticosteroids was expressed in terms of events per patient per year. The low incidence of exacerbations in the study by Drazen et al.[15] is also likely to reflect the fact that patients had mild asthma, as judged by the high forced expiratory volume (FEV_1)% predicted, and the fairly stringent criteria for defining an exacerbation. This included an increase in symptoms

Table 1.1 Exacerbation rates in some large prospective studies in adults

First author, year	FEV₁ (% predicted)	No of subjects	% on ICS on entry	Duration of study (months)	Exacerbations/ subject/year*
Drazen 1996[15]	90	255	0	4	0.26, 0.30
van der Molen 1997[16]	67	239	100	6	0.96, 0.93
Pauwels 1997[2]	76	852	100	12	0.91, 0.67, 0.46, 0.34
Taylor 1998[17]	80	165	92	6	1.2, 1.1, 0.42
Dennis 2000[18]	85†	983	90	12	1.3, 1.25
Tattersfield 2001[19]	74	362	100	3	0.64, 1.06
O'Byrne 2001[20]					
Study a	90	698	0	12	0.29, 0.34, 0.77
Study b	86	1272	100	12	0.36, 0.56, 0.92, 0.96
Ind 2002[21]	76	357	100	3	1.0, 1.15
Pauwels 2003[22]	86	7241††	0	36	0.21, 0.12

ICS, inhaled corticosteroids
*May be underestimate as patients often withdrawn after two or more exacerbations. The different figures relate to different treatment limbs in the various studies
†Peak expiratory flow % predicted
††Includes children

plus either an increase in β-agonist use (by eight puffs a day for 2 days) or a fall in peak flow of 35% from the run-in value. The highest incidence of exacerbations was seen in the TRUST study[18] presumably due to the less exacting criteria for defining an exacerbation, since the patients did not have particularly severe asthma as judged by their FEV₁. The criteria for defining an exacerbation included the addition of oral or an increase in inhaled corticosteroids, or two of the following over 2 days: increase in symptoms, or β-agonist use of three puffs a day or a peak flow 20% below baseline values.

The subjects included in these studies are unlikely to be representative of all patients with asthma, since patients with severe or brittle asthma were usually excluded from such studies, although these patients probably have the highest incidence of exacerbations and often the most severe. At the other end of the spectrum patients with very mild asthma are often excluded from prospective trials of treatment, although they represent the most frequent presentation of asthma in the community. In some studies, such as the FACET and TRUST studies, patients had to have

a 15% response to a bronchodilator or show 15% variability in peak flow readings to enter the study. This would also make the patients less representative of the broad spectrum of subjects with asthma in the community.

The frequency of exacerbations will also be influenced by the medication being taken by the patients. Several studies have shown that the introduction of inhaled corticosteroids reduces exacerbation rates. The FACET study[2] showed that quadrupling the dose of budesonide reduced the frequency of exacerbations, as did the addition of a long-acting β-agonist formoterol; both interventions caused a reduction of roughly 25% and the effect of the two combined was additive. Although the frequency of exacerbations was reduced by whether the patient was taking formoterol or a high or low dose of inhaled corticosteroid, the severity and duration of exacerbations was not affected.[1] Other studies have confirmed that long-acting β-agonists reduce the frequency of exacerbations in patients already taking an inhaled corticosteroid; studies in corticosteroid-naive patients have generally not shown a reduction, however.[23] The frequency of exacerbations may be reduced by other drugs, including the leukotriene antagonists.[24,25]

ASTHMA ATTACKS IN LARGE, RANDOM POPULATION SURVEYS

Studies in random populations are better able to assess the problem from exacerbations as they affect the whole community, though the definition of an exacerbation or attack of asthma is usually not defined. There have been two major international surveys of asthma in adults and children, respectively, designed to measure differences in asthma prevalence in different geographical regions, to explore possible etiological factors and to determine changes over time prospectively using standardized methodology. Although not designed to look at exacerbations specifically, the studies provide some data on the proportion of the population that have attacks of asthma, though less information on the severity of the attacks or the impact they may have on the patient.

The European Community Respiratory Health Survey (ECRHS) has provided data on various measures of asthma amongst large random populations based in 48 centers in Western Europe and in a few instances outside Europe. The initial survey[26] of 11168 people aged 20–44 in 1991–93 found marked variations between centers and between countries for symptoms of asthma, including the question of whether the subject had experienced an attack of asthma in the previous 12 months. The positive response rate to this question was highest in Australia and New Zealand (6.8–9.7%) and within Europe it was highest in centers in England (up to 5.7%) and lowest in centers in Belgium and Germany (1.3%). Centers with a high prevalence of self-reported attacks of asthma also reported more nasal allergies and more waking at night due to breathlessness. A follow-up study 5–11 years[27] later found that, although more people were being treated for asthma, the number reporting asthma attacks in the previous year had increased by only 0.8%.

A similar approach has been taken in children, with over 460000 children aged 13 and 14 years from 56 countries and over 250000 children aged 6 and 7 years from 35 countries participating in phase 1 of the International Study of Asthma and Allergies in Childhood (ISAAC).[28,29] The prevalences of asthma, rhinoconjunctivitis and atopic eczema were assessed using a questionnaire, supported by a video in many centers. Overall, 3.7% of 13- and 14-year-olds had had more than four attacks of asthma in the previous year, although the figure ranged widely from 9.9% for Australia and New Zealand to 1.6% in South East Asia. The mean prevalence for 6- and 7-year-olds experiencing more than four attacks was 3.1%, with similar geographical variations. A further question that is likely to reflect exacerbations in children was about severe wheeze that limited speech; this was reported by 3.8% of 13- and 14-year-olds and by 2.4% of the younger children.

Several other questionnaire studies provide prevalence figures for children reporting attacks of asthma and these again show geographical variations[30] and also changes over time. Between 1982 and 1992 there was a six-fold increase in the number of Australian children having more than four attacks of asthma a year,[31] and a three-fold increase in British children reporting attacks of asthma.[32] Between 1995 and 2002, however, the annual prevalence of speech-limiting attacks of asthma amongst 12–14-year-olds in Britain fell from 9% to 6.8%.[33]

SEVERE EXACERBATIONS

The need for a course of oral prednisolone is a marker of a relatively severe exacerbation of asthma; other markers that identify exacerbations of increasing severity include general practitioner consultations, visits to the accident and emergency department, admissions to hospital and finally death as a result of asthma.

Need for a course of oral corticosteroids

The need for oral prednisolone was assessed in several of the prospective studies described above. Studies based in the community should provide a more global picture of the impact from exacerbations of asthma, since patients with asthma are not included or excluded according to predefined criteria.

In a study in five general practices in 1995[34] covering a population of over 38 000 subjects in and around Nottingham, we were able to assess the need amongst the asthmatic population for a course of oral prednisolone. Of the 3373 patients given a diagnosis of asthma, 12.5% had received one or more courses of prednisolone in the previous year. As expected this occurred more often in patients with more severe asthma, as judged by the amount of treatment they were taking on a regular basis. However, because more patients in the community are taking a β-agonist alone or a β-agonist in combination with a low dose of inhaled corticosteroid, more than half the patients requiring a course of prednisolone were taking either a low dose or no regular inhaled corticosteroid. Extrapolation of these figures to the UK as a whole suggests that in 1995 over half a million patients with asthma were requiring prednisolone for an attack of asthma each year. Of these, 360 000 were only on steps one or two of the UK guidelines, i.e. they were taking only a low dose of inhaled corticosteroid and/or a short-acting β-agonist on a regular basis.

General practitioner consultations

The extent to which general practitioner consultations are due to acute exacerbations of asthma rather than a more general review of asthma management can be difficult to determine. Figures from England and Wales showed an increase in the number of patients consulting their general practitioner for asthma between 1970 and 1981,[35] from around 10 to 18 per 1000 population. Weekly rates for new episodes of asthma in England and Wales (when a patient consults for a new attack or exacerbation) have fallen since peaking in 1993, from around 50 to 40 per week per 100 000 population.[36] In young children consultations are highest in autumn, whereas in older subjects consultation rates tend to be higher in winter.[37]

Visits to accident and emergency departments and hospital admissions for asthma

Measuring the number of visits to an accident and emergency department or hospital admissions for asthma are robust measures of asthma exacerbations in that the data are likely to be reasonably reliable. They do, however, depend on the criteria used by patients to decide to visit an accident and emergency department and those used to admit patients to hospital, and both can change rapidly following a scare or publicity about asthma deaths, for example. Nevertheless, both have implications for patients and their families and cost implications for health services.

In general, patients with more severe asthma are more likely to be admitted to hospital. Nevertheless, a prospective study of over 3000 admissions to 37 accident and emergency departments in France in 1997–98[38] found that amongst patients with life-threatening features only 77% were admitted to hospital compared to 55% and 29% amongst those defined as having severe or moderate to mild asthma, respectively. Some 26% of the patients seen in the emergency room were defined as having life-threatening asthma. A study of children who presented frequently at the accident and emergency department for asthma concluded that, although the children had more severe asthma, the main determinant of attendance appeared to be the parent's conviction that this was the best place to get appropriate treatment.[39]

The annual figures for the number of hospital visits and admissions for exacerbations of asthma have changed over time, with seasonal variations and short-lived epidemics superimposed on longer-term variations in rates for both visits and admissions to hospital. Age is also an important factor, with children under 4 years of age being more likely to be admitted to hospital,[40] though often for only one night.

Data from England and Wales showed an increase in admissions to hospital in the 1980s in both children and adults,[40] some of which may have been related to concerns about asthma deaths at the time. For children under 4 years there was a roughly three-fold increase in hospital admissions between 1979 and 1989, peaking at around 100 per 10 000 before declining to around 60 per 10 000 by 1999. For older children and adults the peak for hospital admissions was also seen in the late 1980s at around 20 and 10 per 10 000, respectively, since when it has shown a gradual decline. Data from Scotland show a similar decline since 1992 in the under-14s.

There are considerable international differences in rates of hospital admission. A study comparing hospital admission for asthma in people under 17 in eight countries found a two- to three-fold higher rate in Finland compared to Greece and Italy.[41] When data from four countries were compared, fewer children in Wales had been admitted to hospital for chest trouble (4.2%) compared to Sweden (6.5%), South Africa (6.8%) and New Zealand (8.5%), although this would include chest problems other than asthma.[42]

Admissions to hospital show seasonal variation, particularly in children, for whom there is a marked increase in September.[43] In older subjects admissions tend to be higher in winter. These data fit with the fact that many exacerbations in adults[44] and even more in children[45] are precipitated by viral infections. This is thought to explain why admissions in children tend to coincide with the beginning of the school term.

Geographically localized epidemics of asthma exacerbations causing a sudden increase in visits and admissions to hospital have been reported at various times,[46] some of the earliest being traced to castor beans. The most notable recent outbreak was in Barcelona[47] where 'epidemic asthma days' were seen at regular intervals after 1979; 12 of these outbreaks, between 1981 and 1986, were investigated carefully. The outbreaks were short-lived and showed geographical clustering in one part of the city suggesting a point source. Careful detective work by a team of epidemiologists eventually identified the culprit as soybean dust, which was released into the atmosphere following unloading of soybeans from boats in the docks. The introduction of silo filters to prevent airborne dissemination of soybean dust when the beans were being unloaded caused a marked reduction in days when admissions to hospital reached epidemic levels.[48]

Sudden increases in visits to accident and emergency departments and in hospital admissions have also been seen in relation to thunderstorms. A well-documented episode occurred in London in June 1994 when 640 patients with asthma attended accident and emergency departments within 30 hours of a thunderstorm, nearly ten times the expected number, and 104 were admitted to hospital.[49] Most patients were aged 20–40, most had hayfever and a third had not had asthma previously. The episode was associated with a fall in temperature and an increase in grass pollen concentration.[50] Similar episodes have been seen in other cities, including Birmingham[51] and Melbourne.[52] The episodes are often short-lived with most patients being discharged within 24 hours. The reason for the association of exacerbations with thunderstorms is still debated, although it has been postulated that the sudden changes in humidity and temperature that occur in association with thunderstorms might disrupt pollen or fungal spores and produce allergenic particles in the respirable range.[53,54] Although some thunderstorms are undoubtedly associated with acute exacerbations of asthma this is not true for all thunderstorms, and it may be that pollen counts need to be high or other climatic conditions need to be present for this to happen.[55,56]

Mortality from asthma

Although the great majority of exacerbations of asthma settle with or in some cases without treatment, a small proportion do not. Mortality from asthma showed a fairly marked increase in many countries, though not all, in the 1960s.[57] The increase in mortality was seen only in countries selling isoprenaline in high doses to patients directly, i.e. over the counter, and the epidemic has been attributed to excessive use of these drugs.[58] A second epidemic of asthma deaths was seen in New Zealand in the 1980s[59] and this was associated with the introduction of another β-agonist, fenoterol, which like isoprenaline was marketed in relatively high doses per puff compared to other inhaled β-agonists on the market.[60]

Apart from these 'epidemics' of asthma deaths, more gradual changes in mortality rates have been documented over the past 50 years in particular.[61] Until the late 1980s asthma mortality rates in England and Wales were running at around 10 per milion for people aged 15–45 and four per million for children under 15 years of age. Mortality then started to decline and by the late 1990s the respective figures were around seven and three per million, respectively. Mortality data from other countries have shown similar figures with a decline in mortality over the past 15 years or so. Although difficult to prove, it is thought that the reduction relates, in part at least, to the greater use of prophylactic medication, and inhaled corticosteroids in particular.

Seasonal variations in asthma deaths and near-fatal attacks are also seen, with a clustering of episodes in North America in autumn when *Alternaria* allergens are at their highest.[62] Asthma mortality in the UK is highest between July and September, peaking in August.[63]

Mortality can also be assessed prospectively from some of the large databases that have identified individuals with asthma. A study of 2499 people with probable or definite asthma in the USA showed no difference in long-term survival compared to the expected rates, except for those with late-onset asthma; only 4% of the deaths were due to asthma.[64] In a large study of 13 540 individuals randomly selected from the general population in Denmark, patients with self-reported asthma had a higher mortality than non-asthmatics although the main cause was cited as chronic obstructive pulmonary disease (COPD).[65] Fewer than 5% of all deaths in the asthmatic cohort were classified as being due to asthma compared to around 10% attributed to COPD. It is not possible from these data to determine the proportion of patients who died following an exacerbation, but it seems unlikely that this was the cause of death in those labeled as having died from COPD. FEV_1 was a strong predictor of mortality and there are data to suggest that atopic patients without asthma may have an increased life expectancy. The findings in a study in Finland[66] that included over 30 000 subjects, mainly twins, were similar in showing an increased mortality in patients labeled as having asthma, but again death was more likely to be attributed to COPD. The database in Saskatchewan[67] has been used to identify and follow-up a cohort of 30 569 patients with asthma, aged 5–44 years. By 1997, 562 patients had died, though only 77 as a result of asthma. Taken together these various studies suggest that, although patients with asthma clearly can die as a result of an acute exacerbation of their asthma, they are considerably more likely to die as a result of progressive chronic lung disease.

FINANCIAL COSTS OF EXACERBATIONS

The financial costs of asthma have been assessed in various countries in different ways.[68,69] In the USA the total cost of illness related to asthma for 1990 was estimated at 6.2 billion dollars (in 1984 dollars) by Weiss *et al.*[70] A second study, by Smith *et al.*,[68] and using costs rather than charges, put the total cost for 1994 at 5.8 billion dollars.

The total costs are higher in the study by Weiss *et al.*, when converted to 1994 dollars (7.78 billion dollars), as detailed in Table 1.2, although the direct costs which include hospital admissions, emergency visits and drugs were similar in the two analyses. Admission to hospital was a major cost burden in both studies, associated with 48% of direct costs in the analysis by Smith *et al.*[68] This fits with recent estimates that the cost of an inpatient admission for asthma in the USA (average duration 3.8 days) is $3102.[69] Other direct aspects of care associated with exacerbations of asthma, such as emergency room use and drugs, also have heavy financial implications. The studies also show that some 80% of the costs of asthma are incurred by the 20% of the asthmatic population with most severe asthma.

Indirect costs in the Smith study[68] are lower in part because no allowance was made for time lost due to premature death. There were also differences in the estimated costs of loss of schooling, which in the Weiss analysis[70] were considerably greater than the costs of loss of work in adults. Other studies have shown that children, including preschool children, consume more resources than adults. Reduced productivity is also a major cost approaching one billion dollars, in the Weiss study.

Studies in other reasonably affluent countries show a roughly similar breakdown of costs.[69,71] Several studies provide data to show that using prophylactic medication to reduce exacerbations is cost effective, at least in economically developed countries. Costs cannot provide a measure of health need in poor countries, where there may be as little as $10 per person a year to spend on health.[72,73] If an exacerbation of asthma is treated, it is likely to be with the cheapest drugs available, which are usually oral β-agonists, theophylline or an oral corticosteroid.

CONCLUSIONS

Exacerbations are a cardinal feature of asthma, representing an exaggeration of the usual

Table 1.2 Direct and indirect costs of asthma in millions of dollars according to two large analyses in the USA by Weiss *et al.*[70] and Smith *et al.*[68] (both in 1994 dollars)

	Weiss *et al.* (%)*	Smith *et al.* (%)*
Direct costs		
Ambulatory visits		
Office and clinic	431 (5.5)	616 (10.6)
Hospital outpatient	262 (3.4)	566 (9.7)
Emergency room	407 (5.2)	348 (6.0)
Hospitalization	2327 (29.9)	2800 (48.1)
Prescribed medicines	1397 (18.0)	817 (14.0)
Total direct costs	4824 (62.0)	5147 (88.4)
Indirect costs		
Housekeeping loss	579 (7.4)	21 (0.4)
Work loss	398 (5.1)	222 (3.8)
School loss	1036 (13.3)	195 (3.3)
Bed days (age 0–4)	N/A	19 (0.3)
Restricted activity loss	N/A	218 (3.6)
Mortality	943 (12.2)	N/A
Total indirect costs	2956 (38.0)	674 (11.6)
Total costs	7780 (100.0)	5821 (100.0)

N/A, not applicable
*% of total costs

fluctuations that characterize asthma. They cause considerable distress and anxiety for patients and their families. Assessing the size of the problem that results from exacerbations requires some measure of their frequency and severity. There is no simple definition of an exacerbation and the frequency with which exacerbations are seen varies indirectly with the severity of exacerbation being assessed. Various indices are therefore used to assess the size of the problem. Estimates based on data from the UK suggest that exacerbations of asthma will be responsible for around 10 000 courses of oral corticosteroids,[34] 20 000 visits to a family doctor[36] and 1000 admissions to hospital[40] per million of the population per year.

Measures such as hospital admissions give hard facts that relate to exacerbations of asthma but do not necessarily measure the personal impact of having an exacerbation or worrying about the possibility of having an exacerbation on the quality of life of a patient or their family. Instruments and scales developed to assess asthma control or quality of life for patients with asthma provide a global measure of the effect of asthma rather than the effect of exacerbations per se. Although it is more difficult to capture the specific effect of exacerbations of asthma in terms of the distress or worry that they cause, there can be little doubt that they are a cause of a great deal of misery and concern for a proportion of patients with asthma.

REFERENCES

1. Tattersfield AE, Postma DS, Barnes PJ, et al. Exacerbations of asthma: a descriptive study in 425 patients. Am J Respir Crit Care Med 1999; 160: 594–9

2. Pauwels RA, Löfdahl C-G, Postma DS, et al. Effect of inhaled formoterol and budesonide on exacerbations of asthma. N Engl J Med 1997; 337: 1405–11

3. Wasserfallen J-B, Schaller M-D, Feihl F, Perret CH. Sudden asphyxic asthma – a distinct entity? Am Rev Respir Dis 1990; 142: 108–11

4. Plaza V, Serrano J, Picado J, Sancho J. Frequency and clinical characteristics of rapid-onset fatal and near-fatal asthma. Eur Respir J 2002; 19: 846–52

5. Kolbe J, Fergusson W, Garrett J. Rapid onset asthma: a severe but uncommon manifestation. Thorax 1998; 53: 241–7

6. Barr RG, Woodruff PG, Clark S, Camargo CA Jr, on behalf of the Multicenter Airway Research Collaboration (MARC) investigators. Sudden-onset asthma exacerbations: clinical features, response to therapy, and 2-week follow-up. Eur Respir J 2000; 15: 266–73

7. Sur S, Crotty TB, Kephart GM, et al. Sudden-onset fatal asthma. Am Rev Respir Dis 1993; 148: 713–19

8. Innes NJ, Reid A, Halstead J, et al. Psychosocial risk factors in near-fatal asthma and in asthma deaths. J R Coll Physicians 1998; 32: 430–4

9. Johnson AJ, Nunn AJ, Somner AR, et al. Circumstances of death from asthma. BMJ 1984; 288: 1870–2

10. Rae HH, Sears MR, Beaglehole R, et al, Lessons from the national asthma mortality study: circumstances surrounding death. NZ Med J 1987; 100: 10–13

11. Hetzel MR, Clark TJH, Branthwaite MA. Asthma: analysis of sudden deaths and ventilatory arrests in hospital. BMJ 1997; 1: 808–11

12. Strunk RC. Deaths due to asthma. Am Rev Respir Dis 1993; 148: 550–2

13. Molfino NA, Nannini LJ, Martelli AN, Slutsky AS. Respiratory arrest in near-fatal asthma. N Engl J Med 1991; 324: 285–8

14. Reddel H, Ware S, Marks G, et al. Differences between asthma exacerbations and poor asthma control. Lancet 1999; 353: 364–9

15. Drazen JM, Elliott I, Boushey HA, et al. Comparison of regularly scheduled with as-needed use of albuterol in mild asthma. N Engl J Med 1996; 335: 841–7

16. van der Molen T, Postma DS, Turner MO, et al. Effects of the long acting β agonist formoterol on asthma control in asthmatic patients using inhaled corticosteroids. Thorax 1997; 52: 535–9

17. Taylor DR, Town GI, Herbison GP, et al. Asthma control during long term treatment with regular inhaled salbutamol and salmeterol. Thorax 1998; 53: 744–52

18. Dennis SM, Sharp SJ, Vickers MR, et al. Regular inhaled salbutamol and asthma control: the TRUST randomized trial. Lancet 2000; 355: 1675–9

19. Tattersfield AE, Löfdahl C-G, Postma DJ, et al. Comparison of formoterol and terbutaline for as-needed treatment of asthma: a randomized trial. Lancet 2001; 357: 257–61

20. O'Byrne PM, Barnes PJ, Rodriguez-Roisin R, et al. Low dose inhaled budesonide and formoterol in mild persistent asthma. Am J Respir Crit Care Med 2001; 164: 1392–7

21. Ind PW, Villasante C, Shiner RJ, et al. Safety of formoterol by Turbuhaler as reliever medication compared with terbutaline in moderate asthma. Eur Respir J 2002; 20: 859–66

22. Pauwels RA, Pederson S, Busse WW, et al. Early intervention with budesonide in mild persistent asthma: a randomized double-blind trial. Lancet 2003; 361: 1071–6

23. Sovani MP, Whale CI, Tattersfield AE. A benefit–risk assessment of inhaled long-acting β-agonists in the management of obstructive pulmonary disease. Drug Saf 2004; 27: 689–715

24. Barnes NC, Miller CJ. Effect of leukotriene receptor antagonist therapy on the risk of asthma exacerbations in patients with mild to moderate asthma: an integrated analysis of zafirlukast trials. Thorax 2000; 55: 478–83

25. Laviolette M, Malmstron K, Lu S, et al. Montelukast added to inhaled beclomethasone in treatment of asthma. Am J Respir Crit Care Med 1999; 160: 1862–8

26. Burney P, for the European Community Respiratory Health Survey. Variations in the prevalence of respiratory symptoms, self-reported asthma attacks, and use of asthma medication in the European Community Respiratory Health Survey (ECRHS). Eur Respir J 1996; 9: 687–95

27. Chinn S, Jarvis D, Burney P, et al. Increase in diagnosed asthma but not in symptoms in the European

Community Respiratory Health Survey. Thorax 2004; 59: 646–51

28. Beasley R, for The International Study of Asthma and Allergies in Childhoood (ISAAC) Steering Committee. Worldwide variation in prevalence of symptoms of asthma, allergic rhinoconjunctivitis and atopic eczema: ISAAC. Lancet 1998; 351: 1225–32

29. Asher MI, for The International Study of Asthma and Allergies in Childhoood (ISAAC) Steering Committee. Worldwide variations in the prevalence of asthma symptoms: the International Study of Asthma and Allergies in Childhood (ISAAC). Eur Respir J 1998; 12: 315–35

30. Pearce N, Weiland S, Keil U, et al. Self-reported prevalence of asthma symptoms in children in Australia, England, Germany and New Zealand: an international comparison using the ISAAC protocol. Eur Respir J 1993; 6: 1455–61

31. Toelle BG, Ng K, Belousova E, et al. Prevalence of asthma and allergy in schoolchildren in Belmont, Australia: three cross sectional surveys over 20 years. BMJ 2004; 328: 386–7

32. Rona RJ, Chinn S, Burney PGJ. Trends in the prevalence of asthma in Scottish and English primary school children 1982–92. Thorax 1995; 50: 992–3

33. Anderson HR, Ruggles R, Strachan DP, et al. Trends in prevalence of symptoms of asthma, hay fever and eczema in 12–14 year olds in the British Isles, 1995–2002: questionnaire survey. BMJ 2004; 328: 1052–3

34. Walsh LJ, Wong CA, Cooper S, et al. Morbidity from asthma in relation to regular treatment: a community based study. Thorax 1999; 54: 296–300

35. Fleming DM, Crombie DL. Prevalence of asthma and hay fever in England and Wales. BMJ 1987; 294: 279–83

36. Fleming DM, Sunderland R, Cross KW, Ross AM. Declining incidence of episodes of asthma: a study of trends in new episodes presenting to general practitioners in the period 1989–98. Thorax 2000; 55: 657–61

37. Fleming DM, Cross KW, Sunderland R, Ross AM. Comparison of the seasonal patterns of asthma identified in general practitioner episodes, hospital admissions, and deaths. Thorax 2000; 55: 662–5

38. Salmeron S, Liard R, Elkharrat D, et al. Asthma severity and adequacy of management in accident and emergency departments in France: a prospective study. Lancet 2001; 358: 629–35

39. O'Halloran SM, Heaf DP. Recurrent accident and emergency department attendance for acute asthma in children. Thorax 1989; 44: 620–6

40. Lung and Asthma Information Agency. Fact sheet 2002/1. Laia@sghms.ac.uk

41. Burney P. The burden of asthma. Eur Respir Rev 1997; 7: 326–8

42. Burr ML, Limb ES, Andrae S, et al. Childhood asthma in four countries: a comparative survey. Int J Epidemiol 1994; 23: 341–7

43. Khot A, Burn R, Evans N, et al. Seasonal variation and time trends in childhood asthma in England and Wales, 1975–81. BMJ 1984; 289: 235–7

44. Nicholson KG, Kent J, Ireland DC. Respiratory viruses and exacerbations of asthma in adults. BMJ 1993; 307: 982–6

45. Johnston SL, Pattemore PK, Sanderson G, et al. The relationship between upper respiratory infections and hospital admissions for asthma: a time trend analysis. Am J Respir Crit Care Med 1996; 154: 654–60

46. Anto JM. Asthma outbreaks: an opportunity for research? Thorax 1995; 50: 220–2

47. Anto JM, Sunyer J, Rodriguez-Roisin R, et al. Toxicoepidemiological committee. Community outbreaks of asthma associated with inhalation of soybean dust. N Engl J Med 1989; 320: 1097–102

48. Anto JM, Sunyer J, Reed CE, et al. Preventing asthma epidemics due to soybeans by dust-control measures. N Engl J Med 1993; 329: 1760–3

49. Davidson AC, Emberlin J, Cook AD, Venables KM. A major outbreak of asthma associated with a thunderstorm: experience of accident and emergency departments and patients' characteristics. BMJ 1996; 312: 601–4

50. Celenza A, Fothergill J, Kupek E, Shaw RJ. Thunderstorm associated asthma: a detailed analysis of environmental factors. BMJ 1996; 312: 604–7

51. Packe GE, Ayres JG. Asthma outbreak during a thunderstorm. Lancet 1985; 2: 199–204

52. Bellomo R, Gigliotti P, Treloar A, et al. Two consecutive thunderstorm associated epidemics of asthma in the city of Melbourne – the possible role of rye grass pollen. Med J Aust 1992; 156: 834–7

53. Knox RB. Grass pollen, thunderstorms and asthma. Clin Exp Allergy 1993; 23: 354–9

54. Marks GB, Colquhoun JR, Girgis ST, et al. Thunderstorm outflows preceding epidemics of asthma during spring and summer. Thorax 2001; 56: 468–71

55. Newson R, Strachan D, Archibald E, et al. Effect of thunderstorms and airborne grass pollen on the incidence of acute asthma in England, 1990–94. Thorax 1997; 52: 680–5

56. Anto JM, Sunyer J. Thunderstorms: a risk factor for asthma attacks. Thorax 1997; 52: 669–70

57. Inman WHW, Adelstein AM. Rise and fall in asthma mortality in England and Wales in relation to use of pressurised aerosols. Lancet 1969; 2: 279–85

58. Stolley PD, Schinnar R. Association between asthma mortality and isoproterol aerosols: a review. Prev Med 1978; 7: 519–38

59. Jackson RT, Beaglehole R, Rea HR, Sutherland DS. Mortality from asthma: a new epidemic in New Zealand. BMJ 1982; 285: 771–4

60. Wong CS, Pavord ID, Williams J, et al. Bronchodilator, cardiovascular and hypokalaemic effects of fenoterol, salbutamol and terbutaline in asthma. Lancet 1990; 336: 1396–8

61. Campbell MJ, Cogman GR, Holgate ST, Johnston SL. Age specific trends in asthma mortality in England and Wales, 1983–95: results of an observational study. BMJ 1997; 314: 1439–40

62. O'Hallaren MT, Yunginger JW, Offord KP, et al. Exposure to an aeroallergen as a possible precipitating factor in respiratory arrest in young patients with asthma. N Engl J Med 1991; 324: 359–63

63. Khot A, Burn R. Seasonal variation and time trends of death from asthma in England and Wales 1960–82. BMJ 1984; 289: 223–4

64. Silverstein MD, Reed CE, O'Connell EJ, et al. Long-term survival of a cohort of community residents with asthma. N Engl J Med 1994; 331: 1537–41

65. Lange P, Ulrik CS, Vestbo J, for the Copenhagen Heart Study. Mortality in adults with self-reported asthma. Lancet 1996; 347: 1285–9

66. Huovinen E, Kaprio J, Vesterinen E, Koskenvuo M. Mortality of adults with asthma: a prospective cohort study. Thorax 1997; 52: 49–54

67. Suissa S, Ernst P, Benayoun S, et al. Low-dose inhaled corticosteroids and the prevention of death from asthma. N Engl J Med 2000; 343: 332–6

68. Smith DH, Malone DC, Lawson KA, et al. A national estimate of the economic costs of asthma. Am J Respir Crit Care Med 1997; 156: 787–93

69. Stanford R, McLaughlin T, Okamoto LJ. The cost of asthma in the emergency department and hospital. Am J Respir Crit Care Med 1999; 160: 211–15

70. Weiss KB, Gergen PJ, Hodgson TA. An economic evaluation of asthma in the United States. N Engl J Med 1992; 326: 862–6

71. Barnes PJ, Jonsson B, Klim JB. The costs of asthma. Eur Respir J 1996; 9: 636–42

72. Watson JP, Lewis RA. Is asthma treatment affordable in developing countries? Thorax 1997; 52: 605–7

73. Parry E. Treating asthma in developing countries: a problem of inaccessible unavailable essential medication. Thorax 1997; 52: 589

Definition of acute asthma exacerbations in adults and children: differentiating asthma exacerbations from poor asthma control

Helen K Reddel and Stephen D Vincent

DEFINITIONS IN THE GUIDELINES

In the Global Initiative for Asthma (GINA) guidelines,[1] exacerbations are defined as '*episodes of rapidly progressive increase in shortness of breath, cough, wheezing, or chest tightness, or some combination of these symptoms. Respiratory distress is common. Exacerbations are characterised by decreases in expiratory airflow that can be quantified by measurement of lung function ...*'. A similar definition is provided in the US guidelines.[2] Apart from the reference to timecourse, these definitions are similar to the guidelines' descriptions of untreated asthma itself. '*In the untreated state, bronchial asthma is recognised by recurrent episodes of airflow limitation ... Depending on severity, the airflow limitation is accompanied by symptoms of breathlessness, wheezing, chest tightness, and cough.*'[1] These features, observed in a patient already on treatment, are referred to as poorly controlled asthma.

Lengthy sections of both of the above guideline documents are devoted to the management of both exacerbations and poorly controlled asthma. However, the similarity of the above clinical manifestations suggests that 'snapshot' views of an exacerbation and of poorly controlled asthma may look very similar. The potential for confusion is highlighted by language in several other sections of the same guidelines, in which the word 'exacerbation' is used to refer to transient symptoms following exercise or hyperventilation,[1,2] or, in the classification of asthma severity,[2] to episodes occurring several times a week. As both exacerbations and poorly controlled asthma are important opportunities for clinical intervention in patients with asthma, contribute substantially to the economic burden of asthma and are the subject of many clinical trials, we need to be able to distinguish these phenomena, both prospectively and retrospectively, in the context of clinical practice, clinical trials and population studies.

WHY DO WE NEED TO DISTINGUISH EXACERBATIONS FROM POORLY CONTROLLED ASTHMA?

Exacerbations and poorly controlled asthma usually represent clinically distinct phenomena

In general medicine, 'exacerbation' is consistently used to refer to episodes of acute or subacute *change from usual or recent state*

(Figure 2.1). This is consistent with usage of 'exacerbations' in other medical conditions such as chronic obstructive pulmonary disease (COPD), Crohn's disease or multiple sclerosis, which are characterized by remissions and relapses of clinical manifestations with some symptoms in between. In asthma, the critical components for an exacerbation appear to be that the rate and magnitude of change in symptoms or airway obstruction are not only outside the normal range of circadian variation, but also outside this patient's recent range of variation. The absolute level of symptoms and airway obstruction which characterize an exacerbation may thus differ substantially from patient to patient, depending on their usual status. A forced expiratory volume (FEV_1) of 50% predicted may be associated with severe dyspnea and hypoxemia for one patient, but be tolerated long term by another. In addition, the levels of symptoms and airway obstruction which are observed during an exacerbation may differ substantially over time for an individual patient, in that, once asthma control improves with treatment, the patient may be considered to be having an exacerbation at levels of symptoms or lung function which are similar to or even better than his/her usual state prior to commencement of treatment (Figure 2.2).

In clinical practice, 'poor asthma control' is used to imply a specific level of clinical manifestations of asthma, i.e. failure to meet absolute criteria. 'Poorly controlled asthma' (Figure 2.3) appears to carry no implication of change from the patient's previous state, as a patient may be described as having had poor asthma control for many years. At present there are no widely accepted criteria for poorly controlled asthma.

Exacerbations and poorly controlled asthma are treated differently

Guidelines for management of poorly controlled asthma recommend a hierarchy of therapeutic interventions, progressing from as-needed β_2-agonist to increasing doses of inhaled corticosteroids, and addition of long-acting

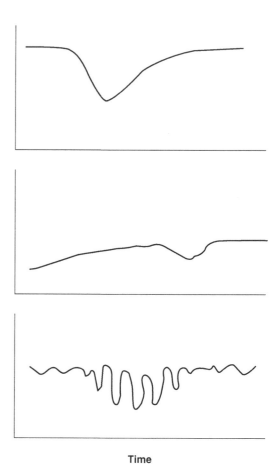

Time

Figure 2.1 Exacerbations represent an acute or subacute change from the patient's usual or recent state. The figure shows stylized representations of three events which could be recognized clinically as exacerbations, with the x-axis representing time, and the y-axis representing any variable such as symptoms, lung function or quality of life

β_2-agonist, leukotriene modifiers, theophylline or oral corticosteroids.[1,2] By contrast, guidelines for the treatment of acute exacerbations focus on frequent/continuous β_2-agonist/anticholinergic agents to relieve acute bronchoconstriction, and oral/systemic corticosteroids to reduce the risk of hospitalization or death. Early treatment of exacerbations, as specified in action plans, focuses on increased use of a short-acting β_2-agonist, and on the use of inhaled or oral

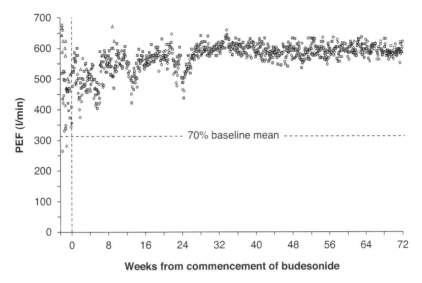

Figure 2.2 In clinical practice, exacerbations are defined by change from usual or recent status, but in clinical trials, the run-in period is often used for comparison. The figure shows electronically recorded PEF data from a subject in a clinical study of inhaled budesonide.[41] The patient (male, 52 years) had long-standing poorly controlled asthma, but symptoms and PEF improved markedly with budesonide. During the study, viral respiratory infections were associated with clearly recognizable exacerbations. None of these would have been identified as exacerbations if the diagnosis had been based on change from run-in values (left of vertical dotted line)

corticosteroids to reduce the risk of progression to a severe exacerbation. There is only limited evidence about the introduction of a long-acting β_2-agonist during exacerbations,[3,4] compared with their established role in poorly controlled asthma. In children with intermittent asthma, viral exacerbations are not prevented by regular inhaled corticosteroids despite an improvement in lung function and airway hyperresponsiveness,[5] but may be reduced by regular treatment with montelukast.[6]

Duration of treatment also differs between exacerbations and poorly controlled asthma. With exacerbations, treatment is usually reduced promptly to maintenance levels once the episode has resolved, usually within a few weeks, whereas for poorly controlled asthma, guidelines recommend that an increased level of treatment should be maintained for ≥ 3 months after achievement of asthma control.[1] There is a less obvious distinction between treatment of mild exacerbations and treatment of poorly controlled

asthma with the management strategy in which the budesonide/formoterol combination is used both as reliever and maintenance treatment.[7]

The clinical distinction between exacerbations and poor asthma control becomes somewhat arbitrary when poor control continues to worsen with time (for example, see Figure 2.3c) to the point where the patient cannot tolerate the symptoms and presents for emergency medical care. At that point, the patient would be considered to be having an exacerbation in terms of immediate treatment needs, but attention would obviously need to be focused on changing long-term management as well, to avoid a recurrence of the problem.

Exacerbations and poorly controlled asthma may have different pathogenesis

The relationship between poorly controlled asthma and exacerbations is complex. If asthma control is defined as a dichotomous measure

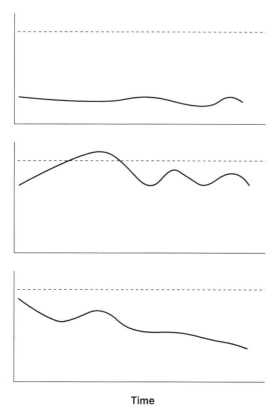

Time

Figure 2.3 Poorly controlled asthma implies failure to meet certain absolute criteria, with no necessary implication of change from the patient's usual state, as a patient may have poorly controlled asthma for many years. The figure shows stylized representations of three patient records which could be recognized clinically as poor asthma control against an absolute criterion (or criteria) indicated by the dotted line. In each case, the x-axis represents time, and the y-axis represents variable(s) such as symptoms, lung function or quality of life. In the third example, asthma control may progressively worsen to the stage that the patient presents for extra care and is diagnosed as having an exacerbation

where poorly controlled asthma represents anything other than perfect control, then exacerbations, being characterized by clinical features which are also manifestations of poor control (symptoms, β_2-agonist use, reduced lung function, etc.) will by definition result in categorization

of the patient as poorly controlled. However, using more widely applicable categorizations of asthma control, there is a strong association between poorly controlled asthma and increased exacerbations,[8,9] and the treatment of poorly controlled asthma reduces the risk of future exacerbations.[10–12] However, some exacerbations still occur despite optimal asthma control,[12,13] particularly in association with viral infection[13] (Figure 2.4); viral exacerbations, although reduced in children who are being treated with inhaled corticosteroids, are not prevented by such treatment.[14,15] An example of the complexity of the relationship is seen in a report which demonstrated that serious exacerbations were increased with regular high-dose formoterol despite an improvement in overall asthma control.[16]

Some of the above observations may be explained by heterogeneity in the causes of exacerbations. Viral exacerbations, or exacerbations which occur despite sustained corticosteroid doses, are characterized by neutrophilic inflammation,[17,18] increased airway responsiveness to methacholine,[18] a sustained decrease in lung function without any increase in diurnal peak expiratory flow (PEF) variability[13] and impaired response to corticosteroids.[19] By contrast, corticosteroid reduction or allergen exposure causes exacerbations with sputum eosinophilia,[17,18,20] increased indirect responsiveness,[18,21] increased diurnal PEF variability[20] and good response to corticosteroids[20] The latter characteristics are also observed in stable (non-exacerbating) patients with poorly controlled asthma.[13] Together, these observations suggest that some exacerbations may occur due to poor asthma control or treatment non-adherence, but that others, including those triggered by viral infections, may also occur independently, unrelated to the level of asthma control or the adequacy of treatment.

Data about exacerbations and poorly controlled asthma are used differently

In clinical practice, if a patient presents because of asthma, information about the timecourse of

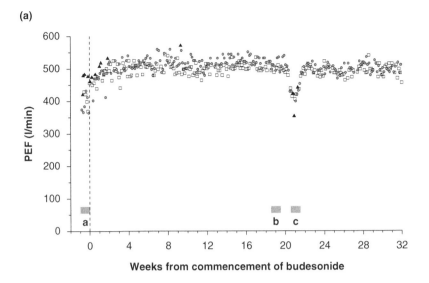

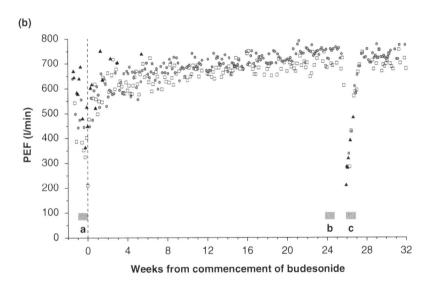

Figure 2.4 Electronically recorded peak expiratory flow (PEF) data from two subjects (a) and (b) in a budesonide study,[41] each over a period of 8 months. Despite good clinical control of asthma as demonstrated by symptoms, reliever use, lung function and normalized airway responsiveness, the subjects experienced asthma exacerbations during typical viral infections

the present problem will usually allow the clinician to judge whether to treat for an exacerbation or for poorly controlled asthma. However, specific diagnostic criteria are needed for the construction of written action plans. Such action plans typically describe 2–4 levels of severity of an exacerbation, with specific treatment for each.[22] The construction of sample action plans in asthma guidelines suggests that they are targeting exacerbations, although guidelines sometimes refer to action plans as assisting patients to recognize when asthma 'goes out of control'.

In clinical trials, diagnostic criteria for exacerbations are needed for several applications during the course of a study. First, exacerbations may be mentioned amongst study inclusion/ exclusion criteria, either by excluding subjects with recent exacerbations to ensure clinical stability at entry, or, less commonly, requiring a certain frequency of exacerbations in order to select a high-risk population.[23,24] Second, clinical asthma studies often utilize a form of action plan, by providing written instructions for when the subject should contact the investigator or commence extra treatment. The specific criteria which are used, via their effect on exacerbation treatment, may have an impact on subsequent efficacy measures relating to asthma control. Third, exacerbations are usually identified as adverse events by subject recall of health-care utilization, courses of oral corticosteroids and time off work. Fourth, several major clinical trials[7,25] have undertaken retrospective analysis of diary data, particularly PEF, to identify unreported episodes which would have qualified as exacerbations. Finally, outcomes relating to exacerbations are also used indirectly as safety measures (e.g. serious exacerbations resulting in hospitalization or death), or, increasingly, as measures of efficacy (numbers of mild, moderate or severe exacerbations, or time to first exacerbation).

In clinical trials, poorly controlled asthma at entry may be specified by the inclusion criteria, although it is often unclear whether the aim is to confirm the diagnosis of asthma or to select patients with the potential to improve. In some previous studies, poor asthma control was deliberately induced by withdrawal of corticosteroids during run-in, sometimes to the point of exacerbation,[20,26] but more commonly, clinical trials require evidence that patients are clinically 'stable' at entry, i.e. not necessarily well controlled, but providing a stable baseline. Many clinical trials use asthma control as a measure of efficacy, often with multiple individual or composite measures, or with subjects categorized into levels of asthma control.[12]

In population studies, there is considerable difficulty in distinguishing between exacerbations and poor control, because of the available datasets. For example, emergency department visits for acute exacerbations cannot be distinguished from those by patients with poorly controlled asthma who use the emergency department for routine sick care.[27]

Exacerbations thus overlap considerably with poor asthma control, in that they are found more commonly in the presence of each other. However, despite this overlap, it is clear from clinical and research usage, evidence for pathogenesis and response to treatment that exacerbations and poorly controlled asthma represent different clinical entities, and that exacerbations are not entirely a subset of poor asthma control.

TOOLS USED FOR DIAGNOSIS OF EXACERBATIONS

Multiple different tools are currently available to the clinician and the researcher to diagnose and assess both exacerbations and poor asthma control. An overview of different types of diagnostic tool is given in the following pages. The choice of diagnostic tool will depend on the context of its use. Some tools are suited for prospective use, and others for retrospective use, and some are suited for clinical practice and others only for the carefully documented environment of a clinical trial. All of these tools should be evaluated in the light of awareness that asthma itself is a heterogeneous condition, so any measure of worsening asthma will also give heterogeneous outcomes.

Physician assessment

Physical examination

Guidelines about exacerbations list multiple physical findings such as respiratory rate, pulse rate and pulsus paradoxus, primarily for classification of severity rather than for diagnosis. It was established long ago in adults[28,29] and in children[30] that physical findings, apart from use of accessory muscles, lack specificity for the detection of severe airway obstruction or arterial desaturation, both of which are predictive of outcome,[31] yet clinicians still appear to be heavily influenced by physical signs.[32] A Pulmonary Score, incorporating respiratory rate, wheezing and retractions, has been found to correlate with PEF during the emergency department assessment of asthma exacerbations in children, but once again, the associations are only moderate,[33] so some exacerbations will be under- or overtreated if objective markers such as lung function or oxygen saturation are not measured.

There is some overlap between physical findings of exacerbations and poorly controlled asthma, as accessory muscle use and widespread wheezing may be observed in some patients with chronically poorly controlled asthma. The medical history will readily establish whether this is a change from usual status.

Global physician assessment

Insight into clinical reasoning about the diagnosis of exacerbations and asthma control was obtained from a recent survey of French clinicians (general practitioners, allergologists, respiratory physicians and emergency care physicians), who were asked to nominate the three criteria which were most important for the diagnosis of mild and severe exacerbations and for the assessment of asthma control.[34] The criteria which were most commonly nominated first, second and third for diagnosis of mild exacerbations were 2 days of increased dyspnea/reliever use (30%), dyspnea affecting daily activities/sleeping (26%) and reduced response to reliever (24%). For severe exacerbations, the three criteria were hospitalization (59%), >30% reduction in PEF on ≥2 days (29%) and use of systemic corticosteroids (23%). For the assessment of asthma control, the clinicians primarily nominated normal PEF or FEV$_1$

(25%), minimum of rescue therapy (29%) and normal daily activity (19%). Ironically, 'normal PEF or FEV$_1$' was most commonly nominated by the groups who were said to be least likely to have a spirometer in their clinical practice (general practitioners and emergency physicians). This study provides useful insight, although the results may not reflect actual clinical decisions, and the very low response rate (7%) limits generalizability.[34]

During the development of the Asthma Control Questionnaire (ACQ),[35] 91 'international opinion leaders' were asked to rank 10 asthma symptoms for their importance in the assessment of asthma control. They were advised that questions about β$_2$-agonist use and lung function would be included. The clinicians were provided with a definition of asthma control which, unlike current guidelines, focused on impact on the patient, ranging from '"well controlled", in which the patient is totally unimpaired and unlimited ... to "extremely poorly controlled", which is a "life-threatening state"'. This implies an assumption by the authors that exacerbations represent extremely poor control. In the responses, the highest-ranked symptoms were night waking, limitation of daily activities, symptoms on awaking, dyspnea and wheeze. The authors then worded the final ACQ questions with text responses, some referring to symptom frequency, some to symptom intensity and some to symptom magnitude, with a recall period of 1 week. It is not widely recognized that, because of its development method, the ACQ was intended to reflect clinicians' assessment of both asthma control and exacerbations as part of a presumed continuum.

Indirect measures

Use of oral corticosteroids

In clinical trials in adults, prescription or use of oral corticosteroids is now commonly used to define exacerbations. This was initially included in study protocols as a safety measure, to ensure that clinically serious episodes, e.g. of rapid onset, were treated. At first sight, use of oral corticosteroids represents a pragmatic proxy for clinician judgment about the presence and severity of an exacerbation. The frequency of its citation in the French survey[34] indicates the extent to which this concept has penetrated into clinical practice. However, use of oral corticosteroids is only useful for *retrospective* diagnosis of exacerbations – for example, number of courses of steroids in the previous 12 months. Use of oral corticosteroids cannot be used as a prospective diagnostic criterion, because of the implicit circular argument: '*I am prescribing oral corticosteroids because this is the accepted treatment for severe asthma exacerbations; this episode is a severe exacerbation because I think it needs treatment with oral corticosteroids*'. Defining exacerbations by oral corticosteroid use is obviously also meaningless for randomized controlled trials of other treatments for acute exacerbations.

In some clinical trials, a high proportion of exacerbations are diagnosed by use of oral corticosteroids, suggesting either real or perceived inadequacy of other diagnostic criteria specified in the same protocols. In the FACET study,[25] in which severe exacerbations were defined either by use of oral corticosteroids or by a 30% fall in PEF for ≥ 2 days, 73% of exacerbations were diagnosed by oral corticosteroid use, and these exacerbations had more symptoms and a lower fall in PEF than those diagnosed by the PEF criterion (Figure 2.5). In clinical trials involving children, the definition of exacerbations by prescription of oral corticosteroids appears considerably less common, and, when this criterion is used, it often also includes inhaled corticosteroids.[6,7]

In reality, the relationship between exacerbation severity or frequency and the use of oral corticosteroids may be weak. Before prescribing oral corticosteroids, the clinician not only assesses exacerbation presence and severity, but also whether the episode is likely to resolve with increased reliever alone (natural history), whether oral corticosteroids will speed recovery

(efficacy) and whether 'costs' (dollars and side-effects) for this patient are outweighed by the potential benefits. Similarly, before the patient takes the medication, he/she goes through a similar evaluation, with perhaps more emphasis on the risk of perceived side-effects than on perceived efficacy.[36,37] 'Steroid phobia' may be a major factor in under-usage of asthma action plans.

Many clinicians have only limited experience with objective measures of lung function such as spirometry or peak flow monitoring, so their assessment of exacerbations is likely to be driven primarily by symptoms. However, it was demonstrated almost 30 years ago that the personalities of both patient and physician had a significant effect on prescribed doses of corticosteroids.[38] This study involved long-term hospitalized patients with frequent infective exacerbations and marked airway hyperresponsiveness. Patients who scored high on a Panic–Fear scale were prescribed an average of 5 mg/day prednisone more than patients who scored low or moderate on the same scale, and empathic physicians prescribed higher doses of prednisone relative to lung function,[38] even after adjustment for Panic–Fear symptoms.[39] Further work on the interactions between patient and physician leave no doubt that prescription of oral corticosteroids is a highly subjective marker of exacerbations, albeit responsive to treatment at a group level.[10]

Oral corticosteroid use cannot necessarily be used to distinguish exacerbations from poorly controlled asthma in retrospective analysis, as, in the past, oral corticosteroids were often used for initiation of treatment for poorly controlled asthma. This was recommended in the 1995 British Thoracic Society guidelines, to ensure rapid symptomatic relief and reduction of risk.[40] This approach has become less common in recent years with use of long-acting β_2-agonists and with awareness of the rapidity of onset of action of inhaled corticosteroids.[26,41,42]

The prescription of antibiotics has occasionally been used in clinical trials to identify

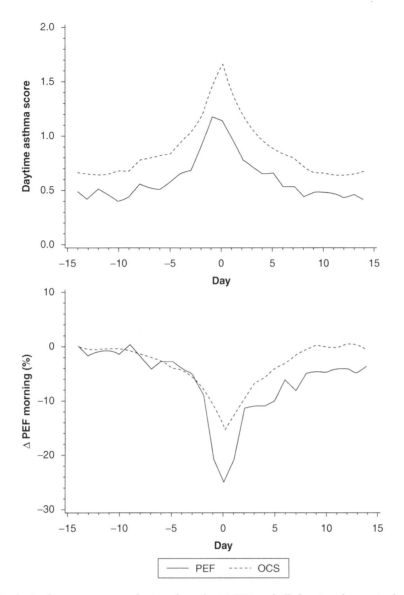

Figure 2.5 Analysis of 425 severe exacerbations from the FACET study,[25] showing changes in daytime asthma score and morning peak expiratory flow (PEF) in relation to whether the exacerbation was diagnosed by the need for oral corticosteroids (OCS; *n* = 311) or by a 30% fall in PEF (PEF; *n* = 114). Reproduced with permission from reference 25

asthma exacerbations,[43] but this definition is not generally accepted, and is likely to disappear as the lack of efficacy of antibiotics for viral respiratory infections is more widely known.[44]

Health-care utilization

Unscheduled health-care utilization is often used as *de facto* evidence of asthma exacerbations, particularly for acute in-hospital studies,

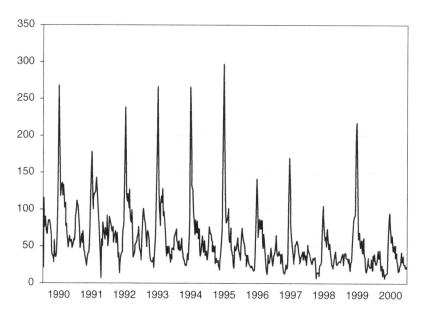

Figure 2.6 Number of hospitalizations of children aged 5–15 years by week of the year in Ontario from 1990 to 2000, showing the peak each year shortly after the end of the summer school vacation, which is believed to be associated with rhinovirus infection. Reproduced with permission from reference 14

e.g. β_2-agonist by nebulizer vs. puffer/spacer.[45] Emergency department presentations and hospitalizations are important outcomes as they contribute a large proportion of health-care costs for asthma, and indicate patients at increased risk of death.[46] It is often assumed that a stepwise increase in severity is indicated by unscheduled primary care visits, emergency department visits and hospital admissions, respectively. Given the frustrations of hospital waiting rooms, and economic restraints on admissions, this appears plausible.

In population studies, health-care utilization is used as a proxy for exacerbation frequency because of the accessibility of these data. Use of such data has allowed recognition of the role of viral infections in childhood asthma exacerbations[47] including post-vacation epidemics[14] (Figure 2.6) and recognition of the specific meteorological phenomena associated with thunderstorm asthma epidemics.[48] Doctor visits are considerably less robust as a marker for exacerbations in population studies, due to

difficulty in distinguishing scheduled from unscheduled visits.

There are several disadvantages in using health-care utilization to diagnose exacerbations, in either adults or children. First, in clinical practice, health-care utilization is primarily useful only for retrospective analysis of exacerbations, because of the same circular argument as for oral corticosteroids (see above). Second, some emergency department asthma presentations are for routine sick care,[49] and patient-related factors such as gender,[50] perception of airway obstruction,[51] anxiety and self-efficacy[52] and attitudes to medical care and medications[27] may influence the decision to present for medical care. Third, there may be important social, economic and health system differences between regions or countries, or over time, which will affect emergency department presentations and hence apparent rates of asthma exacerbations. For example, patients presenting to an emergency department in Uruguay had a mean FEV_1 at entry of approximately 0.8 l,[53] whereas in a Canadian

26

study, the mean FEV_1 was 1.6 l.[54] Fourth, emergency department visits exclude most mild exacerbations, and, although some patients with even mild recent-onset asthma will require emergency department presentation or hospitalization,[55] such health-care utilization does not necessarily reflect changes in mild asthma in the community. Finally, increased health-care utilization may be a marker of improved asthma management, if patients using a written action plan present for medical review before asthma is severe.[56] Exacerbations which occur without health-care utilization are important, as late presentation[57] is a factor in many asthma deaths.

The relationship between health-care utilization, exacerbations and poor asthma control is complex. First, emergency department presentation is undoubtedly more common in patients with features of poor asthma control. For example, daily reliever use was found to be associated with increased risk of emergency department presentation within the next 12 months (relative risk 2.2),[58] and emergency department attendance was found to be increased in patients with lower use of inhaled corticosteroids and with poor inhaler technique.[59] Second, some emergency department attendances follow a period of worsening asthma control, particularly when the patient has few social supports at home. In one study, 20–25% of adult patients with near-fatal asthma or hospital admission for asthma had symptoms for > 21 days prior to presentation.[60] Third, long-term risks for poorly controlled asthma may interact with short-term triggers, as in the study by Green and colleagues which showed increased risk of hospitalization for patients who were sensitized and exposed to an allergen and also had a viral respiratory infection.[61]

Patient or parent assessment

Language about exacerbations

The word 'exacerbation', which is widely used in clinical practice guidelines and occasionally in questionnaires,[62] fails all of the cardinal rules for effective communication with patients – it has five syllables, is difficult to pronounce and, outside medicine, is found only in erudite contexts. Some patients refer to 'exasperations', which seems remarkably apt. The simplest synonym for 'exacerbation' is 'attack'. This word is part of the GINA definition of exacerbation, and two widely used epidemiological questionnaires for adults[63] and children[64] include the question 'How many asthma attacks have you had in the last 12 months?'. However, responses to this question range from 'one' to '365 times a year' and 'Don't know'. In a qualitative study, Aroni and colleagues[65] found that the response to this question was associated with patients' interpretation of the meaning of 'attack', with some using it for minor symptoms, and others reserving its use for intensive care unit episodes. Vincent and colleagues found that patients experiencing an exacerbation would sometimes use the word 'attack' to work colleagues or strangers to avoid ambiguity, but would mostly avoid its use to family members, in order to avoid alarm or criticism.[66] Ironically in the present context, Aroni and colleagues concluded that the most useful expression for referring to severe episodes which required emergency medical review was 'out of control'.[65]

Patient or parental assessment

In order to use symptom-based action plans, or present for medical care, patients must be able to recognize worsening asthma. It is now well recognized that patients vary in their ability to detect airway obstruction. Rubinfeld and Pain found that about 15% of subjects experienced no symptoms during methacholine challenge despite a > 15% fall in FEV_1.[67] Rapid-onset airway obstruction was more readily identified, suggesting that poor perception may be relevant to chronically poorly controlled asthma as well as to exacerbations. Poor perception cannot be predicted by age, sex or previous duration of asthma,[68] but may be more common with indirect rather than direct challenges,[69] or in patients with moderate/severe asthma.[70] The above conclusions from bronchial challenge studies have been confirmed in emergency department studies, which showed no relationship between $FEV_1\%$ predicted and patient assessment of exacerbation severity.[32] Patients with previous near-fatal asthma were found to have poor perception of and responses to hypoxia, even when in clinical remission.[71] These studies raise concerns about the reliability of symptom-driven exacerbation diagnosis, and suggest that poor perception, if undetected, may predispose to the risk of severe attacks by reducing the chance of early intervention.

Parental report is an important component of exacerbation diagnosis for children, and, for young children, a repeatedly observed change in behavior or activity may indicate an impending exacerbation.[72] Parental report is also essential for the evaluation of asthma control. However, formal studies have demonstrated little relationship between parental report and the magnitude of exercise-induced bronchoconstriction[73] or the frequency of symptoms[74] in their children.

Spirometry

Lung function predicts outcome in patients presenting to hospital with acute asthma exacerbations.[31] In clinical practice guidelines and clinical trials, FEV_1 or PEF is used primarily to categorize exacerbations by severity, rather than to diagnose them. Typical cut-off points are >80% predicted or best for mild, 60–80% for moderate and <60% for severe exacerbations.[1] However, these same cut-off points are used within the same guidelines for the categorization of asthma control outside the context of an exacerbation.[1] Thus, lung function alone cannot be used to distinguish between exacerbations and poor control.

Symptom-based criteria for exacerbations

A very large number of symptom criteria have been used for diagnosis of exacerbations, but few publications have examined their performance characteristics. Many publications fail to specify the criteria which were used, suggesting lack of awareness of the potential impact on outcomes. Some criteria refer to worsening/increase in symptoms, or loss of response to a β_2-agonist,[75] relying on the patient's subjective judgment that there has been a significant change.[76] Onset of night waking is often included as an absolute criterion, but has poor sensitivity for exacerbations.[25] The above criteria do not require a daily symptom diary, and are feasible for clinical practice, but they are usually subjective. All symptom criteria are subject to problems with perception of airway obstruction and impact of personality (as above). Osman and colleagues showed that patients 'dislike' cough and dyspnea more than wheeze or night waking,[77] and one can perhaps extrapolate to assume that the former symptoms will be more likely to result in presentation for medical care. In pediatric studies, the symptom criteria for diagnosis of exacerbations tend to be far more pragmatic than those in adult studies, often using parental assessment of significant change.

For clinical asthma trials in which a daily symptom diary is recorded, symptom criteria are usually based on the run-in period. This requires immediate analysis of run-in data, which may be difficult with paper diaries. Scores may vary in their components (generic 'asthma symptoms' or individual symptoms of cough, wheeze, dyspnea, chest tightness), the symptom attribute (frequency, intensity or impact on daily activities) and the range of available scores, considered separately or added to give a total symptom score. Change is variously characterized by simple arithmetic calculation as an absolute or percentage change in score from baseline, or a specific score level. None of these can be regarded as equivalent, and none appear to take into account the level of variability in the subjects' baseline level of symptoms. In some studies, the symptom score criterion for a change in treatment may be within the range of run-in data.[78] There is little clarity in the literature about the impact of different scoring systems on diagnostic accuracy, and they are sometimes, inappropriately, used interchangeably.

Bronchodilator use

Multiple absolute and relative criteria for an as-needed β_2-agonist have been utilized for the diagnosis of exacerbations. There is no consistent approach as to whether use of a β_2-agonist before exercise should be included, and many publi cations do not state how this issue has been handled. Marked differences in β_2-agonist use may be found between different countries. For example, in a study of acute severe asthma in Uruguay, only 60% of patients had used a β_2-agonist in the previous 24 hours,[53] whereas in a Canadian study, the proportion was almost 90%.[54]

As with symptom scores, β_2-agonist criteria are primarily identified by simple arithmetic calculation from baseline. A wide range of criteria have been used, from two to seven[7,79] extra puffs per day, or a 70% increase[80] over baseline. The impact of such differences, and the effect of different levels of baseline usage, have not been examined. The concept of defining exac-erbations as change from baseline (rather than change from recent status) is problematic if, as often occurs, β_2-agonist usage falls after the subject commences active treatment.

Although reliever use is easily quantified, it is primarily driven by symptoms, and is there-fore subject to limitations of over- and under-perception, and the impact of personality and beliefs about medication.[36] In an early study, patients with high Panic–Fear ratings requested more as-needed medications even when lung function was normal, and patients with low Panic–Fear ratings rarely requested as-needed medications, even when their lung function was reduced.[39] β_2-Agonist use may also be influenced by habitual use, unreported changes in exercise frequency, anticipatory use for very mild symp-toms or differences over time. Twenty years ago, eight puffs of β_2-agonist per day would have been

standard management, whereas now it could characterize either an exacerbation or poorly controlled asthma.

PEF-based criteria

Given that the definition of exacerbation includes both symptoms and airflow obstruction, exacerbation definitions for adults often include an objective measure of lung function, usually PEF. In clinical practice, for patients undertaking regular monitoring, a PEF criterion gives the opportunity to identify objective 'change from usual status', from either a chart or a diary. Some patients only start monitoring when symptoms increase, although this approach is dependent on good perception. For children, although lung function measurements have important prognos-tic significance, PEF monitoring does not appear to be practicable for detection of exacerbations,[81] because of poor technique and poor adherence.[82]

Because of the efffects of age, height and gen-der on PEF, the criteria for exacerbations are calculated from a PEF reference value. In clini-cal trials, this is usually established during the run-in period, but again this only allows identi-fication of exacerbations as '*change from base-line status*' rather than '*change from recent status*'. The run-in period is suitable as a base-line for diagnosis of exacerbations if subjects have well-controlled asthma at entry.[83] However, a far more common situation is that subjects are recruited with poorly controlled asthma and the PEF subsequently increases (Figure 2.2). In the latter instance, the greater is a subject's post-randomization increase in PEF, the greater is the percentage fall from recent status that the subject would need to experience in order to satisfy a PEF criterion based on run-in data. Basing PEF criteria on run-in data is likely to increase the apparent dissociation between PEF and symp-toms (and hence prescription of oral cortico-steroids) in clinical trials.

Clinical practice guidelines recommend that the reference value for PEF criteria should be predicted or personal best PEF. Action plans based on personal best PEF are associated with better health outcomes, including hospitalization, than those based on predicted PEF.[22] This presumably reflects better customization of the PEF criterion to the patient. Personal best PEF is defined in guidelines as the highest PEF over 2–3 weeks of pre- and post-bronchodilator monitoring during a period of good asthma control.[2] However, many patients present for care only when their asthma is poorly controlled, and some measures of asthma control continue to improve for many months after commencement of treatment.[41] By contrast, it has been shown that personal best PEF from twice daily monitoring reaches a plateau after only 3 weeks of high-dose inhaled corticosteroid treatment.[84] Thus, exacerbation criteria based on personal best PEF can be established early in treatment, while the patient is still motivated to return.

Rather than basing PEF criteria on personal best or predicted PEF, clinical trials typically use mean PEF or mean morning PEF as the reference value (for example, see references 10 and 78). Mean PEF has not been evaluated in this role. However, the difference between mean morning PEF and personal best is substantially greater during poor asthma control than when asthma is well controlled.[84] Thus, for studies in which subjects enter with poorly controlled asthma, and in which a percentage criterion is used, mean morning PEF may be an inappropriate reference value for diagnosis of exacerbations.

In both clinical practice guidelines and clinical trials, the PEF criterion for exacerbations is usually calculated for convenience as a percentage of the reference value. Multiple different percentages have been used; in their meta-analysis of action plans, Gibson and Powell found studies using 70%, 75%, 80% and 85% of personal best or predicted PEF.[22] Several authors have found a criterion of <70% of baseline mean to be too stringent, with most patients requiring medical intervention before this point is reached.[25,75,85] Gibson and colleagues[86] had earlier examined the performance characteristics of cut-off points of 80% and 60% of best or predicted PEF, using 43

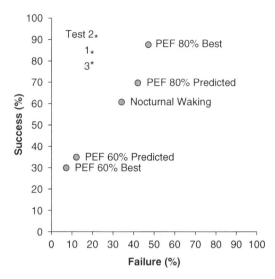

Figure 2.7 Performance characteristics of published action points (filled circles) and action points derived from quality-control analysis of peak expiratory flow (PEF) records (stars). Success and Failure refer to the ability of the given action point to identify 43 exacerbations defined by need for oral corticosteroids. Test 1 was satisfied if a single PEF value was below mean − 3 standard deviations (SD); Test 2 was satisfied if 2 of 3 consecutive values were below mean − 2SD; and Test 3 was satisfied if 4 of 5 consecutive values were below mean − 1SD. The quality control action points had a low failure rate, e.g. Test 2 had 23% failures (false positives) compared with 47% for an action point of 80% personal best, $p = 0.002$. Reproduced with permission from reference 86

exacerbations defined from respiratory physician assessment of increase in symptoms/reliever use and fall in lung function. The sensitivity and specificity of percentage criteria were poor (Figure 2.7), because of interpatient differences in baseline PEF variability (Figure 2.8). Use of percentage PEF criteria would therefore lead to both undertreatment and overtreatment of exacerbations. In the same study, much better sensitivity and specificity were obtained using 'quality control' cut-off points,[87] based on standard deviation fall below the mean.[86] However,

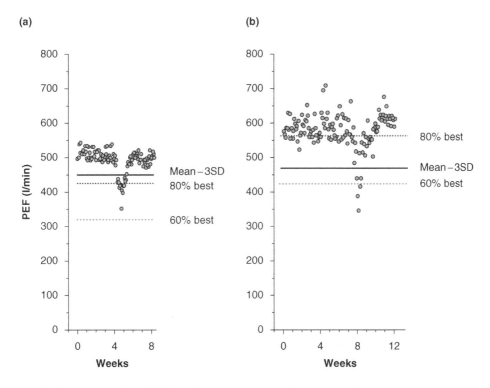

Figure 2.8 Peak expiratory flow (PEF) data before, during and after a viral asthma exacerbation in two patients (a) and (b), from electronic monitoring. The figure shows a difference in baseline PEF variability between the two patients, and the resulting poor performance of standard percentage criteria (60% and 80% of personal best) for identifying both exacerbations. By contrast, the quality control action point (mean – 3 standard deviations [SD]) was able to identify both exacerbations. Reproduced with permission from reference 93

this type of analysis requires computerized processing, which is not usually feasible within the constraints of a consultation or clinical trial visit. It is ironic that in clinical trials in which sophisticated statistical analysis methods are used to assess PEF as an outcome measure, and in which exacerbations are an important outcome variable, exacerbations are still diagnosed on the basis of percentage PEF criteria. Electronic monitoring will obviously facilitate the integration of more statistically appropriate exacerbation diagnosis into both clinical practice and clinical trials.

In the assessment of asthma control, the most commonly used PEF index is diurnal variability, calculated daily as amplitude per cent mean or maximum, and averaged over 1–2 weeks.[88] Increased diurnal variability, as a marker of poor asthma control, is a significant predictor of subsequent severe exacerbations.[25] However, under present-day monitoring conditions, 'increased' levels of diurnal variability (>20%[1]) are now only rarely seen, because of the underestimation of diurnal variability when PEF is recorded only twice daily.[89] Few studies have examined diurnal variability during exacerbations. Diurnal variability of >25% at discharge from hospital was found to be associated with increased risk of early relapse and readmission.[90] Diurnal variability is known to increase following withdrawal of inhaled corticosteroid.[20] However, diurnal variability does not increase during even severe viral exacerbations

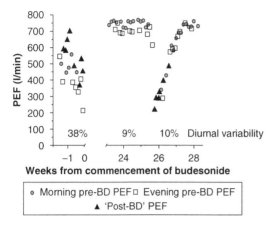

Figure 2.9 Three sections of peak expiratory flow (PEF) data from Figure 2.4(a), from the run-in period (poorly controlled asthma), good asthma control and viral exacerbation. During the exacerbation, there was a sustained fall in PEF with loss of normal daytime recovery and of response to a β_2-agonist (budesonide; BD), but with no increase in diurnal PEF variability compared with during good asthma control. Reproduced with permission from reference 13

compared with good asthma control, despite a substantial decrease in overall PEF[13] (Figure 2.9).

Percentage PEF criteria are also included in the assessment of asthma control for both clinical practice and clinical trials, with cut-off points of >80%, 60–80% and <60% predicted/personal best for mild, moderate and severe persistent asthma,[1] respectively. These points are the same as those sometimes used for the categorization of exacerbations as mild, moderate and severe.[1] Thus, cross-sectional PEF data cannot distinguish between exacerbations and poorly controlled asthma.

Relationship between symptoms, PEF and medication

Even during stable asthma, there is not a strong relationship within individuals between symptoms and airway obstruction, although both are characteristic of asthma. During

exacerbations, group mean data demonstrate an apparently good relationship over time between symptoms and PEF.[25,75,91] Even small changes can be identified if the date of exacerbation onset is precisely known, as in experimental rhinovirus studies.[92] However, the relationships between symptoms and PEF within individual patients are more variable. Some of this variation is due to overlap with other conditions causing symptoms which mimic asthma, e.g. upper airway dysfunction, obesity, obstructive sleep apnea.

Several studies have examined the relationship between symptoms and lung function during asthma exacerbations. Gender appears to be a factor, with women reporting greater impact of symptoms for a given fall in PEF.[50] For severe exacerbations in the FACET study, symptoms, reliever use and PEF showed parallel time-courses,[25] although, as previously mentioned, symptoms were greater for exacerbations identified by oral corticosteroid use than for those identified by a >30% fall in PEF for 2 days. In the case–control study by Chan-Yeung and colleagues[75] (Figure 2.10), exacerbations were defined (day 0) by any of multiple features: unscheduled doctor visit or emergency department presentation, 2 days of increased daytime and night-time symptoms not responding to usual medication, a >30% fall in PEF or commencement/doubling of oral/inhaled corticosteroids. Retrospective analysis of diary data showed that PEF began to fall on day –6, although the difference, when analyzed as percentage change from baseline, was not significant until day 2. Symptom score did not begin to change until day –2, and the difference from baseline was significant on day 0.[75]

Interestingly, this study is often incorrectly quoted as reporting that change in symptoms during exacerbations precedes change in PEF; however, change in PEF was analyzed only as percentage fall from baseline (days –9 to –7).[86] A more sensitive criterion using standard deviation analysis[86] may thus be able to improve the early detection of exacerbations. Electronic

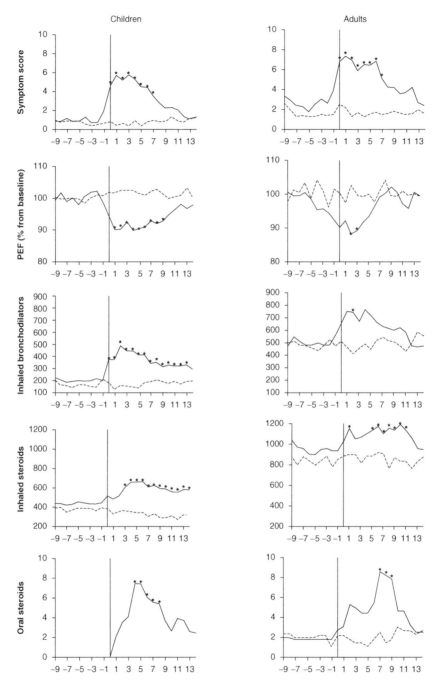

Figure 2.10 The relationship in time between symptoms, peak expiratory flow (PEF), β_2-agonist use, inhaled corticosteroid and oral corticosteroid use, during exacerbations (solid lines) and in control patients for the same period (broken lines), for children (left panel) and adults (right panel). *The value on that day is significantly different from baseline (days −9 to −7). Reproduced with permission from reference 75

monitoring will be needed before this approach can be widely applicable, but early changes may be able to be identified by visual inspection of horizontally compressed PEF charts.[93]

The impact of poor adherence with medication on the retrospective diagnosis of exacerbations, and the relationship between symptoms and PEF, has not been examined. PEF falls by 24 hours after a dose of formoterol, although bronchoprotection is still present,[94] indicating some residual symptom protection. With washout following regular treatment, the fall in PEF is somewhat slower.[95] Intermittent poor adherence with a long-acting β_2-agonist could result in asymptomatic 'exacerbations' appearing on retrospective analysis. Human nature being what it is, clinical trial subjects, regardless of study instructions, may be less likely to contact the investigator for a PEF below their trigger point if they suspect that it is related to missed study medication.

Likewise, the impact of poor adherence or data falsification on the retrospective diagnosis of exacerbations has not been examined. There is irrefutable evidence that data falsification affects around 25% or more of paper PEF data,[96] as well as paper diaries of inhaler adherence[97] and symptoms.[98] The characteristics of falsified data have not been studied, but many patients cannot accurately predict their PEF,[99] so falsified PEF data are unlikely to reflect their actual status at the time of the missing measurement. Retrospectively completed symptom diaries may be more accurate, because of recall of actual events, again increasing the potential for discordance between symptom and PEF data.

Clinicians have considerable expertise in assessing the importance of changes in asthma symptoms, but many have little experience with PEF monitoring. In addition, they may see PEF data in many different formats. Reddel and colleagues observed a seven-fold variation in the horizontal-to-vertical scale of currently available PEF charts.[93] This variation has a major impact on retrospective visual recognition of exacerbations (Figure 2.11), and would be likely to affect prospective recognition of worsening asthma. Variation in the way in which PEF data are presented means that clinicians have not been able to develop pattern recognition skills for changes in lung function. This is likely to increase reliance on symptoms – and hence, the influence of patient personality[38] – in deciding whether to prescribe additional medication. All of the above features will contribute to some of the apparent weaknesses in the relationship between symptoms, PEF and prescription of oral corticosteroids during exacerbations.

Composite scores

Exacerbation days and poor control days

An asthma exacerbation day is a day (or one of a pair of days) that meets one or more criteria for symptoms, bronchodilator use and PEF, as well as major events such as emergency department presentations. Exacerbation days are reported as percentage of total days. Multiple different definitions for exacerbation days are in circulation; most include night waking. The relationship between 'exacerbation days' and clinically recognizable exacerbations appears weak, particularly because only 1–2 days are considered together. The criteria for 'exacerbation days' are almost identical with those for 'poor control days' examined in other studies,[11] and the latter name probably better reflects what is being captured.

As can be seen from the material in the preceding sections, none of the individual components of 'exacerbation days' has been standardized for the diagnosis of exacerbations, so combining several criteria magnifies the variability. A graphic example was reported by Vaquerizo and colleagues,[100] in a study that compared the addition of montelukast or placebo to budesonide. The primary outcome variable was 'asthma-exacerbation days'. In a *post hoc* analysis, the authors also analyzed the same dataset using two additional definitions of exacerbation days. The proportion of exacerbation days in the

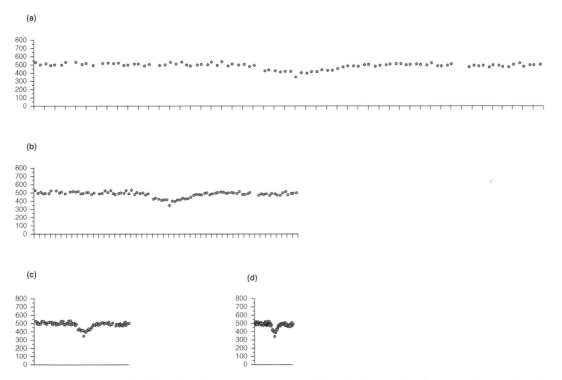

Figure 2.11 Seven weeks of data from the patient in Figure 2.4(a), including a viral asthma exacerbation, plotted on the scale of four different peak expiratory flow (PEF) charts. (a) Allersearch chart; (b) Mini-Wright chart; (c) Prototype clinic chart; (d) Standard occupational asthma scale chart. On horizontally expanded charts (a and b), the exacerbation onset and resolution are difficult to identify, and the exacerbation appears to be very mild, but on horizontally compressed charts (c and d), the baseline PEF data form a solid 'band', from which the exacerbation stands out clearly. Reproduced with permission from reference 93

placebo group was 4.8%, 21.1% and 13.0% with the three definitions, respectively, and these differences are of obvious clinical importance. Differences in exacerbation days between the montelukast and placebo groups for the three definitions were not as marked (35%, 37% and 32%, respectively). Surprisingly, the differences between the actual criteria for the three definitions were fairly subtle (Table 2.1). The high rates with the second of these definitions probably related to the inclusion of an absolute change in PEF of 100 l/min; and an absolute rather than relative β_2-agonist criterion (≥ 4 puffs/day, on a baseline of 3.3 puffs/day). This study[100] highlights the critical importance of

the details of individual criteria for composite scores.

Pediatric studies have also incorporated composite measures of exacerbations, although usually without PEF criteria. For example, Bisgaard and colleagues[6] used a complex definition of 'asthma exacerbation episodes' defined as any three consecutive days with daytime symptoms (average of four symptom questions > 1.0 on each day) and at least two uses/day of β_2-agonist, or rescue with oral/inhaled corticosteroids during ≥ 1 days, or hospitalization. The end of an episode was a day out of the hospital with no daytime symptoms (average of four symptom questions ≤ 0.25) and < 2 uses of

35

EXACERBATIONS OF ASTHMA

Table 2.1 Analysis of 'exacerbation days' using three different criteria for the definition of 'exacerbation days'. From reference 100

Component	'Defined by Laviolette[80]'	'Similar to Wilding[101]' and 'Chan-Yeung[75]'	'Similar to Pauwels' mild exacerbations[10]'
No. of days	1 day	2 consecutive days for all criteria, or 'attack'	1 day, but not single isolated days
PEF	Dec. from baseline of >20% in a.m. PEF OR a.m. PEF <180 l/min	Dec. from baseline of >30% OR dec. from baseline of >100 l/min OR daily PEF variability of >20%	Dec. from baseline of >20% in a.m. PEF
Symptoms	Inc. from baseline symptom score of >50%	Inc. from baseline symptom score of >50%	
Night waking	Awake all night (= awake all night or recurrent episodes of awakening)	Nocturnal waking	Nocturnal waking because of asthma
Short-acting β$_2$-agonist	Inc. from baseline of >70% AND inc. from baseline of ≥2 puffs/day	Use of ≥4 puffs/day	Inc. from baseline of ≥3 puffs
Other	'Asthma attack' = unscheduled medical care for asthma	'Asthma attack'	
Rate in placebo group, median (95% CI)	4.8% (3.5–6.3)	21.1% (15.7–28.2)	13.0% (9.7–18.2)
Rate in montelukast group, median (95% CI)	3.1% (2.0–4.2)	13.4% (9.9–18.0)	8.9% (6.3–12.2)
Difference	35% ($p=0.03$)	37% ($p=0.05$)	32% ($p=0.07$)

PEF, peak expiratory flow; dec., decrease; inc., increase

Vaquerizo et al.[100] analyzed a clinical trial dataset for 'exacerbation days', using three different definitions derived from other publications. Differences in criteria between the three definitions, although apparently small, resulted in major differences in the observed frequency of 'exacerbation days'

β_2-agonist, and no oral corticosteroids. The longer minimum period (3 days) makes this definition fall somewhere between the previously mentioned exacerbation days, and a clinically recognizable exacerbation.

CONCLUSIONS

Exacerbations of asthma can be life-threatening, and, even at a less severe level, they contribute substantially to the burden of asthma to the patient and to the community. There is a major incentive to diagnose exacerbations when they are early or mild, as late presentation for medical care increases the risks to the patient. The impetus for early treatment increases the need for better diagnostic criteria. Written action plans, when part of self-management education and regular review, are associated with substantially improved health outcomes,[22] although they have utilized surprisingly diverse diagnostic criteria and treatment instructions. Despite the importance of diagnosing exacerbations, our current knowledge – and our ability to improve on current knowledge – is significantly limited by the current practice of combining heterogeneous exacerbation data. We need to be particularly cautious about referring to the sensitivity and specificity of existing diagnostic criteria for exacerbations when there is no gold standard for their definition, particularly when current criteria are heavily influenced by subjective factors.

In both medical and non-medical usage, the word 'exacerbation' refers to 'worsening of an existing state'. Diagnosis of exacerbations is thus dependent on a clear characterisation of asthma itself. However, the definition of asthma is multifactorial, comprising multiple clinical, physiological and pathological features, none of which is both necessary and sufficient for the diagnosis of asthma. As a result, asthma itself is a markedly heterogeneous condition. There are several known sub-groups, particularly relating to the type of inflammatory process, and these are known to demonstrate at least some differences

in clinical characteristics and response to treatment. In addition, the clinical manifestations of asthma overlap with other conditions such as COPD, vocal cord dysfunction and obesity. Heterogeneity in the diagnosis of asthma inevitably leads to heterogeneity in the diagnosis of exacerbations.

In addition, identification of exacerbations is, by definition, relative to the patient's usual or recent state. The level of symptoms and airway obstruction differs markedly between patients, either associated with or independent of pharmacological treatment. Thus an absolute level of symptoms or airway obstruction that is the usual status of one patient will be an exacerbation for another or even for the same patient later in the course of treatment (Figure 2.2). Likewise, variation in symptoms and airway obstruction differs from patient to patient, so a percentage or absolute change from a reference value will represent a significant worsening for one patient but will be within the usual range of variation for another (Figure 2.8). In clinical trials, we should expect to apply the same level of statistical rigor to the detection of change from usual status within individuals that we take for granted in the detection of change in outcomes at a group level. The current approach in clinical trials of diagnosing exacerbations on the basis of change from baseline status, rather than change from recent status, is seriously flawed in concept.

The situation is further complicated by the often unacknowledged poor quality of much of the available clinical trial diary data for symptoms, reliever use and PEF, due to poor adherence and data falsification. In one covert study, only 54% of paper diary entries were present, and 22% of these had been falsified,[96] and other studies have confirmed similar results. Diary data offer the best opportunity for prospective diagnosis and retrospective analysis of exacerbations, but we would not accept an error rate of this magnitude in any other outcome variable for clinical trials. Use of electronic monitoring devices will markedly improve data quality.

Based on the above observations, clarification of the definition of exacerbations needs to focus initially on establishing scientifically valid criteria for their diagnosis. This should involve a three-step process. First, there is a 'straightforward' statistical task of identifying the point at which a measure would become *statistically significantly different* from the patient's previous status, i.e. outside the patient's usual range of variation. This process should be carried out for multiple different variables, particularly the clinically relevant characteristics related to symptoms and airway obstruction, with observation of their relative timecourses. The second step is to establish which of these criteria identify episodes that are *clinically important*, i.e. that cause distress and/or risk to the patient. This information can be obtained from re-analysis of studies which include records of morbidity and of patient-centered outcomes, e.g. quality of life.

The third step is to identify the point at which patients would *benefit from treatment*, which is a separate issue from the question of whether or not an exacerbation has occurred. At present, this question cannot be readily answered because of heterogeneity of the diagnostic criteria in existing studies. This can be improved by retrospectively examining the response to treatment of exacerbations identified by each of several different criteria (developed as above), from a large dataset. For example, rather than looking at the overall effect of a particular treatment for exacerbations, one would look at the response of episodes identified by night waking, episodes identified by various symptom scores, episodes identified by health-care utilization, etc., in order to determine which criteria best predicted response to treatment.

Although, in clinical practice, there is clear recognition of both exacerbations and poorly controlled asthma in their more severe incarnations, neither of these phenomena is dichotomous, and each forms part of an ill-defined continuum, with overlapping manifestations. It may be unrealistic to expect that a single criterion or set of criteria could be established for diagnosis of exacerbations, and it may be more appropriate to develop separate criteria for early identification of exacerbations which would or would not respond to corticosteroid and/or long-acting β_2-agonist treatment.

RECOMMENDATIONS

Firm recommendations for the diagnosis of exacerbations are difficult because of the heterogeneity of existing data, and there is an urgent need for standardization in this area. If possible, the requirements for diagnosis of occurrence of exacerbation should be considered separately from the requirements for diagnosis of 'need to treat'.

For the purposes of clinical trials or population studies, oral corticosteroid use and emergency department presentations will capture the majority of severe exacerbations. In these contexts, a certain degree of misclassification is acceptable, and may not significantly impact on the responsiveness of the measure. However, misclassification is obviously far less acceptable at the level of the individual patient, whether a participant in a clinical trial or in clinical practice, because of the risks of undertreatment and overtreatment.

For clinical practice, the diagnosis at present will need to continue to rely on physician judgment about a history of change from usual status in symptom frequency and reliever use, but such evaluations should always be accompanied by a measurement of lung function. Provided this is done, clinicians will be able to enhance their clinical pattern recognition skills for the relationship between subjective and objective features, and will be able to identify poor perceivers. More work needs to be done before recommendations can be made about the design of written action plans, for both the diagnostic criteria and the therapeutic adjustments which are involved. However, the known benefits of action plans despite the heterogeneity of their content suggests that their specific design features may not be critical for at least some benefit to occur.

Some current criteria appear on existing evidence to be substantially flawed, and cannot be recommended. These include criteria for diary data such as symptoms, reliever use and PEF which are determined by percentage or absolute change without taking baseline variation into account, and/or which use run-in data to determine the level for comparison. In addition, composite criteria appear very problematic because of the multiple cut-off points which are involved.

In ongoing clinical trials, there should be an emphasis on improving the quality of the data which are collected. This should include documenting the exact criteria by which a patient is considered to be having an exacerbation, recording lung function during the evaluation of any possible exacerbation and noting any available evidence about the etiology of exacerbations, e.g. symptoms of viral infection, so that heterogeneity in their clinical manifestations and treatment responses can be investigated. Electronic monitoring will obviously assist in the long-term implementation of scientifically valid and clinically relevant diagnostic criteria, both for clinical trials and, hopefully, for clinical practice. It will be particularly relevant to implementation of future clinical diagnostic algorithms for use with time-trend data.

With reliable data and appropriate analysis tools, the relationships between the various diagnostic criteria for exacerbations can then be confidently explored, and the modifications that would be needed for use of these diagnostic criteria in clinical practice can be established.

ACKNOWLEDGMENTS

HR is supported by the Asthma Foundation of NSW, and SV is supported by the Australian Government and the Cooperative Research Centre for Asthma.

REFERENCES

1. GINA (Global Initiative for Asthma). Workshop Report. Global strategy for asthma management and prevention. NIH Publication No 02–3659, 2002
2. National Asthma Education and Prevention Program Expert Panel Report 2. Guidelines for the diagnosis and management of asthma. NIH Publication 97–4051. Bethesda, MD: NHLBI, NIH 1997
3. Peters JI, Shelledy DC, Jones AP Jr et al. A randomized, placebo-controlled study to evaluate the role of salmeterol in the in-hospital management of asthma. Chest 2000; 118: 313–20
4. Boonsawat W, Charoenratanakul S, Pothirat C, et al. Formoterol (OXIS) Turbuhaler as a rescue therapy compared with salbutamol pMDI plus spacer in patients with acute severe asthma. Respir Med 2003; 97: 1067–74
5. Doull IJ, Lampe FC, Smith S, et al. Effect of inhaled corticosteroids on episodes of wheezing associated with viral infection in school age children: randomised double blind placebo controlled trial. BMJ 1997; 315: 858–62
6. Bisgaard H, Zielen S, Garcia-Garcia ML, et al. Montelukast reduces asthma exacerbations in 2- to 5-year-old children with intermittent asthma. Am J Respir Crit Care Med 2005; 171: 315–22
7. O'Byrne PM, Bisgaard H, Godard PP, et al. Budesonide/formoterol combination therapy as both maintenance and reliever medication in asthma. Am J Respir Crit Care Med 2005; 171: 129–36
8. Fuhlbrigge AL, Adams RJ, Guilbert TW, et al. The burden of asthma in the United States: level and distribution are dependent on interpretation of the national asthma education and prevention program guidelines. Am J Respir Crit Care Med 2002; 166: 1044–9
9. Vollmer WM, Markson LE, O'Connor E, et al. Association of asthma control with health care utilization: a prospective evaluation. Am J Respir Crit Care Med 2002; 165: 195–9
10. Pauwels RA, Lofdahl C-G, Postma DS, et al. Effect of inhaled formoterol and budesonide on exacerbations of asthma. N Engl J Med 1997; 337: 1405–11
11. O'Byrne PM, Barnes PJ, Rodriguez-Roisin R, et al. Low dose inhaled budesonide and formoterol in mild persistent asthma: the OPTIMA randomized trial. Am J Respir Crit Care Med 2001; 164: 1392–7
12. Bateman ED, Boushey HA, Bousquet J, et al. Can guideline-defined asthma control be achieved? The Gaining Optimal Asthma ControL study. Am J Respir Crit Care Med 2004; 170: 836–44
13. Reddel H, Ware S, Marks G, et al. Differences between asthma exacerbations and poor asthma control [erratum in Lancet 1999; 353: 758]. Lancet 1999; 353: 364–9

14. Johnston NW, Johnston SL, Duncan JM, et al. The September epidemic of asthma exacerbations in children: a search for etiology. J Allergy Clin Immunol 2005; 115: 132–8

15. Corne JM, Marshall C, Smith S, et al. Frequency, severity, and duration of rhinovirus infections in asthmatic and non-asthmatic individuals: a longitudinal cohort study. Lancet 2002; 359: 831–4

16. Mann M, Chowdhury B, Sullivan E, et al. Serious asthma exacerbations in asthmatics treated with high-dose formoterol. Chest 2003; 124: 70–4

17. Wark PA, Johnston SL, Moric I, et al. Neutrophil degranulation and cell lysis is associated with clinical severity in virus-induced asthma. Eur Respir J 2002; 19: 68–75

18. in't Veen JC, Smits HH, Hiemstra PS, et al. Lung function and sputum characteristics of patients with severe asthma during an induced exacerbation by double-blind steroid withdrawal. Am J Respir Crit Care Med 1999; 160: 93–9

19. Green RH, Brightling CE, Woltmann G, et al. Analysis of induced sputum in adults with asthma: identification of subgroup with isolated sputum neutrophilia and poor response to inhaled corticosteroids. Thorax 2002; 57: 875–9

20. Gibson PG, Wong BJO, Hepperle MJE, et al. A research method to induce and examine a mild exacerbation of asthma by withdrawal of inhaled corticosteroid. Clin Exp Allergy 1992; 22: 525–32

21. Leuppi JD, Salome CM, Jenkins CR, et al. Predictive markers of asthma exacerbation during stepwise dose reduction of inhaled corticosteroids. Am J Respir Crit Care Med 2001; 163: 406–12

22. Gibson PG, Powell H. Written action plans for asthma: an evidence-based review of the key components. Thorax 2004; 59: 94–9

23. Holgate S, Bousquet J, Wenzel S, et al. Efficacy of omalizumab, an anti-immunoglobulin E antibody, in patients with allergic asthma at high risk of serious asthma-related morbidity and mortality. Curr Med Res Opin 2001; 17: 233–40

24. FitzGerald JM, Becker A, Sears MR, et al. Doubling the dose of budesonide versus maintenance treatment in asthma exacerbations. Thorax 2004; 59: 550–6

25. Tattersfield AE, Postma DS, Barnes PJ, et al. Exacerbations of asthma: a descriptive study of 425 severe exacerbations. The FACET International Study Group. Am J Respir Crit Care Med 1999; 160: 594–9

26. Meijer RJ, Kerstjens HA, Arends LR, et al. Effects of inhaled fluticasone and oral prednisolone on clinical and inflammatory parameters in patients with asthma. Thorax 1999; 54: 894–9

27. Wasilewski Y, Clark NM, Evans D, et al. Factors associated with emergency department visits by children with asthma: implications for health education. Am J Public Health 1996; 86: 1410–15

28. McFadden ER Jr, Kiser R, DeGroot WJ. Acute bronchial asthma. Relations between clinical and physiologic manifestations. N Engl J Med 1973; 288: 221–5

29. Shim CS, Williams MH Jr. Evaluation of the severity of asthma: patients versus physicians. Am J Med 1980; 68: 11–13

30. Kerem E, Canny G, Tibshirani R, et al. Clinical–physiologic correlations in acute asthma of childhood. Pediatrics 1991; 87: 481–6

31. Brenner B, Kohn MS. The acute asthmatic patient in the ED: to admit or discharge. Am J Emerg Med 1998; 16: 69–75

32. Atta JA, Nunes MP, Fonseca-Guedes CH, et al. Patient and physician evaluation of the severity of acute asthma exacerbations. Braz J Med Biol Res 2004; 37: 1321–30

33. Smith SR, Baty JD, Hodge D 3rd. Validation of the pulmonary score: an asthma severity score for children. Acad Emerg Med 2002; 9: 99–104

34. Demoly P, Crestani B, Leroyer C, et al. Control and exacerbation of asthma: a survey of more than 3000 French physicians. Allergy 2004; 59: 920–6

35. Juniper EF, O'Byrne PM, Guyatt GH, et al. Development and validation of a questionnaire to measure asthma control. Eur Respir J 1999; 14: 902–7

36. Osman LM, Russell IT, Friend JA, et al. Predicting patient attitudes to asthma medication. Thorax 1993; 48: 827–30

37. Boulet LP. Perception of the role and potential side effects of inhaled corticosteroids among asthmatic patients. Chest 1998; 113: 587–92

38. Dirks JF, Horton DJ, Kinsman RA, et al. Patient and physician characteristics influencing medical decisions in asthma. J Asthma Res 1978; 15: 171–8

39. Dahlem NW, Kinsman RA, Horton DJ. Requests for as-needed medications by asthmatic patients. Relationships to prescribed oral corticosteroid regimens and length of hospitalization. J Allergy Clin Immunol 1979; 63: 23–7

40. The British Thoracic Society. The National Asthma Campaign and The Royal College of Physicians of London in association with the General Practitioner in Asthma Group, The British Association of Accident and Emergency Medicine, The British Paediatric Respiratory Society and the Royal College of Paediatric and Child Health. The British Guidelines on Asthma Management. 1995 Review and Position statement. Thorax 1997; 52 (Suppl 1): S1–S21

41. Reddel HK, Jenkins CR, Marks GB, et al. Optimal asthma control, starting with high doses of inhaled budesonide [erratum in Eur Respir J 2000; 16: 579]. Eur Respir J 2000; 16: 226–35

42. Gibson PG, Saltos N, Fakes K. Acute anti-inflammatory effects of inhaled budesonide in asthma: a randomized controlled trial. Am J Respir Crit Care Med 2001; 163: 32–6

43. Ayres JG, Higgins B, Chilvers ER, et al. Efficacy and tolerability of anti-immunoglobulin E therapy with omalizumab in patients with poorly controlled (moderate-to-severe) allergic asthma. Allergy 2004; 59: 701–8

44. Arroll B, Kenealy T. Antibiotics for the common cold. Cochrane Database Syst Rev 2002; 3: CD000247

45. Cates CC, Bara A, Crilly JA, et al. Holding chambers versus nebulisers for beta-agonist treatment of acute asthma. Cochrane Database Syst Rev 2003; 3: CD000052

46. Crane J, Pearce N, Burgess C, et al. Markers of risk of asthma death or readmission in the 12 months following a hospital admission for asthma. Int J Epidemiol 1992; 21: 737–44

47. Johnston SL, Pattemore PK, Sanderson G, et al. The relationship between upper respiratory infections and hospital admissions for asthma in adults and children: a time trend analysis. Am J Respir Crit Care Med 1996; 154: 654–60

48. Marks GB, Colquhoun JR, Girgis ST, et al. Thunderstorm outflows preceding epidemics of asthma during spring and summer. Thorax 2001; 56: 468–71

49. Halfon N, Newacheck PW, Wood DL, et al. Routine emergency department use for sick care by children in the United States. Pediatrics 1996; 98: 28–34

50. Cydulka RK, Emerman CL, Rowe BH, et al. Differences between men and women in reporting of symptoms during an asthma exacerbation. Ann Emerg Med 2001; 38: 123–8

51. Magadle R, Berar-Yanay N, Weiner P. The risk of hospitalization and near-fatal and fatal asthma in relation to the perception of dyspnea. Chest 2002; 121: 329–33

52. Nouwen A, Freeston MH, Labbe R, et al. Psychological factors associated with emergency room visits among asthmatic patients. Behav Modif 1999; 23: 217–33

53. Rodrigo GJ, Rodrigo C. Rapid-onset asthma attack: a prospective cohort study about characteristics and response to emergency department treatment. Chest 2000; 118: 1547–52

54. FitzGerald JM, Grunfeld A, Pare PD, et al. The clinical efficacy of combination nebulized anticholinergic and adrenergic bronchodilators vs nebulized adrenergic bronchodilator alone in acute asthma. Canadian Combivent Study Group. Chest 1997; 111: 311–15

55. Pauwels RA, Pedersen S, Busse WW, et al. Early intervention with budesonide in mild persistent asthma: a randomised, double-blind trial. Lancet 2003; 361: 1071–6

56. Ignacio-Garcia JM, Gonzales-Santos P. Asthma self-management education program by home monitoring of peak expiratory flow. Am J Respir Crit Care Med 1995; 151: 353–9

57. Janson S, Becker G. Reasons for delay in seeking treatment for acute asthma: the patient's perspective. J Asthma 1998; 35: 427–35

58. Cowie RL, Underwood MF, Revitt SG, et al. Predicting emergency department utilization in adults with asthma: a cohort study. J Asthma 2001; 38: 179–84

59. Dalcin PT, Piovesan DM, Kang S, et al. Factors associated with emergency department visits due to acute asthma. Braz J Med Biol Res 2004; 37: 1331–8

60. Turner MO, Noertjojo K, Vedal S, et al. Risk factors for near-fatal asthma. A case–control study in hospitalized patients with asthma. Am J Respir Crit Care Med 1998; 157: 1804–9

61. Green RM, Custovic A, Sanderson G, et al. Synergism between allergens and viruses and risk of hospital admission with asthma: case–control study [erratum appears in BMJ 2002; 324: 1131]. BMJ 2002; 324: 763

62. Cai Y, Carty K, Henry RL, et al. Persistence of sputum eosinophilia in children with controlled asthma when compared with healthy children. Eur Respir J 1998; 11: 848–53

63. Burney PG, Luczynska C, Chinn S, et al. The European Community Respiratory Health Survey. Eur Respir J 1994; 7: 954–60

64. The International Study of Asthma and Allergies in Childhood Steering Committee. Worldwide variations in the prevalence of asthma symptoms: the International Study of Asthma and Allergies in Childhood (ISAAC). Eur Respir J 1998; 12: 315–35

65. Aroni R, Goeman D, Stewart K, et al. Enhancing validity: what counts as an asthma attack? J Asthma 2004; 41: 729–37

66. Vincent SD, Toelle BG, Aroni RA, et al. 'Exasperations' of asthma. A qualitative study of patient language about worsening asthma. Med J Aust 2006; 184: 451–4

67. Rubinfeld AR, Pain MCF. The perception of asthma. Lancet 1976; 1: 882–4

68. Boulet LP, Cournoyer I, Deschesnes F, et al. Perception of airflow obstruction and associated breathlessness in normal and asthmatic subjects: correlation with anxiety and bronchodilator needs. Thorax 1994; 49: 965–70

69. Sont JK, Booms P, Bel EH, et al. The severity of breathlessness during challenges with inhaled methacholine and hypertonic saline in atopic asthmatic subjects. The relationship with deep breath-induced bronchodilation. Am J Respir Crit Care Med 1995; 152: 38–44

70. Chetta A, Gerra G, Foresi A, et al. Personality profiles and breathlessness perception in outpatients with different gradings of asthma. Am J Respir Crit Care Med 1998; 157: 116–22

71. Kikuchi Y, Okabe S, Tamura G, et al. Chemosensitivity and perception of dyspnea in patients with a history of near-fatal asthma. N Engl J Med 1994; 330: 1329–34

72. Peterson-Sweeney K, McMullen A, Yoos HL, et al. Parental perceptions of their child's asthma: management and medication use. J Pediatr Health Care 2003; 17: 118–25

73. Panditi S, Silverman M. Perception of exercise induced asthma by children and their parents. Arch Dis Child 2003; 88: 807–11

74. Lara M, Duan N, Sherbourne C, et al. Differences between child and parent reports of symptoms among Latino children with asthma. Pediatrics 1998; 102: E68

75. Chan-Yeung M, Chang JH, Manfreda J, et al. Changes in peak flow, symptom score, and the use of medications during acute exacerbations of asthma. Am J Respir Crit Care Med 1996; 154: 889–93

76. Zanconato S, Scollo M, Zaramella C, et al. Exhaled carbon monoxide levels after a course of oral prednisone in children with asthma exacerbation. J Allergy Clin Immunol 2002; 109: 440–5

77. Osman LM, McKenzie L, Cairns J, et al. Patient weighting of importance of asthma symptoms. Thorax 2001; 56: 138–42

78. Harrison TW, Oborne J, Newton S, et al. Doubling the dose of inhaled corticosteroid to prevent asthma exacerbations: randomised controlled trial. Lancet 2004; 363: 271–5

79. Taylor DR, Town GI, Herbison GP, et al. Asthma control during long-term treatment with regular inhaled salbutamol and salmeterol [erratum appears in Thorax 1999; 54: 188]. Thorax 1998; 53: 744–52

80. Laviolette M, Malmstrom K, Lu S, et al. Montelukast added to inhaled beclomethasone in treatment of asthma. Montelukast/Beclomethasone Additivity Group. Am J Respir Crit Care Med 1999; 160: 1862–8

81. Brand PL, Roorda RJ. Usefulness of monitoring lung function in asthma. Arc Dis Child 2003; 88: 1021–5

82. Kamps AW, Roorda RJ, Brand PL. Peak flow diaries in childhood asthma are unreliable. Thorax 2001; 56: 180–2

83. Busse W, Koenig SM, Oppenheimer J, et al. Steroid-sparing effects of fluticasone propionate 100 microg and salmeterol 50 microg administered twice daily in a single product in patients previously controlled with fluticasone propionate 250 microg administered twice daily. J Allergy Clin Immunol 2003; 111: 57–65

84. Reddel HK, Marks GB, Jenkins CR. When can personal best peak flow be determined for asthma action plans? Thorax 2004; 59: 922–4

85. Wensley D, Silverman M. Peak flow monitoring for guided self-management in childhood asthma: a randomized controlled trial. Am J Respir Crit Care Med 2004; 170: 606–12

86. Gibson PG, Wlodarczyk J, Hensley MJ, et al. Using quality-control analysis of peak expiratory flow recordings to guide therapy for asthma. Ann Intern Med 1995; 123: 488–92

87. Boggs PB, Wheeler D, Washburne WF, et al. Peak expiratory flow rate control chart in asthma care: chart construction and use in asthma care. Ann Allergy Asthma Immunol 1998; 81: 552–62

88. Ryan G, Latimer KM, Dolovich J, et al. Bronchial responsiveness to histamine: relationship to diurnal variation of peak flow rate, improvement after bronchodilator, and airway calibre. Thorax 1982; 37: 423–9

89. Gannon PFG, Newton DT, Pantin CFA, et al. Effect of the number of peak expiratory flow readings per day on the estimation of diurnal variation. Thorax 1998; 53: 790–2

90. Udwadia ZF, Harrison BD. An attempt to determine the optimal duration of hospital stay following a severe attack of asthma. J R Coll Physicians Lond 1990; 24: 112–14

91. Matz J, Emmett A, Rickard K, et al. Addition of salmeterol to low-dose fluticasone versus higher-dose fluticasone: an analysis of asthma exacerbations. J Allergy Clin Immunol 2001; 107: 783–9

92. Grunberg K, Timmers MC, de Klerk EP, et al. Experimental rhinovirus 16 infection causes variable airway obstruction in subjects with atopic asthma. Am J Respir Crit Care Med 1999; 160: 1375–80

93. Reddel HK, Vincent SD, Civitico J. The need for standardisation of peak flow charts. Thorax 2005; 60: 164–7

94. Rabe KF, Jorres R, Nowak D, et al. Comparison of the effects of salmeterol and formoterol on airway tone and responsiveness over 24 hours in bronchial asthma. Am Rev Respir Dis 1993; 147: 1436–41

95. van der Molen T, Postma D, Turner M, et al. Effects of the long-acting beta agonist formoterol on asthma control in asthmatic patients using inhaled corticosteroids. Thorax 1997; 52: 535–9

96. Verschelden P, Cartier A, L'Archeveque J, et al. Compliance with and accuracy of daily self-assessment of peak expiratory flows (PEF) in asthmatic subjects over a three month period. Eur Respir J 1996; 9: 880–5

97. Rand CS, Nides M, Cowles MK, et al. Long-term metered-dose inhaler adherence in a clinical trial. Am J Respir Crit Care Med 1995; 152: 580–8

98. Stone AA, Shiffman S, Schwartz JE, et al. Patient noncompliance with paper diaries. BMJ 2002; 324: 1193–4

99. Silverman BA, Mayer D, Sabinsky R, et al. Training perception of air flow obstruction in asthmatics. Ann Allergy 1987; 59: 350–4

100. Vaquerizo MJ, Casan P, Castillo J, et al. Effect of montelukast added to inhaled budesonide on control of mild to moderate asthma [erratum appears in Thorax 2003; 58: 370]. Thorax 2003; 58: 204–10

101. Wilding P, Clark M, Coon JT, et al. Effect of long-term treatment with salmeterol on asthma control: a double blind, randomised crossover study. BMJ 1997; 314: 1441–6

CHAPTER 3

The socioeconomic impact of asthma exacerbations

Todd A Lee

As the costs of health care continue to grow, more of an emphasis is placed on understanding the sources of cost increases and examining techniques to control the growth. While individuals consuming health care want the most recent and frequently most expensive advances available to them, this may be at odds with those providing and financing health care. The financers and providers frequently need to make decisions on how to provide health care to the most people in which the most amount of good is done for the smallest amount of resources consumed. That is, they are interested in providing care in the most efficient manner so that they are getting the most bang for the buck. This requires an understanding of the value of interventions so that those making decisions can do so rationally while incorporating both the costs and outcomes associated with new interventions. A current approach that allows for the comparison of the relative value of different interventions in health care is cost-effectiveness analysis. The increased reliance on cost effectiveness results for informing decisions related to the provision and financing of health care places more importance on understanding the social, functional and economic burden of illness and the cost and outcomes of interventions.

The awareness of health-care costs and the realization that continued growth at the current rate may not be sustainable has contributed to more information being examined when making funding decisions regarding a new intervention. Now, rather than relying solely on the efficacy and safety of an intervention to determine whether or not the intervention is worthwhile, decision-makers also consider costs and the value of the intervention when making judgments about the intervention. These additional information requirements have led to more extensive technology assessment. In addition to safety and efficacy, decision-makers may require information on the clinical epidemiology of the disease, the total cost of the disease, the budgetary impact of the intervention and the cost effectiveness of the intervention.

The objective of this chapter is to review the evidence on the burden related to acute exacerbations in patients with asthma. The chapter is divided into five sections. The first section briefly discusses issues of measuring disease burden and cost of illness. The following two sections contain a review of the literature with regard to the overall costs of asthma followed by a specific focus on studies that have examined the direct costs associated with acute events. The next section summarizes the social burden of acute exacerbations. Finally, the evidence with regard to cost-effective interventions in asthma is discussed.

MEASURING THE BURDEN OF DISEASE

The burden of a disease can be characterized using several metrics. Disease burden can include measures of the incidence and prevalence of the disease, the mortality rate associated with the disease or the expected duration of the disease. Seminal work on the burden of asthma in terms of estimating the prevalence and non-cost of impact throughout the world has recently been published.[1] However, understanding the health-care resources that are used by those with the disease is also an important measure of the disease burden. For example, knowing the number of hospitalizations, emergency department (ED) visits or unscheduled outpatient visits may be important indicators of the burden of the disease. The health-care utilization can also be measured in economic terms in order to understand how much the disease costs. Finally, disease burden can also be measured by the impact on overall health and quality of life.

Economic estimates of the disease burden are most typically referred to as cost-of-illness studies. These studies can be conducted from various perspectives in order to understand the cost of the disease from a particular point of view. For example, cost-of-illness studies can be performed to measure the disease burden from the perspective of the family, health plans, communities, countries or the world.

Cost-of-illness studies can include estimates of the direct and indirect costs that are attributable to the disease. Direct medical costs are those associated with the consumption of health-care resources for a specific condition and include things like the cost of hospitalizations, ED visits, office visits, medications, procedures and laboratory tests. The term 'indirect costs' is typically used to denote costs not associated with the use of medical resources and mostly refers to costs attributed to lost or decreased productivity as a result of the medical condition or its treatment. Thus, in asthma exacerbations the concept of indirect costs is an important one as exacerbations, whether in an adult or a child, may result in days missed from work or school, which would be included in estimates of the indirect costs of a disease.

THE ECONOMIC BURDEN OF ASTHMA

The total cost of a disease is related to the health-care resources consumed during the treatment of the illness, the indirect costs attributable to the disease and the prevalence of the disease in the population. Because of the prevalence of asthma, the episodic nature of the disease that leads to acute events that result in the use of intense health-care services, the need for chronic treatment and the impact on indirect costs, asthma imparts a large economic burden on society. Because of this, the total costs of asthma have been examined in several countries throughout the world. In order to understand the economic burden of asthma exacerbations, it is important to have a frame of reference for the costs of disease as a whole. Several papers have reviewed the cost-of-illness studies in asthma.[2–4] The following sections provide several examples of the asthma cost-of-illness studies from throughout the world.

North America

One of the first studies in the USA to look at the economic burden of asthma was based on the treatment of asthma in 1985.[5] The analysis indicated that 53% of the total costs of asthma were related to direct costs of treating asthma. The estimated total cost of asthma in the USA in 1985 was $4.5 billion. When those costs are adjusted to 2004 dollars using the Medical Care component of the Consumer Price Index, the estimated costs of asthma in the USA would be $6.49 billion in direct costs and $5.72 billion in indirect costs for a total cost of disease of $12.2 billion.

However, much in the way of asthma management and epidemiology has changed since 1985. New medications are available and the focus is

Table 3.1 Estimates of the overall economic burden of asthma in North America (in billions)

	Weiss et al. 1992[5]	Smith et al. 1997[7]	Weiss et al. 2000[6]	Krahn et al. 1996[11]
Country	USA	USA	USA	Canada
Year	1985	1987	1994	1990
Direct costs	$6.5	$8.0	$16.7	$0.5
Indirect costs	$5.7	$1.4	$12.7	$0.3
Total costs	$12.2	$9.4	$29.4	$0.8
Cost per asthma patient	$1371	$2000	$2070	NR

NR, not reported
All costs adjusted to 2004 US dollars using Medical Care component of the Consumer Price Index and average exchange rate for results reported in non-US currency
Year indicates time for data used in analysis

on control and management of the disease rather than on treating exacerbations. Thus, an update to this analysis confirmed that costs related to the treatment of asthma shifted between 1985 and 1994.[6] In 1985, medications accounted for about 16% of the direct medical costs for asthma; however, by 1994 almost 23% of the direct medical costs were due to the costs of prescription medications. When both the 1985 and 1994 estimates were adjusted to 2004 US dollars, the total cost of asthma in 1994 was more than double the costs based on analysis of 1985 patterns of care. The estimated total cost of asthma from analyzing 1994 data was $29.4 billion (2004 US dollars) with 57% due to direct medical costs and 43% from indirect costs (Table 3.1).

A final study in the USA on the overall economic burden of asthma estimated that indirect costs were only 15% of the total cost of asthma.[7] Based on data collected in 1987, Smith et al. reported that the total burden of asthma was $3.5 billion. When adjusted to 2004 dollars, the total costs for asthma were $9.4 billion. Of the total, $8 billion were attributed to direct medical costs and $1.4 billion were attributed to indirect costs. Thus, the estimates of direct medical costs were consistent with those from Weiss et al., using 1985 data.[5] However, there were large differences in the indirect costs that were reported between the analysis of Smith et al.[7] and the two papers from Weiss et al.[5,6] The largest factor in the differences in indirect costs were a result of Weiss and colleagues assigning a cost to

premature death in persons with asthma, while Smith et al. did not account for asthma mortality in their analysis. There were also differences in the magnitude of costs reported for work lost and school days missed between the Weiss et al. papers and the Smith et al. paper.

Regardless of the precision of the indirect cost estimates, a clear picture of the burden of asthma in the USA is provided by these three analyses.[5–7] Asthma imparts a substantial burden on the US health-care system and the costs are continuing to increase. Importantly, the estimated costs of asthma have more than doubled in a 10-year period. This is probably due to several factors that include an increasing prevalence of the disease,[8] an increased number of therapeutic alternatives and clearly defined consensus guidelines.[9,10] Each of these factors contributes to increasing costs over time in different ways. An increasing prevalence of asthma results in higher costs simply due to having more persons with the disease. More therapeutic alternatives can lead to an increase in total costs because new medications cost more than older medications. Even though these new medications may be more effective than older alternatives, the increase in costs is not likely to be totally offset by savings from preventing hospitalizations and ED visits, which would still result in a net increase in total costs. Finally, consensus guidelines may increase costs, as more providers are educated as to the problem of asthma and the appropriate treatment of patients

45

with asthma. This could lead to identification of more patients with asthma, the use of more medications in these patients and the prevention of premature mortality, again resulting in a net increase in the overall costs of the disease.

In Canada, Krahn *et al.* estimated the direct and indirect costs of asthma.[11] Adjusted to 2004 US dollars, the total cost of asthma in Canada was $0.8 billion. Direct costs were responsible for 61% of the total costs whereas indirect costs accounted for 39% of the total costs. Medication costs were the largest component of the direct costs, while lost productivity was the largest component of indirect costs.

European Union

There are several studies from countries in the European Union that have estimated the economic burden of asthma. Van den Akker-van Marle *et al.* provided a comprehensive overview of the economic burden of asthma in children in the 25 countries of the European Union.[12] They summarized the reported evidence from several countries of the European Union and assigned missing values to the remaining countries. Importantly, many of the estimates came from various sources and used various methods to estimate costs. In 2004 US dollars, the average cost per child with asthma was estimated to be $761 (613 euros) per year. The average annual cost per child ranged from a low of $176 (142 euros) in Estonia to a high of $1899 (1529 euros) in Hungary. Based on estimates of self-reported asthma prevalence, the average cost of asthma in children for European Union countries is $3.7 billion (3.0 billion euros). The cost in each country ranges from $1.2 million (1 million euros) in Estonia to $581.3 million (468 million euros) in Italy. The five countries with the highest economic burden for children with asthma were Italy, Germany ($491 million), Poland ($487 million), the UK ($446 million) and France ($364 million).

Rutten van-Molken and colleagues estimated the direct costs of asthma in The Netherlands.[13]

Using data from 1993, they estimated that asthma cost was $293 per patient, which equals $90.6 million. Adjusted to 2004 US dollars, the cost of asthma in The Netherlands was $139.5 million. A total of 45% of the costs were attributed to the costs of medications. Inpatient hospitalizations contributed 27% of the total costs while physicians were responsible for 13% of the direct costs. They also projected the costs of asthma and chronic obstructive pulmonary disease (COPD) to 2010 based on prevalence and incidence rates, current treatment patterns and smoking patterns; however, they only provided aggregate estimates for asthma and COPD combined, and did not report the costs for either individually.

In Denmark, the costs of asthma were estimated by Sorensen *et al.*[14] in 1995 and were updated to 2000 by Mossing and Nielsen.[15] When these estimates are adjusted to 2004 US dollars, the total cost of asthma in Denmark was $279 million in 2000. Direct costs were responsible for $162 million (58%) and indirect costs contributed $117 million (42%).

Barnes *et al.* and Jonsson summarized the cost estimates from several other cost-of-illness studies from throughout the world.[2,16] Adjusting the estimates reported by Jonsson to 2004 US dollars, the estimated cost of asthma in the UK would be between $2.6 billion and $3.5 billion. These studies were based on populations studied in the 1990s and, given the changing prevalence and treatment patterns for asthma, they would be likely to represent underestimates of the current cost of asthma in the UK.

Regardless of the country, evidence indicates that the overall cost of asthma is substantial. Additionally, from the studies in the USA, the cost of asthma did not decrease as more treatment options became available. Rather, there appeared to be a shifting in the major components of the costs. The shifting in costs from urgent care for asthma exacerbations to medications used to prevent exacerbations and control the disease represent an improvement in overall asthma care. However, hospitalizations and ED visits remain a major component of the direct costs for asthma. Closer examination of the costs for hospitalizations and ED visits allows us to understand the impact that asthma exacerbations have on the overall burden of the disease.

One additional point on the overall burden of asthma warrants mention. Nearly all of the data on the cost of illness for asthma comes from developed countries. Very little is known about the burden of asthma in developing countries. While asthma may not be high on their current health-care priority list, it is likely to become an important one as the country develops. As Masoli *et al.* point out, much work still needs to be done to understand the rates of asthma prevalence and mortality in these countries before examining the economic impact of asthma.[1] However, as health-care systems mature in developing countries, the economic burden of asthma will warrant examination.

Finally, all of the studies that examine the cost of illness of asthma from the national perspective rely on data and treatment patterns that are 10–20 years old. These studies provide information on the historical burden of asthma and may provide information on trends during that period. However, it is not clear how applicable these older studies may be in terms of the current costs of asthma. It is likely that the trends observed in these studies, showing that medications are becoming a larger part of the overall costs of asthma, continue to hold. The relevant question becomes whether or not increasing use of medications continues to decrease the costs of ED visits and hospitalizations. Additionally, the use of case management and disease management programs has become an important component of asthma care. Again, the impact of these interventions on the overall costs of asthma is not clear. The only means by which these interventions would not be increasing the total costs of asthma would be if savings in costs due to acute events offset the costs of the program. Replicating these studies using more contemporary treatment patterns and data would provide information on the current economic burden of asthma and how that relates to historical numbers. This information can be used to help set priorities in terms of research and health-care dollars but is not as valuable in decision making as economic evaluations that explore the value of interventions.

THE ECONOMIC BURDEN OF EXACERBATIONS

To understand the role of acute exacerbations on the economic burden of asthma as a whole, one can examine the costs of hospitalizations and ED or urgent care visits. Consumption of these resources does not reflect standard outpatient care of asthma, but rather indicates an acute event for which the patient needs care. Thus, these are good indicators of the direct costs of asthma exacerbations. Medications may also be used to treat exacerbations; however, relative to medications used for disease control, those used to treat exacerbations (oral steroids) would contribute very little to the overall cost of the disease because of their low acquisition cost. Visits to physicians could either be due to an acute exacerbation or be part of routine follow-up care. Therefore, in studies that examine national or administrative data it is difficult to attribute physician costs to routine care or to being part of an exacerbation.

In addition to examining the costs attributable to hospitalizations and ED visits from national cost-of-illness studies, examinations of smaller populations of patients can provide information on the economic burden of acute exacerbations. Micro-costing studies of exacerbations provide information on the specific resources that are consumed during an exacerbation.[17] These studies can identify what resources are used during a typical exacerbation treated in the ED and/or hospital. Second, studies in smaller populations can provide information similar to the national cost of illness studies as to what proportion of costs are a result of acute exacerbations.[18–21]

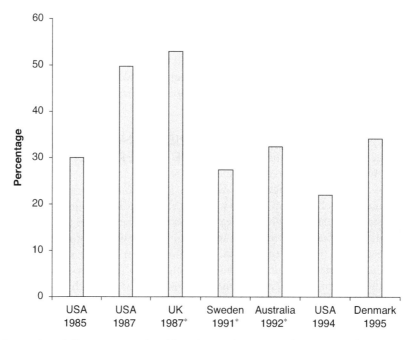

Figure 3.1   Proportion of direct costs attributable to hospitalizations and emergency department visits. *Data adapted from reference 2

Direct costs

In the national burden of illness studies, the proportion of direct costs attributable to ED visits and hospitalizations ranged from 22% in the USA based on 1994 costs and utilization to 53% in the UK based on 1987 costs. Figure 3.1 shows the proportion of the direct costs that were due to ED visits or hospitalizations for several national cost-of-illness studies. In the figure, the studies are ordered from the oldest to the most recent. For both the USA and the UK the proportion of costs related to acute events was about 50% in 1987. From 1991 forward the proportion of costs attributed to hospitalizations and ED visits in each of the studies was between 22% and 34%. This decrease in the proportion of costs due to acute events could be an indication of better asthma management in terms of preventing exacerbations. However, differences could also exist for many other reasons, one example being changes in the delivery of health care. Regardless,

the trends are encouraging but yet leave much room for improvement, because a significant proportion of costs are still related to acute events.

In addition to the national cost-of-illness studies, several studies have examined the costs of asthma on a per patient basis. These studies can also provide estimates of the proportion of costs in asthma patients that are attributable to acute events. In a cohort of patients in Spain, Serra-Batlles *et al.* estimated the costs of asthma for 333 patients stratified by asthma severity based on lung function measures.[20] The average annual direct cost was $1245 (2004 US dollars) per patient. A total of 38.5% of those costs were related to hospitalizations or ED visits. The proportion of costs attributable to acute events increased as the severity of disease worsened. In patients with mild asthma, a total of 28.9% of their direct costs were due to hospitalizations or ED visits. For patients with moderate disease, 40.4% of their costs were for the treatment of acute events. In the severe patients, the proportion of total direct costs due to hospitalizations or ED visits was 43.5%. What is not clear from these cost comparisons across the severity classifications is why the costs are different across the groups. The costs could be higher as severity worsens as a result of an increased number of acute exacerbations with worsening severity or exacerbations that are more severe. It is likely that both factors play into the higher costs associated with more severe disease. Patients in the severe group may have more frequent exacerbations and may have exacerbations that require more resources for the treatment of the events. Therefore, strategies to reduce the number of exacerbations as well as reducing the severity of the exacerbation may result in decreased costs associated with asthma exacerbations.

In addition to showing differences in direct costs for acute events based on asthma severity, Serra-Batlles et al. also showed differences based on gender.[20] Females had higher average annual direct costs for asthma care than males ($1419 vs. $937). Additionally, females had a higher proportion of their direct costs that were associated with hospitalizations and ED visits (42.4%) than did males (27.8%).

In France, Godard et al. also found a relationship between asthma severity and treatment for acute events.[18] In their analysis of 234 patients with asthma, none of the patients with intermittent or mild persistent asthma had a hospitalization during the 1-year follow-up period. Those with moderate persistent asthma spent an average of 1.24 days in the hospital and patients with severe persistent asthma averaged 6.08 inpatient days.

Focusing on children with asthma, Lozano and colleagues found, based on national data, that acute events were responsible for 61.7% of the overall costs of asthma-related expenditures.[22] Of those costs, 51.2% were for hospitalizations and 10.5% for ED visits. The analysis was based on data from 1987 and, like changes in the data reported by Weiss et al.[6] from 1985 to 1994, one may expect that a shift would have occurred from costs for acute events to a larger

share of costs for medications if the analysis were to be repeated using contemporary data.

Other regional studies in the USA using more recent data have shown that acute events are still a large part of the overall costs of care in patients with asthma. Using data from 1992, Grupp-Phelan et al. showed that urgent care and hospitalizations were responsible for 34.8% of all health-care costs in children with asthma.[19] Of those costs, 61.2% were for inpatient care, while the remaining 38.8% were for urgent care visits. Similarly, based on 1996 data, Piecoro and colleagues reported that 38.6% of costs for asthma care were due to inpatient care.[23]

Stanford et al. examined the resources that were consumed during an acute exacerbation of asthma.[17] They used data from 27 hospitals in the USA to determine how patients presenting to an ED or admitted to a hospital for an acute exacerbation of asthma were treated in 1996 and 1997. The 3223 patients they studied were required to have an ED visit for asthma at one of the study hospitals, of which 33% were also admitted for their exacerbation. Adjusting the costs to 2004 US dollars, the average cost of an ED visit for patients who were not subsequently admitted to the hospital was $310. The average cost of a hospitalization for patients with an acute exacerbation was $4101 (Figure 3.2).

In those patients who where not admitted to the hospital, the majority of the costs were for ED services (53%). The next two highest categories were respiratory therapy (11%) and radiology (10%). Medication costs accounted for only 6% or just over $18 of the total cost of the ED visit. For those patients who were admitted to the hospital, the medication costs were a higher percentage of their overall costs. In hospitalized patients, medications accounted for around 10% of the overall cost of care. The largest proportion of costs was due to nursing care provided during the hospitalization (44%). The average length of stay was just under 4 days with 93% of the hospitalizations lasting no longer than 7 days.

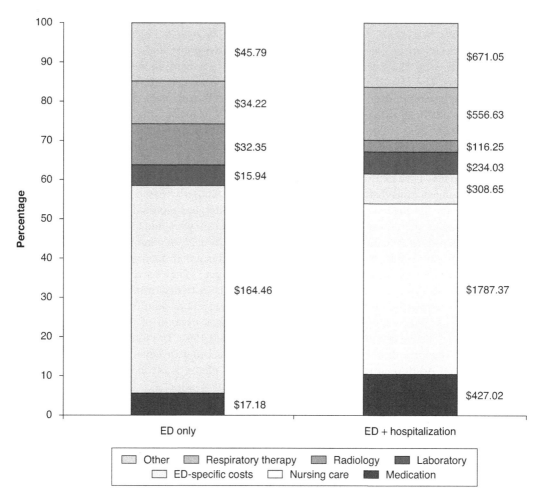

Figure 3.2 Resources consumed during emergency department (ED) visits and hospitalizations from asthma. *Data adapted from reference 17

Pendergraft and colleagues studied the most severe exacerbations that resulted in hospitalizations.[24] They reported that, for patients requiring intubation, the length of stay was 4.5 days longer and the additional costs of hospital care were $11 000 compared to a non-intensive care unit (ICU) asthma admission. Patients who were not intubated but admitted to the ICU had one additional day in the hospital on average and $3000 in additional costs compared to non-ICU asthma admissions. Thus, one admission for a severe exacerbation that results in an ICU admission will significantly increase the costs of treating patients with asthma.

Indirect costs

In addition to the impact of acute asthma exacerbations on the direct costs of asthma, exacerbations also have an impact on the indirect costs. As noted above, indirect costs include costs related to decreased productivity, work days missed for adults and school days missed for children as a result of asthma. It is uncertain exactly what fraction of indirect costs is due to acute asthma exacerbations. However, in asthma the indirect costs would seemingly be related to three factors. Indirect costs could be due to an acute exacerbation which requires missed time from work and/or school. Indirect costs could be due to uncontrolled disease where asthma symptoms are decreasing productivity while at work but may not result in time missed from work or school. Finally, indirect costs could be attributed to asthma treatments or routine care. Indirect costs could result from adverse effects of treatments, although with asthma treatments this is probably a rarity, or from interventions that may require patients to miss work or school (e.g. patient education interventions) or from routine follow-up visits.

In the asthma literature, the indirect costs of asthma are reported as a single category and not reported by the reason for the indirect cost. Therefore, it is not possible to attribute indirect costs solely to exacerbations. Examination of the indirect costs may still provide some insight into the burden caused by exacerbations. The largest component of the indirect costs is likely to be a result of acute exacerbations due to the severity and duration of the event. However, uncontrolled symptoms certainly play an important role in the overall estimate of indirect costs.

Estimates of indirect costs reported in the literature range from 15% to nearly 70% of the overall costs of asthma. In Figure 3.3, the proportion of overall costs resulting from indirect costs is reported for several studies. The smallest estimate of indirect costs is from the study of Smith et al. that estimated asthma costs in the USA.[7] They reported that indirect costs were associated with 15.4% of the overall costs of asthma. The majority of the other studies reported that indirect costs were between 40% and 60% of the overall asthma costs. The exceptions were an analysis from Spain that reported that indirect costs were nearly 70% of the total costs of asthma and an analysis from Switzerland that reported that indirect costs were 36% of total costs.[20,21]

One important reason for differences in the proportion of overall asthma costs due to indirect costs is the inconsistent inclusion of indirect costs from premature mortality attributed to asthma. Many of the national studies include an estimate of lost productivity and thus an indirect cost if someone with asthma dies prematurely.[5,6,14,15,20] Others, however, do not include this cost when estimating the indirect costs associated with the disease.[7,21] Thus, there are large differences in the indirect costs when their estimates were based on the costs that were included. This makes it difficult to compare results across countries and settings when different methods are used for estimating the costs. Attribution of indirect costs to asthma for patients who die prematurely is difficult and the primary reason most analyses will not include an indirect cost for years of life lost. With most data used to generate burden-of-illness studies, it is difficult if not impossible to determine the cause of death. Therefore, if patients have more than one disease, assigning an indirect cost of the same amount to each disease would seem to be overcounting the true burden of illness. That is, if an individual has both asthma and another unrelated co-morbidity such as diabetes and dies prematurely, and cost-of-illness studies are conducted for both diseases, should that individual's costs be included in both diseases? If so, that would seem to be double counting the lost producitivty due to that person. This and other methodological difficulties with regard to assigning costs to premature mortality may be the primary reason the majority of the studies estimating indirect costs do not include a cost for years of life lost due to the disease.

THE SOCIAL BURDEN

In addition to examining the burden of a disease in economic terms, one can also look at the impact of the disease on disability or quality of life to understand the overall disease

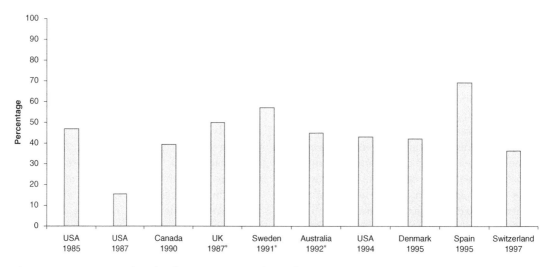

Figure 3.3 Proportion of total asthma costs reported as indirect costs. *Data adapted from reference 2

burden. Disability adjusted life-years (DALYs) are a metric that has been used to compare the relative impact of diseases around the world. DALYs were used in the Global Burden of Disease study to compare disease burden in terms of impact on mortality and disability and rank the relative burden of diseases.[25–28] DALYs are a measure of the years of life lost and the years lived with disability that is weighted by severity due to a disease.[26,29] The more DALYs that are attributed to a disease the worse is the overall burden of that disease.

In 1990, asthma was ranked 30th in terms of number of overall DALYs.[26] It was estimated to be responsible for 10.8 million DALYs worldwide. Asthma ranked immediately behind HIV (11.2 million) and diabetes (11.1 million) on the list that compared the leading causes of DALYs. By 2001, asthma was ranked as the 25th leading cause of DALYs.[1] Asthma was estimated to cause 15.0 million DALYs.

Similar to indirect costs, it is impossible to determine what proportion of DALYs is due to acute exacerbations. Living with uncontrolled asthma is again going to contribute to the measure of DALYs related to the disease. However, given that exacerbations are the acute event most linked to an asthma-related death, one could speculate that the majority (if not all) of the life years lost attributed to asthma is a result of acute exacerbations.

Acute exacerbations of asthma also have an impact on the overall quality of life of patients with asthma. Most asthma-related quality of life instruments are aimed at assessing the impact of asthma on the day-to-day experiences of patients with asthma. They are not intended to measure the impact of acute exacerbations but rather to assess the impact of uncontrolled symptoms on quality of life. However, Juniper and colleagues have modified their original AQLQ scale to be used in cases of acute exacerbations.[30] The measure was administered to patients presenting to the emergency department with an acute asthma exacerbation. The instrument was moderately correlated with patient's self-reported symptom severity and the change in symptoms following treatment.[30] Importantly, the study shows that acute exacerbations of asthma not only impact upon a patient in terms of their symptoms but also have an impact on emotional factors related to overall asthma-related quality of life.

Exacerbations impact not only asthma-related quality of life but also overall health-related quality of life. Andersson *et al.* asked patients about the effect of mild and severe exacerbations on their overall quality of life.[31] Patients with asthma were asked to rate their current health and then rate a mild and severe exacerbation all on a scale from 0 (death) to 100 (perfect health). The average overall quality of life for the patients was 81, while the average quality of life for a mild exacerbation was rated as 62 and a severe exacerbation as 26. Thus, on average, mild exacerbations decrease overall health-related quality of life by 25% and severe exacerbations decrease overall health-related quality of life by about 75%.

It is understandable that there are relatively few studies of the impact of an acute exacerbation on overall quality of life. An acute exacerbation can be an impractical time to measure quality of life, as it is more relevant to care for the patient at the time of their exacerbation. Therefore, measurements need to rely on patient recall of symptoms or descriptions of hypothetical situations. This is in contrast to a vast literature on the overall impact of asthma on health-related quality of life. However, even though few studies have evaluated the impact of exacerbations, they show that exacerbations affect more than physical symptoms for patients and that the severity of the exacerbation is related to the magnitude of the impact.

ECONOMIC EVALUATIONS

Understanding the overall economic burden of a disease can be valuable for setting spending priorities and tracking the overall trends in health-care costs. For example, in asthma the costs of care are shifting from the majority of direct costs related to hospitalizations to the majority related to medication. This could be considered a gross indicator as to the overall quality of asthma care, in that more patients are being appropriately treated with medications to manage their disease. However, it could also be an indicator of the continued shifting of care away from inpatient care with more of an emphasis on short lengths of stay and more care in the outpatient setting. Regardless, these studies provide context to the overall burden of the disease. In order for decisions to be made about resource allocation relative to interventions, it becomes important to understand the relative value of the interventions.

Economic evaluations compare the incremental value of interventions by comparing the costs and effects of two alternatives. In asthma, it is not possible to evaluate the cost effectiveness of interventions for treatment or control of acute exacerbations. The cost effectiveness of interventions needs to be considered for the treatment of the chronic condition as a whole and not just be focused on acute exacerbations. The cost effectiveness of interventions in asthma has been extensively reviewed.[3,32] The following are some general conclusions regarding economic evaluations in asthma.

Medications have been the most extensively studied interventions with regard to their cost-effectiveness in treating asthma patients. The medications that have been most rigorously evaluated include inhaled corticosteroids (ICS), long-acting β-agonists (LABA) and leukotrienes. A variety of methods have been used in the evaluations, including cost-effectiveness analyses alongside clinical trials and health economic models. The primary limitations of cost-effectiveness analyses of medications for asthma have been the study duration and the study population, both of which impact the generalizability of the results and the ability to understand the long-term implications of using the medications.

With those caveats in mind, ICS have been shown to represent good value for money in treating patients with asthma. One of the first health economic evaluations in asthma compared ICS to short-acting β-agonists (SABA) only. Over a 1-year period, the incremental cost-effectiveness ratio (ICER) of ICS compared to SABA was $5.35 per symptom-free day (SFD) gained.[33] In a 3-year study of initial treatment with ICS, the ICER for ICS was $3.70 per

SFD gained from the societal perspective and $11.30 per SFD gained from the health-care payer perspective in the US analysis.[34] Finally, a long-term evaluation of ICS using a health ecomomic model showed that, in patients with mild to moderate asthma, the ICER for ICS was $7.50 per SFD gained.[35] The ICER from this study was also calculated in terms of quality-adjusted life years (QALYs) gained and was $13 500 per QALY gained for ICS compared to no ICS. Thus, the evidence is solid that ICS represent good value for money in patients with asthma.

In addition to ICS, the cost effectiveness of LABA has also been assessed. Andersson *et al.* showed that the addition of LABA to ICS compared to ICS alone in patients with uncontrolled asthma resulted in ICERs of between 4.67 euros and 6.60 euros per SFD gained.[36] The long-term safety of the use of LABA was not examined in this analysis and that could ultimately impact the cost effectiveness of the combination of ICS and LABA. Additionally, there is no evidence that ICS and LABA are cost effective as a first-line agent in the treatment of asthma. Finally, the evidence on the cost effectiveness of leukotrienes is limited by the duration of the studies that have included cost-effectiveness analyses.

In comparison to medications, there are relatively few randomized, controlled trials that included a cost-effectiveness analysis of disease management programs or health system interventions that focus on asthma. Lee and Weiss reviewed the recent studies.[3] Many economic evaluations of disease management programs have been before and after studies that rely on a quasi-experimental design. The majority of these analyses showed cost savings following the intervention. That is, those receiving the intervention cost less following the implementation of the intervention than they did prior to the intervention. With these designs it is difficult to attribute the effect solely to the intervention and there are concerns about regression to the mean when identifying a high-risk group of patients with asthma based on their prior health-care utilization experience.

There have been a few evaluations of asthma interventions alongside large clinical trials that did not focus on medications. These studies provide valuable evidence as to the cost effectiveness of these sorts of intervention. Sullivan and colleagues examined the cost effectiveness of a social worker-based intervention in children in an inner city.[37] In 2 years of follow-up, they found that the social worker intervention compared to no social worker resulted in an ICER of $9.20 per SFD gained.

In the Pediatric Asthma Care Patient Outcomes Research Team II (PAC-PORT) study, Sullivan *et al.* compared a physician leader intervention and a practice redesign to usual care in a 2-year study.[38] Both interventions increased the overall costs relative to usual care. The ICER for the physician leader intervention compared to usual care was $18.31 per SFD gained. The ICER for the practice redesign compared to usual care was $68.20 per SFD gained.

The cost effectiveness of disease management, patient education and practice-based interventions in asthma is not extensively studied in formal economic evaluations in comparison to medications. The value of the intervention appears to be dependent on the type of intervention as well as the population in which the intervention is to be implemented. In other words, identifying asthma patients with the worst control and doing anything for those patients probably represents good value, but the key is finding cost-effective interventions in a wider group of patients. Finally, the before and after studies of asthma interventions frequently show cost savings; however, the attribution of these results to the intervention being studied is questionable.

CONCLUDING REMARKS

Regardless of the origin of the study or the timeframe of the analysis, the burden of asthma is remarkable. Importantly, acute exacerbations remain a significant portion of the overall burden of the disease. This is despite the fact that there are effective medications for improving asthma control and reducing the number of acute exacerbations.

Improvements have been made in the proportion of asthma costs that are attributable to acute events; however, there is much room left for reducing the economic burden of acute exacerbations of asthma. It remains imperative for providers and decision-makers to identify and use cost-effective interventions appropriately in patients with asthma, to reduce the burden due to uncontrolled disease.

REFERENCES

1. Masoli M, Fabian D, Holt S, Beasley R. The global burden of asthma: executive summary of the GINA Dissemination Committee report. Allergy 2004; 59: 469–78

2. Barnes PJ, Jonsson B, Klim JB. The costs of asthma. Eur Respir J 1996; 9: 636–42

3. Lee TA, Weiss KB. An update on the health economics of asthma and allergy. Curr Opin Allergy Clin Immunol 2002; 2: 195–200

4. Weiss KB, Sullivan SD. The health economics of asthma and rhinitis. I. Assessing the economic impact. J Allergy Clin Immunol 2001; 107: 3–8

5. Weiss KB, Gergen PJ, Hodgson TA. An economic evaluation of asthma in the United States. N Engl J Med 1992; 326: 862–6

6. Weiss KB, Sullivan SD, Lyttle CS. Trends in the cost of illness for asthma in the United States, 1985–1994. J Allergy Clin Immunol 2000; 106: 493–9

7. Smith DH, Malone DC, Lawson KA, et al. A national estimate of the economic costs of asthma. Am J Respir Crit Care Med 1997; 156: 787–93

8. Mannino DM, Homa DM, Akinbami LJ, et al. Surveillance for asthma – United States, 1980–1999. MMWR Surveill Summ 2002; 51: 1–13

9. Guidelines for the diagnosis and management of asthma. National Heart, Lung, and Blood Institute. National Asthma Education Program. Expert Panel Report. J Allergy Clin Immunol 1991; 88: 425–534

10. Guidelines for the diagnosis and management of asthma: Expert Panel Report 2. NIH Publication 97–4051, 1–153. Bethesda, MD: National Institutes of Health, National Heart, Lung, and Blood Institute, 1997

11. Krahn MD, Berka C, Langlois P, Detsky AS. Direct and indirect costs of asthma in Canada, 1990. Can Med Assoc J 1996; 154: 821–31

12. van den Akker-van Marle, Bruil J, Detmar SB. Evaluation of cost of disease: assessing the burden to society of asthma in children in the European Union. Allergy 2005; 60: 140–9

13. Rutten-van Molken MPMH, Postma MJ, Joore MA, et al. Current and future medical costs of asthma and chronic obstructive pulmonary disease in The Netherlands. Respir Med 1999; 93: 779–87

14. Sorensen L, Weng S, Weng SL, et al. The costs of asthma in Denmark. Br J Med Econ 1997; 11: 103–11

15. Mossing R, Nielsen GD. [Cost-of-illness of asthma in Denmark in the year 2000]. Ugeskr Laeger 2003; 165: 2646–9

16. Jonsson B. Measuring the economic burden in asthma. In Weiss KB, Buist AS, Sullivan SD, eds. Asthma's Impact on Society: Social and Economic Burden. New York, NY: Marcel Dekker, 2000: 251–67

17. Stanford R, McLaughlin T, Okamoto LJ. The cost of asthma in the emergency department and hospital. Am J Respir Crit Care Med 1999; 160: 211–15

18. Godard P, Chanez P, Siraudin L, et al. Costs of asthma are correlated with severity: a 1-yr prospective study. Eur Respir J 2001; 19: 61–7

19. Grupp-Phelan J, Lozano P, Fishman P. Health care utilization and cost in children with asthma and selected comorbidities. J Asthma 2001; 38: 363–73

20. Serra-Batlles J, Plaza V, Morejon E, et al. Costs of asthma according to the degree of severity. Eur Respir J 1998; 12: 1322–6

21. Szucs TD, Anderhub H, Rutishauser M. The economic burden of asthma: direct and indirect costs in Switzerland. Eur Respir J 1999; 13: 281–6

22. Lozano P, Sullivan SD, Smith DH, Weiss KB. The economic burden of asthma in US children: estimates from the National Medical Expenditure Survey. J Allergy Clin Immunol 1999; 104: 957–63

23. Piecoro LT, Potoski M, Talbert JC, Doherty DE. Asthma prevalence, cost, and adherence with expert guidelines on the utilization of health care services and costs in a state Medicaid population. Health Serv Res 2001; 36: 357–71

24. Pendergraft TB, Stanford RH, Beasley R, et al. Rates and characteristics of intensive care unit admissions and intubations among asthma-related hospitalizations. Ann Allergy Asthma Immunol 2004; 93: 29–35

25. Murray CJ, Lopez AD. Alternative projections of mortality and disability by cause 1990–2020: Global Burden of Disease Study. Lancet 1997; 349: 1498–504

26. Murray CJ, Lopez AD. Global mortality, disability, and the contribution of risk factors: Global Burden of Disease Study. Lancet 1997; 349: 1436–42

27. Murray CJ, Lopez AD. Regional patterns of disability-free life expectancy and disability-adjusted life expectancy: Global Burden of Disease Study. Lancet 1997; 349: 1347–52

28. Murray CJ, Lopez AD. Mortality by cause for eight regions of the world: Global Burden of Disease Study. Lancet 1997; 349: 1269–76

29. Murray CJ. Quantifying the burden of disease: the technical basis for disability-adjusted life years. Bull World Health Organ 1994; 72: 429–45

30. Juniper EF, Svensson K, Mork AC, Stahl E. Measuring health-related quality of life in adults during an acute asthma exacerbation. Chest 2004; 125: 93–7

31. Andersson F, Borg S, Stahl E. The impact of exacerbations on the asthmatic patient's preference scores. J Asthma 2003; 40: 615–23

32. Sullivan SD, Weiss KB. Health economics of asthma and rhinitis. II. Assessing the value of interventions. J Allergy Clin Immunol 2001; 107: 203–10

33. Rutten-van Molken MP, Van Doorslaer EK, Jansen MC, et al. Costs and effects of inhaled corticosteroids and bronchodilators in asthma and chronic obstructive pulmonary disease. Am J Respir Crit Care Med 1995; 151: 975–82

34. Sullivan SD, Buxton M, Andersson LF, et al. Cost-effectiveness analysis of early intervention with budesonide in mild persistent asthma. J Allergy Clin Immunol 2003; 112: 1229–36

35. Paltiel AD, Fuhlbrigge AL, Kitch BT, et al. Cost-effectiveness of inhaled corticosteroids in adults with mild-to-moderate asthma: results from the asthma policy model. J Allergy Clin Immunol 2001; 108: 39–49

36. Andersson F, Stahl E, Barnes PJ, et al. Adding formoterol to budesonide in moderate asthma – health economic results from the FACET study. Respir Med 2001; 95: 505–12

37. Sullivan SD, Weiss KB, Lynn H, et al. The cost-effectiveness of an inner-city asthma intervention for children. J Allergy Clin Immunol 2002; 110: 576–81

38. Sullivan SD, Lee TA, Blough DK, et al. A multisite randomized clinical trial of the effects of physician education and organizational change in chronic asthma care: cost-effectiveness analysis of the Pediatric Asthma Care Patient Outcomes Research Team (PAC-PORT). Arch Pediatr Adolesc Med 2005; 159: 428–34

CHAPTER 4

Seasonal patterns of asthma exacerbations

Neil W Johnston and Malcolm R Sears

INTRODUCTION

This chapter describes variation in the risks or severity of asthma exacerbations related to seasons of the year, global differences in seasonal cycles of asthma, factors that have been associated with them and implications of this information for asthma management and control. We also examine temporal trends in annual cycles of asthma exacerbations and the possible causes of these.

Seasons are changes in average temperature and length of day that result from the tilt of the Earth's axis with respect to the plane of its orbit. While there is no clear evidence that temperature and light may directly affect the risk of asthma exacerbations they are important for their indirect effects on exposure to factors such as pollens and mold spores. Other apparently seasonal patterns of asthma exacerbation may occur because of administrative decisions, driven by seasonal considerations, that create conditions fostering exposure to exacerbation factors. For example, the most striking annual peak in asthma exacerbations occurs in the Northern Hemisphere after children return to school in late August or early September. The summer has traditionally been the season for the major school vacation but the length and timing of this are purely administrative decisions and the epidemic is probably unrelated to season per se.

In addition to seasonal variation in the risks of asthma exacerbation leading to hospital treatment within years, asthma exacerbation cycles vary in form and amplitude between years. While some of this variation may be due to changing patterns of health service use, it is also possible that differences in climate, aeroallergen burden, viral pathenogenicity or other factors between years may have profound effects.

OBJECTIVES

The objectives of this chapter are:

- To provide a comprehensive review of studies that have documented and investigated the causes of seasonal variation in asthma exacerbations, both globally and locally
- To examine the distinctions between temporal variations in asthma exacerbations caused primarily by seasonal weather patterns, those secondarily associated with seasons such as aeroallergens and those apparently only coincidentally associated, such as respiratory viral infections (RVIs)
- To assess the importance of seasonal patterns of risk factors for asthma exacerbations in the development of asthma management plans for patients

METHODS

In general, studies of the seasonality of asthma exacerbations fall into two groups: those that identify a short-term fluctuation in asthma exacerbations and then seek to explain it by examining coincident changes in one or more variables; and those that set out to examine the relation of cycles of variation in asthma morbidity to specific risk factors. Typically studies of the first type are based on hospital case series while the latter are usually population based. While valuable information is contributed by the former group, many such studies are limited by not recognizing the cyclic nature of variation in rates of asthma exacerbations or the full range of variables that may contribute to them.

The majority of published reports of seasonal cycles of asthma exacerbations have analyzed hospitalization or emergency room (ER) visit data. Patterns of health service use for asthma have changed significantly over the past two decades with consumption of many increasing, while inpatient hospitalization rates have declined. These changes may be related to multiple factors, the direction and magnitude of whose effects can only be conjectured, including a possible increase in disease prevalence, increased use of asthma control medications, lower propensity of physicians to admit to hospital and administrative incentives in some countries to reduce inpatient hospitalization.

The secondary use of data extracted from hospital charts should impose caution in their interpretation in epidemiology, particularly when temporal changes are being evaluated. The nuances of the International Classification of Diseases are beyond the scope of this chapter, but methods used to assign diagnoses vary between jurisdictions and are influenced by many factors including methods of reimbursement for hospital services. They also change over time. Very few studies have systematically audited hospital charts to verify diagnoses. The relation of asthma exacerbations to respiratory viral infections is complex and differential diagnosis is not always straightforward. Few studies have obtained data for both asthma and respiratory tract infections,

and determined the degree of coincidence of their cycles and how such coincidence varies with age.

While asthma in children under the age of 2 years is of great medical importance, there are no published reports of seasonal variation in asthma exacerbations in this group. They may experience the same cycles as older children but this remains to be established.

We have used previously unpublished figures to illustrate asthma cycles where these improve clarity or enable more comprehensive international comparisons to be made. Data to prepare these were obtained, following ethical approvals, from the Canadian Institute for Health Information, the Australian Institute for Health and Welfare, the New Zealand Health Information Service and the Small Area Health Statistics Unit (Imperial College, London, UK).

HISTORY OF OBSERVED SEASONAL VARIATION IN EXACERBATIONS OF ASTHMA

Descriptions of asthma have been recorded since the time of Hippocrates.[1] The earliest explicit reference to seasonal influences on asthma is found in ben Maimon's *Treatise on Asthma* written in the 12th century.[2] Referring to asthma patients, he writes: 'Then should be considered his age and habits as well as the season of the year.' Even more propitiously, ben Maimon continues 'From what I have heard from others and as is known to your highness, I conclude that this disorder starts with a common cold, especially in the rainy season and the patient is forced to gasp for breath day and night'.

Sir John Floyer, a 17th century physician and himself severely asthmatic, in his *A Treatise of the Asthma*[3] observed from his own diary entries that his asthma and that of his patients showed seasonal cycles and that exacerbations were more frequent before storms.

OVERVIEW OF STUDIES OF ASTHMA EXACERBATION CYCLES

While most studies of seasonal cycles of asthma exacerbation have analyzed hospital admissions or emergency room presentations, some have examined patterns of visits to general practitioners. Only a very few provide data on symptoms collected prospectively from cohort studies.

Seasonal cycles of asthma exacerbation requiring hospital treatment have been reported in many Northern Hemisphere countries, including Canada,[4–7] the USA,[8–11] the UK,[12–14] Mexico,[15] Israel,[16] Finland[17] and Trinidad, West Indies.[18] All of these describe an annual peak that occurs in the late summer or early fall. Those that have examined different age groups report that this peak is of greatest magnitude in children, less in younger adults and barely detectable in the elderly. In the Southern Hemisphere, one report each from Australia[19] and New Zealand[20] also described a consistent late summer peak in asthma hospitalization.

In the UK, using data from the Weekly Returns Service of the Royal College of General Practitioners, Fleming et al.[12] have shown annual cycles of general practitioner visits for asthma that are quite consistent in timing with those observed for hospitalizations in children and young adults. Interestingly, the cycles for general practitioner visits and hospitalizations are almost identical except in the early fall, when the peak in general practitioner visits is of lower intensity than that for hospitalization, suggesting that at that time patients may experience more sudden or severe symptoms and bypass their general practitioner to go straight to hospital.

The National Cooperative Inner-City Asthma Study (NCICAS),[10] in addition to tracking hospital and ER use by a cohort of asthmatic children, also collected data on asthma symptoms of children. The frequency of reported wheeze showed a seasonal pattern very similar to that for unscheduled hospital and ER use.

CHARACTERISTICS OF SEASONAL VARIATION IN ASTHMA EXACERBATIONS IN DIFFERENT COUNTRIES

United Kingdom

Reports of asthma exacerbation cycles in the UK all show four or five minor peaks in children and less distinctly in adults throughout the year and a major peak in the early fall following a trough over the summer. Data from four published reports[12–14,21] analyzing hospitalization and general practitioner visits show consistency in the form and magnitude of the cycles. One report[21] examined 1 year of data, and the others multiple years, but only one[14] showed cycles within multiple years. There is clearly some variation from year to year in the annual cycles, more in the magnitude than apparent timing of the peaks and troughs. The latter report also suggests some differences in the timing of the major peak in children's asthma hospitalization in the fall between Scotland and England and Wales.

Annual cycles of asthma hospitalization for children aged 5–15, and adults aged 16–49 and over 50 in England and Wales are shown in Figure 4.1. These graphs use data for all hospitalizations for asthma that occurred in England and Wales in 1998 and 1999.

In children aged 5–15, peaks can be seen at approximately weeks 5, 11, 25, 38 and 46 with that at week 38 of greatest magnitude. In adults aged 16–49 there is some coincidence in the form of the cycle to that for children but much less extreme variation over the year. There is, however, a significant peak spread over weeks 51 and 52 and 1 that is not seen in children. In adults over 50 there are no obvious peaks except for those during weeks 51 and 52 and 1.

North America

Three reports from Canada,[4–6] one using national data and two data for the Province of Ontario,

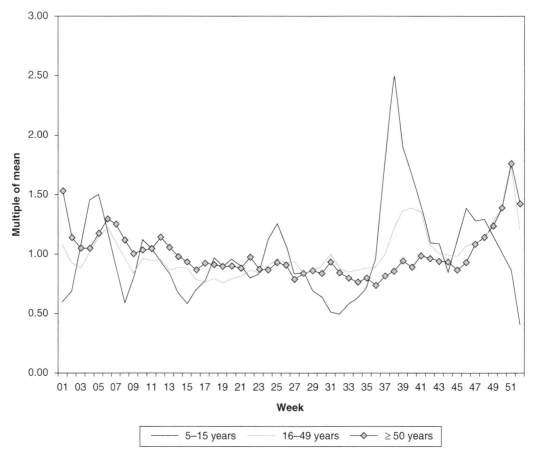

Figure 4.1 Hospitalization for asthma in England and Wales (combined data for 1998 and 1999) by age group and week of the year

show cycles of asthma hospitalizations in multiple years. One report[5] presents data for multiple age groups and two reports present data only for children.[4,6] Asthma admissions in children in Canada show a slight rise in the spring and a major peak in the early fall following a trough during the summer (Figure 4.2). In adults aged 16–49 the early fall peak is smaller than in children and in general the cycle is flatter but, in contrast to children, a peak occurs in December and January. In adults over 50 the peak in early fall is smaller again and that in early winter larger than in younger adults. One US study using national data[11] and two using local data,

from Maryland[8] and New York City,[9] show admission cycles in children and adults similar to those in Canada.

Patterns of ER presentation for asthma reported from Mexico[15] show similar patterns to the rest of North America, although the data are limited. Children have the most distinct cycles and greatest early fall peaks, and older adults the smallest.

The major difference between North America and the UK in asthma hospitalization cycles is that the series of four small peaks, most noticeable in school-age children in the UK, do not occur in Canada or the USA.

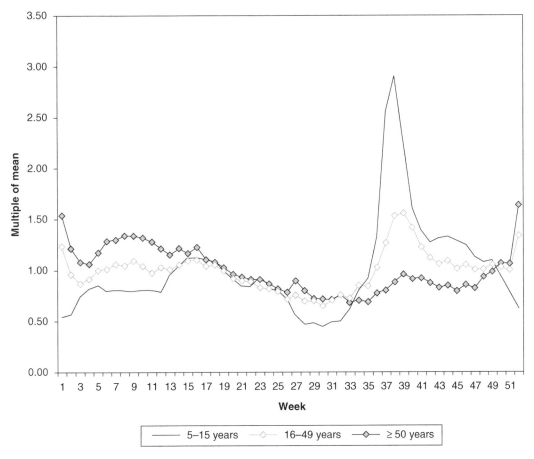

Figure 4.2 Hospitalization for asthma in Canada (combined data for 1990–2000) by age group and week of the year

Finland

Data aggregated for all pediatric asthma hospitalizations in Finland from 1972 to 1992[17] show troughs in the winter months and in July and August. A peak in May is similar to the spring rise in North America but of greater amplitude and the early fall peak is of similar magnitude to those seen in the UK and North America.

Trinidad

A report from Trinidad of ER presentations during 1997[18] shows cycles very similar to those

reported from the UK, with multiple peaks more like the pattern in England and Wales than those in North America (Figure 4.3). The early fall peak appears to be identical in timing to those in the UK and Canada. In adults aged 16–64 there is a much smaller peak in September but more hospitalization in the winter months than in children. This pattern too is similar to those observed in North America and England and Wales.

Australia and New Zealand

Two published reports, one each from Australia[19] and New Zealand,[20] have examined cycles of

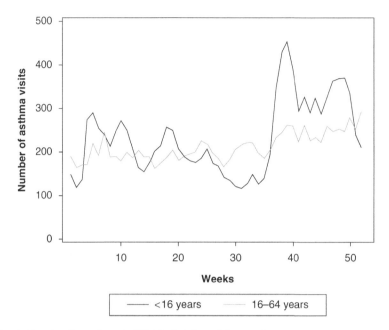

Figure 4.3 Hospitalization for asthma in Trinidad. Adapted from reference 18

asthma exacerbations in the Southern Hemi-sphere. There is a peak of asthma hospital atten-dances during February in Sydney, and peaks at this time have been recurrent across New South Wales. The New Zealand study examined hospi-talization data for the whole country over an 18-year period. Data were aggregated and analyzed by month, which may have limited sensitivity to subtle fluctuations, but, in children, the low-est point in the cycle occurred in the summer months, December and January, while a peak occurred in the fall. In adults aged 15–44 the cycle was of similar form but less extreme than in children. In adults over 45 the highest hospital-ization rates were observed in mid-winter and the lowest in the summer months.

Figure 4.4 shows the yearly cycle of asthma hospitalization in New Zealand using data aggre-gated from 1995 to 1999. The first major peak in children occurred in weeks 7–10 and a second in week 18. In the late spring and summer there was a sharp decline followed by two or three further peaks. The cycle in adults aged 16–49 shows some similarity to that in children but is

smoother, rising to a high point in the winter with low rates in summer. The pattern in adults aged over 50 is similar to that of the younger adults. Even allowing for obverse seasons the patterns observed in New Zealand show little comparability to those in the Northern Hemi-sphere. The possibility that the week 7–10 peak in New Zealand children and the late summer peak in the Northern Hemisphere are linked directly to school return after the summer vaca-tion will be discussed in a subsequent section.

While the quality and comprehensiveness of the studies reviewed varied, the results are highly consistent.

- In children in both the Northern and Southern Hemispheres there is an annual cycle of asthma exacerbations requiring hospital treatment which peaks in the late summer and early fall
- The annual peak of asthma exacerbations in children follows a trough that occurs in the summer months. The summer trough is also present in young adults but is most apparent in children

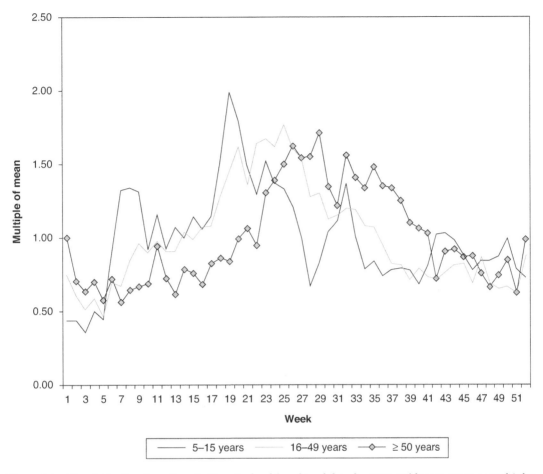

Figure 4.4 Hospitalization for asthma in New Zealand (combined data for 1995–99) by age group as multiples of the weekly mean number by week of the year

- Across all the countries examined, the magnitude of the annual late summer and early fall peak in weekly rates of hospital service use in children is between two and four times the average weekly rates observed in the remainder of the year
- Similar cycles to those in children are observed in adults under age 50, with a peak in the late summer or early fall, but these are of lesser magnitude than those in children
- In winter months, peaks in asthma exacerbations are observed in young adults but rarely in children
- In older adults the early fall peak is barely detectable but the winter peak is striking

- Reported cycles of general practitioner visits or asthma symptoms are consistent with those for hospital service use, but of smaller amplitude

VARIATION IN ASTHMA EXACERBATION CYCLES BETWEEN YEARS

While the overall form of asthma exacerbation cycles is similar between years, there are significant differences in their amplitude at different times. Figure 4.5 shows the cycles of

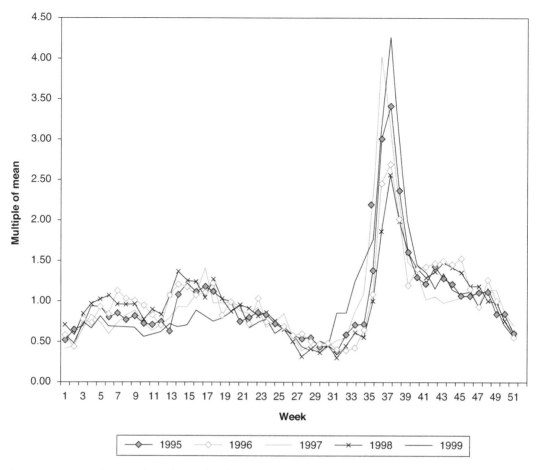

Figure 4.5 Hospitalization for asthma of children aged 5–15 in Canada (excluding Quebec) for individual years from 1995 to 1999 expressed as multiples of the within-year weekly mean number

asthma hospitalization in Canada from 1995 to 1999 in children aged 5–15. The timing of the early fall peak is almost identical in each year (week 38, September 17–24, in 4 years and in week 37 in 1996); however, the magnitude of the peak (expressed as multiples of the within-year weekly mean number of hospitalizations) varied from a multiple of 2.5 to almost 4.5. Differences in the rest of the year are less obvious but, for example, in 1999 the spring rise was markedly lower than in the other years shown.

FACTORS ASSOCIATED WITH SEASONAL CYCLES OF ASTHMA

While some reports simply describe seasonal patterns of asthma exacerbation, most have attempted to relate the observations to one or more causal factors. Among the factors considered to explain asthma exacerbation cycles are air pollution, weather patterns, seasonal allergens, school attendance, respiratory viral infections, patterns of medication use and prescribing and intrinsic factors.

Air pollution

A critical challenge in the evaluation of the effects of ambient and domiciliary air pollution on cycles of asthma exacerbations is how to distinguish these from the effects of multiple co-variables when all may coincide but vary in the magnitude of their effects at different times of the year. The relations of ambient air pollution, aeroallergens and climatic factors are hard to dissect from each other and their possible interactions. There is also epidemiological and experimental evidence that concurrent exposure to atmospheric and domiciliary air pollutants may worsen asthma symptoms during respiratory viral infections,[22] but to date few studies examined have considered this possible effect. This is important as respiratory viral infections are associated with the majority of asthma exacerbations.[23,24] Some of the methodological issues in studies of the relation of aeroallergens and climatic factors to asthma exacerbations, particularly those relating to the use of time series analysis, have been documented by Atkinson and Strachan,[25] who noted the inherent difficulties, given the relatively short periods in which aeroallergens may have their effects and the coincident variation in confounding factors such as weather patterns, of attributing effects to individual insults.

The evidence associating increases in levels of ambient air pollutants with worsened asthma morbidity is strong, although the absolute magnitude of their effects may be modest. It is also possible that the distinct contribution of ambient air pollutants, and/or their interaction with other causal factors, to asthma exacerbations varies over the life cycle.

Bates et al.[7] found that, while there was an overall relation of ER presentations for asthma in Vancouver to levels of air pollutants, no relation was present during the September peak period in asthma exacerbations. The NCICAS, a prospective study of a large cohort of inner-city children aged 4–12, found no relation between wheeze, ER visits or inpatient hospitalizations and ambient air pollutants or indeed domiciliary environmental tobacco smoke.[10] Families were contacted bi-monthly and asked to recall episodes of wheezing or hospital treatment. The units within which events were related to air pollution levels were months, and as the effects of changes in levels of air pollutants on asthma hospitalization appear shortly after they occur, this study may not have had adequate sensitivity to detect them. The cycle of levels of atmospheric sulfur dioxide, but not other pollutants, coincided with the observed cycles of asthma symptoms and hospital treatment. In a cohort study of asthmatic adults in Denver, Colorado conducted over a 3-month period from December 1987 to February 1988,[26] Ostro et al. found a weak relation of diary-recorded cough, but not asthma severity rating, to atmospheric hydrogen ion (H+) concentration (acidity). A regression model that included symptoms on the previous day and exposure to gas stoves in the domestic environment explained 44% of the overall variation observed in symptoms, with the strongest effect from gas stove exposure. Other than H+ concentration the only other detectable effect of an ambient air pollutant was for sulfate on shortness of breath. In a subsequent analysis[27] of the effects of domiciliary air quality, Ostro and colleagues found that use of a gas stove on a given day increased the likelihood of experiencing either cough or shortness of breath by 10.4 and 9.2%, respectively, among non-smokers. The increases in the likelihood of cough or shortness of breath related to environmental tobacco smoke were 1.9 and 4.6%, respectively. This finding of an effect of domiciliary tobacco smoke in adults is in contrast to the finding of no such relation in the NCI-CAS study[10] of a much larger cohort of children aged 4–12 years.

A relation of ambient sulfur dioxide to hospitalization of children for asthma has been observed in the APHEA (Air Pollution and Health: a European Approach) studies.[28] Admissions of children aged 0–14 increased by 1.3% (95% CI 0.4–2.2) for every increase of $10 \, \mu g/m^3$ of atmospheric sulfur dioxide, but not other pollutants. No increase in asthma hospitalization attributable to ambient air pollutants was observed in adults aged 15–64.

Jamason et al.[29] categorized the nature of air masses and their associated air pollution characteristics by day for an 11-year period in New York City from 1982 to 1992. Air mass characteristics and their associated pollution burdens were related to daily variation in asthma hospitalization. The association of air masses during which the highest rates of asthma hospitalization occurred varied in their coincidence with levels of air pollutants, being strongly associated with high levels of air pollution in summer, but not in fall and winter, suggesting that the contribution of ambient air pollutants to asthma exacerbations may be of variable magnitude at different points in the seasonal cycle. The results also emphasize the possibility that the interaction effects of weather and ambient air pollution on asthma exacerbations may vary over the annual cycle. The overall form of the annual cycles of asthma hospitalizations observed in this study were very similar to those found in other studies (Figures 4.1–4.3).

A study of the relation of general practitioner visits for asthma to ambient air pollution in London, England from 1992 to 1994[30] found a weak association *overall* to a 10–90th centile change in ambient levels of nitrogen dioxide and carbon monoxide in children, and with airborne particulate matter of less than 10 μm diameter (PM_{10}) levels in adults. When the effects of air pollutants were analyzed within seasons, defined as warm (April to September) or cold (October to March), a strong seasonal effect was found. In the warm season daily general practitioner visits for asthma in children aged 0–14 increased by 13.2% (95% CI 5.6–21.3) for a 10–90th centile change in nitrogen dioxide, 11.4% (95% CI 3.3–20) for carbon monoxide and 5.8% for sulfur dioxide (95% CI 1.6–10.2). In adults a 10–90th centile increase in PM_{10} was associated with a 9.2% increase (95% CI 3.7–15.1) in general practitioner visits for asthma in the warm season. No associations

between ambient air pollutant levels and general practitioner visits for asthma were found in the cold season in children or adults.

A similar study[31] examined the relation of ER visits for asthma and other respiratory morbidity to changes in levels of ambient air pollution in London from 1992 to 1994 and found an even stronger relation, particularly in children, than for general practitioner visits. A 10–90th centile change in nitrogen dioxide and for sulfur dioxide levels was associated, respectively, with a 19.7% (95% CI 10.61–29.53) and a 9.9% (95% CI 4.8–15.3) increase in ER visits for asthma. Again the effect was much stronger during the April to September 'warm season' than in the October to March 'cold season'. In adults, only increases in levels of PM_{10} produced a significant increase in ER visits. A study of a cohort of moderately to severe asthmatic children in Denver, Colorado[32] over three winter periods from 1999 to 2002 found no significant association of changes in forced expiratory volume (FEV_1), peak expiratory flow (PEF) or asthma exacerbations with ambient air pollution levels, but a highly significant relation to upper respiratory tract infections. This study may have lacked adequate power to detect effects of air pollution on the selected outcomes, and the effects of air pollutants on asthma symptoms may have been moderated by co-variables in that study period. However, the results emphasize the challenge of attributing fractions of observed morbidity to individual causal factors with relatively small effects.

In summary the contribution of exposure to individual air pollutants to asthma exacerbations is complex. The attribution of their effects is confounded by the interrelationship of ambient air pollutants, weather patterns and aeroallergens. The magnitude and specificity of effects differ between adults and children and between cold and warm seasons. The study by Jamason et al.[29] is particularly interesting as it documents an effect of weather pattern categories that appear to have different effects even when air pollution levels are similar. As these differences occurred between cold and warm seasons, pollens and spores which appear in spring and summer may be responsible. Domiciliary air quality too may play a significant role in asthma morbidity and, particularly in colder regions, have seasonal effects as people spend more time confined indoors.

Overall the influence of ambient air pollution on cycles of asthma exacerbations is probably a short-term effect which varies in amplitude with seasonal changes in weather patterns and the burden of aeroallergens. It is likely that exposure of asthmatics to combinations of high risk atmospheric conditions and/or domiciliary air pollution during respiratory viral infections may increase the risk of exacerbation. The nature of the effects of either domiciliary or ambient air pollution during RVIs in asthmatics is a subject requiring further research.

Climate, pollens and fungal spores

In most parts of the world, climate is defined by the seasons and much human behavior is dictated by them. Many of the factors associated with cycles of asthma exacerbations such as pollens, molds and fungal spores tend to occur at specific times of the year. As weather patterns have been specifically implicated in the risk of exposure to aeroallergens the effects of these will be considered together.

Asthma exacerbation cycles in the Northern Hemisphere are strikingly similar in countries with quite dissimilar climates (Figures 4.1–4.3). Trinidad is located 10 degrees above the equator and experiences very mild weather throughout the year, albeit with high risks of violent storm activity in the hurricane season. England and Wales in general have winters and summers that are milder and wetter than those in almost every part of Canada. The factors associated with the similarities in asthma cycles in these countries will be explored later, but the role of climate per se is probably small. As in the case of ambient air pollution, climate may influence short-term variation within yearly cycles of

asthma exacerbations. The synoptic effect described by Jamason,[29] where air masses associated with high rates of asthma hospitalization vary by season in their association with air pollutants, is one example of how this may occur. Another is thunderstorm activity.

One of the earliest studies reporting an association of asthma exacerbations to thunderstorm activity examined ER visits during a severe thunderstorm in the city of Birmingham, England.[33] Visits for asthma increased to three or four times their usual levels in the rest of June and July. Unusual patterns and peaks of levels of fungal spores and pollens were observed in the area and were hypothesized to have caused the epidemic. Marks et al.[34] observed an epidemic of hospital presentations for asthma following a severe thunderstorm in south-eastern Australia. Almost all of the victims were allergic to grass pollens. In a retrospective analysis of thunderstorm activity and asthma hospital presentations conducted in the region, thunderstorm days were associated with 13 of 39 asthma epidemic days but only 5 of 155 non-epidemic days (odds ratio 15.0, 95% CI 6.0–37.6). Grass pollen concentrations were observed to be eight times higher at the time of the thunderstorms than in the previous 9 hours.

A relation of thunderstorms to asthma exacerbations has also been shown in London, England. Two studies[35,36] examined hospital presentations for asthma that occurred during severe thunderstorm activity on 24 June 1994. The latter study found ER presentations for asthma that were 10 times the number expected. Both reported that grass pollen counts were particularly high in the period immediately following the storm and during the hospital presentation epidemic. A further intriguing study of the thunderstorms of 24 June 1994 examined records of call-centers in the UK established to enable patients of general practitioners to obtain home visits out of office hours.[37] Calls were categorized as being for asthma or other causes, and call-centers were categorized as having asthma epidemics or not and to be in a thunderstorm-affected area or not. The pattern of calls recorded during the night of the thunderstorm was compared to that which occurred during a control night 1 week earlier. In the thunderstorm-affected areas the odds ratio for calls for asthma on thunderstorm days was 6.36 (95% CI 5.0–8.3) and in the areas unaffected by thunderstorms 1.01 (95% CI 0.8–1.3).

Anderson et al.[38] examined the relation of thunderstorm days, hospital admissions for asthma and aeroallergen concentrations in Cardiff, Wales between 1990 and 1996. Thunderstorm days were compared to date-matched control days. Asthma admissions on thunderstorm days were found to be 30% higher than on control days (incident rate ratio 1.3, 95% CI 1.01–1.68). No association of the thunderstorm effect was found with aeroallergen levels. It is possible, however, that thunderstorms in the Cardiff area during the study period were not as intense as those that produced the extreme effects observed in the London and Australian epidemics.

A comprehensive study in Ottawa, Canada related children's ER presentations for asthma at a tertiary care hospital from 1993 to 1997 to thunderstorm activity, levels of grass and ragweed pollen and fungal spores.[39] The investigators performed adjustments for the effects of seasonal variation in children's asthma exacerbations, possibly related to viral epidemics, air pollution and climate as well as weekly patterns of ER use. Atmospheric concentrations of fungal spores doubled during thunderstorms, which were also associated with increases in levels of ozone, nitrogen dioxide and haze. No effects of weed, grass or tree pollens or of air pollution levels on emergency visits for asthma during periods of thunderstorm activity were found. Overall, on thunderstorm days there was a 15% increase in the average number of ER visits for asthma compared to non-thunderstorm days.

A study of hospitalization for asthma in ten major cities across Canada by Dales et al.[40] examined the relation of spore and pollen levels (basidiomycetes, ascomycetes, deuteromycetes, weeds, trees and grasses) to daily admissions.

Adjustments were made for long-term trends, within-week hospitalization cycles, climate variables and ambient air pollution levels. Increases in spore and pollen levels of double the mean daily values were associated with increases in daily asthma hospitalizations ranging from 3.3% (95% CI 2.3–4.1%) for basidiomycetes to 2.0% (95% CI 1.1–2.8%) for grasses.

A study of severe asthma attacks leading to respiratory arrest and two deaths in 11 patients in the US Midwest compared their skin-test reactivity to *Alternaria alternata* to that of 99 matched controls with no history of respiratory arrest.[41] Ten cases (91%) were sensitive to *A. alternata* compared to 31% of the controls ($p < 0.001$). Serum levels of IgE antibodies to *A. alternata* in nine of 11 cases tested were elevated. All of the cases of respiratory arrest occurred in the summer or early fall. Campbell et al.[42] analyzed all deaths from asthma occurring in the UK in 1983–95. In people under the age of 45 there was a clear peak of deaths in the summer months. Between the ages of 45 and 64 the risk of death shifted toward the winter months, but still with an identifiable peak in the summer. In people over 65 there was no summer peak and a large one in the winter. This pattern is consistent with a hypothesis that asthma deaths in children and young adults may be related to aeroallergen exposure, with those in older adults more likely related to winter viral infections. A similar phenomenon has been reported in the USA[11] with children and young adults at greatest risk of death during an asthma exacerbation in the summer and adults over 65 during the winter.

It is reasonable to conclude that climate and aeroallergen levels have significant short-term effects on the risk of asthma exacerbations. Their effects are also inextricably associated in complex ways with those of individual ambient air pollutants and possibly their interactions. As aeroallergens generally appear for a specific period of the year, they probably manifest their effect on a seasonal basis as does climate. Modest associations of individual climate factors, particularly temperature and relative humidity, are also associated with short-term variation in asthma hospitalization. The possibility that summer aeroallergen exposure may pose a particular risk of life-threatening exacerbations for children and young adults is an area requiring further study, particularly since asthmatics are less likely to take control medications in the summer months.[4]

Thunderstorms are associated with some short-term epidemics of asthma exacerbations that may be striking, but the majority of epidemics are not.[43] As thunderstorms are more frequent at certain times of year, particularly the summer in North America and Europe, the epidemics, when they occur, are largely seasonal.

The magnitude of the combined effects of aeroallergens, ambient air pollution and climate on asthma is uncertain and probably has different effects in different age groups. Atkinson and Strachan[25] conclude their assessment of the methodological issues facing studies in this area as follows. *'The possible roles of meteorological conditions and other environmental factors in determining the nature of any of the health effects of pollens are not fully understood, although it seems that thunderstorms in particular are associated with striking epidemics of asthma in which aeroallergens may play a role. Further studies in other locations with different environmental situations are required to provide the variability in confounding factors and coincident exposures in order to clarify which aeroallergen species can have a detrimental effect on the health of asthmatics and under what conditions.'*

No studies have been identified that have examined the possibility that cumulative exposure to seasonal aeroallergens affects asthma symptoms. The emphasis in the studies reviewed of the short-term associations of aeroallergens and climate with asthma exacerbations is understandable. All of the studies reviewed have related discrete events such as hospital admissions to environmental conditions. The effects of cumulative seasonal exposures on individual asthmatics is an area where further investigation may be valuable.

Viral infections

Worsened symptoms during respiratory infections have been recognized in asthmatics since medieval times and are pathognomonic of the disease.[2] The incidence of asthma exacerbations shows a strong seasonal effect, being greater in the fall and winter months, coinciding with periods in which RVIs also most commonly occur.

Viral respiratory tract infections, particularly of rhinoviruses, are associated with the great majority of exacerbations of asthma in children[23,24,44] and almost half of them in adults.[23,44,45] Respiratory syncytial virus (RSV) infection of infants with asthma or chronic wheezing appears to be associated with the majority of exacerbation episodes.[46] RSV has also been implicated in the genesis of the asthma phenotype.[47]

In older children picornaviruses, particularly rhinoviruses, are predominantly associated with asthma exacerbations.[24] Johnston et al.[23] detected viruses in 80–85% of episodes of exacerbations of asthma symptoms in children in a year-long study. Picornaviruses, almost all probably rhinoviruses, were detected in 65%, coronaviruses in 17%, influenza and parainfluenza in 9% each and RSV in 5%.

In adults with asthma exacerbations, infections with rhinovirus are also those most commonly found, although influenza and parainfluenza infections are more frequent than in children. None of the studies reviewed explicitly examined the relation of RVIs to asthma exacerbations in older adults, an area deserving further research.

In a study of adults with asthma and chronic obstructive pulmonary disease (COPD) exacerbations requiring hospital treatment, Tan et al.[48] found that 48% of the asthmatics had respiratory viral infections, 62% of which were picornaviruses or adenovirus and 21% influenza A or B. Teichtahl et al.[49] found evidence of recent RVI in 37% of patients requiring hospitalization for asthma compared with 9% of patients in hospital for elective surgery in Melbourne, Australia. Of the 29 asthma patients with evidence of RVI, influenza A or B viruses were

Table 4.1 Viruses detected in asthma exacerbations in Houston, Texas, 1998. The values in parentheses are the percentages of each virus relative to the total number of viruses detected in the group. From reference 51

Virus detected	Cohort (n=29)	ER visit (n=122)
Picornavirus	24 (39)	53 (56)
Coronaviruses	10 (16)	21 (22)
Influenza A and B	11 (18)	12 (13)
Parainfluenza	16 (26)	0 (0)
RSV	0 (0)	4 (4)
Adenovirus	1 (1)	1 (1)
Cytomegalovirus	0 (0)	3 (3)

ER, emergency room; RSV, respiratory syncytial virus

detected in 15, rhinovirus in nine and RSV and adenovirus in one each.

Nicholson et al.[50] followed a cohort of 138 asthmatic adults with a mean age of 33 years between October 1990 and August 1992 (average participation period 54.5 weeks). A total of 84 asthma exacerbations were documented. Specimens for virological testing were obtained in 61 (73%) of these and viruses were detected in 27 (44%). Rhinoviruses were present in 16/61 (26%), coronaviruses in 4/61 (7%), parainfluenza in 3/61 (5%) and influenza, RSV and dual viral infections in one each.

Atmar et al.[51] combined a 30-month prospective study of 29 adults (mean age 37.8 years) with an average length of follow-up of 19.5 months with a study of asthmatic patients treated in an ER. The method used to select the ER patients was not described. Asthma exacerbations were associated with a RVI in 44% of the prospective group and 55% in the ER group. The spectrum of viruses detected in each group is shown in Table 4.1.

Several, mostly earlier, studies of the coincidence of RVIs and asthma exacerbations in adults had reported lower frequencies of infection. These have been hypothesized to be due to the lower sensitivity of the earlier methods used for viral detection compared to the polymerase chain reaction (PCR) used in the reports cited in

this section. The four studies summarized above show consistent results with 48%, 37%, 44% and 44% of adult asthma exacerbations coinciding with RVIs. In the adult studies, with the exception of that by Nicholson et al.,[50] influenza viruses were more commonly found in adults than in children. It is possible, in addition, that all of these studies may have underestimated the role of influenza, because they did not specifically include periods in which influenza epidemics occurred. Further studies of adult asthmatics of all ages, particularly during influenza epidemics of diverse strains, would be of great help in understanding the risks these pose for exacerbations of asthma.

Seasonality of respiratory viral infections

The four major respiratory virus types associated with asthma exacerbations are the picornaviruses including rhinovirus, RSV, influenza A and B and parainfluenza. Infections with rhinovirus are most common in the fall months in the Northern Hemisphere[52–54] while RSV, influenza and parainfluenza infections occur predominantly in the late fall and winter months. Adenovirus, whilst generally tested for in studies of the role of RVIs in asthma exacerbations, is uncommonly associated with them. While its role in asthma exacerbations in older adults remains to be established, rhinovirus is the infectious agent most commonly associated with asthma exacerbations in both children and younger adults.

In a seminal study of patterns of rhinovirus transmission in a cohort of insurance company workers over a 3-year period from 1963 to 1966, Gwaltney et al.[52] demonstrated that both detections of the virus and respiratory symptoms associated with them followed a consistent pattern, with extreme peaks in the early fall and smaller ones in the spring. The cycles, with 3 years of data for the frequency of 'rhinovirus illnesses' and the percentage of those with rhinovirus infections condensed to a 1-year period, are shown in Figure 4.6. A similar pattern of rhinovirus infection, with the early fall peak beginning 2.27 days

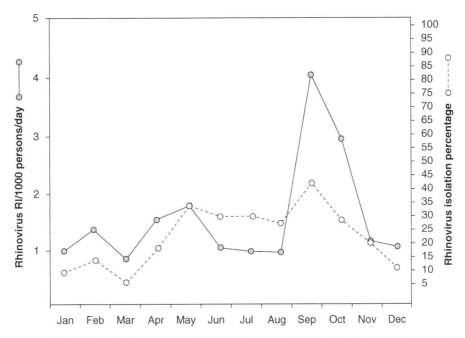

Figure 4.6 Combined data for the 3-year period, March 1963 to March 1966, depicting the seasonal variation in the percentage of sampled respiratory illnesses yielding rhinoviruses and in the rate of rhinovirus illness derived by application of this percentage to the total rate of respiratory illness. Data from reference 52

after school return after Labor Day, was observed by Longini *et al.*[55] in an analysis of data from the Tecumseh study[56] of respiratory virus transmission. The report also documented the distinction between the seasons for rhinovirus and those for influenza A (strain H3N2) beginning in early December and for influenza A (H1N1) and B beginning in late January. RSV infections also peak in the winter months. In a 4-year study of Medicaid beneficiaries in Tennessee, Griffin *et al.*[57] showed that RSV was detected over a longer period than influenza, beginning in early November and ending as late as mid-April. In all 4 years the period for RSV began earlier than that for influenza and ended later. A similar pattern has been reported by Monto.[58]

Given that rhinovirus infections are associated with approximately 80% of asthma exacerbations in children and 50% in young adults,[23,24] it is to be expected that their cycles will coincide to some extent. As shown in Figures 4.1–4.3, this is indeed the case with a peak of asthma

hospitalization occurring in the early fall coinciding with the time reported for peak occurrences of rhinovirus infection. The early fall peak of asthma exacerbations in adults is smaller, reflecting the lesser role of rhinovirus reported in this group. Exacerbations for adults, however, show increased levels in the winter months, suggesting a greater role for influenza viruses or possibly RSV, although this has not been reported.

Figure 4.7 shows the superimposition of the chart of asthma hospitalization for 5–15-year-old children taken from Figure 4.2 onto the chart in Figure 4.6. There is a remarkable coincidence of both form and the overall nature of the cycles, particularly given that these data were collected three decades apart in different age groups.

The role of schools in cycles of rhinovirus

School-age children have been shown to introduce rhinovirus infections into their families

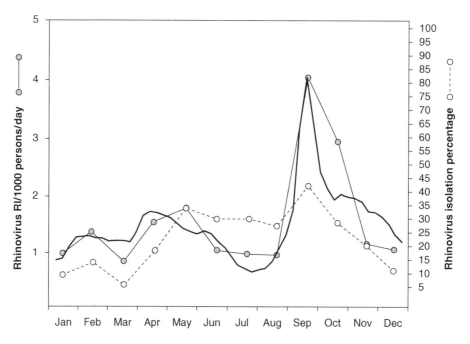

Figure 4.7 Data from Figure 4.2, showing the annual cycle of asthma hospitalization from 1990 to 2000 in children aged 5–15 in Canada (bold line) superimposed on Figure 4.6 from reference 52

three times more frequently than working adults.[59] During the 3-week September asthma exacerbation peak period in 2001, in a major city in Ontario, over 60% of all school-age children presenting to ERs with asthma had viral infections, predominantly of rhinovirus.[4] In a control group of subjects in the community with asthma of comparable severity not experiencing exacerbation, 42% had respiratory viral infections during this period, with rhinoviruses again predominating.

Across Canada, hospitalization of children for asthma reaches an annual peak in September of every year.[4,5] The peak occurred in week 38 (17–24 September) from 1990 to 2000 except in 1992, when it was in week 39 and in 1997 when it was in week 37.[6] Labor Day was at its latest possible date in 1992 and its earliest in 1997, suggesting that the peak is related in time to school return which is on the Tuesday after Labor Day each year. This possibility is supported by the observation

made by Longini et al.[55] that the annual rhinovirus infection peak begins shortly after Labor Day.

Using mathematical modeling we have demonstrated that the September asthma epidemic peak occurs 17.9 (95% CI 16.8–19.0) days after Labor Day (range 15.5–20.3 days) in school-age children, 19.6 (95% CI 18.6–20.6) days after Labor Day (range 17.5–21.7 days) in preschool children and 23.7 (95% CI 21.9–25.5) days after Labor Day (range 21.3–30.9 days) in adults.[6]

These findings strongly support those discussed earlier that viral infections, predominantly rhinovirus, are an important cause of exacerbations during the most extreme period of risk. The consistent timing in relation to Labor Day and sequence of the epidemic peaks in September in Canada also suggest that the annual cycle of rhinovirus infections is a consequence of conditions encountered by children upon return to school rather than an independent biological event.

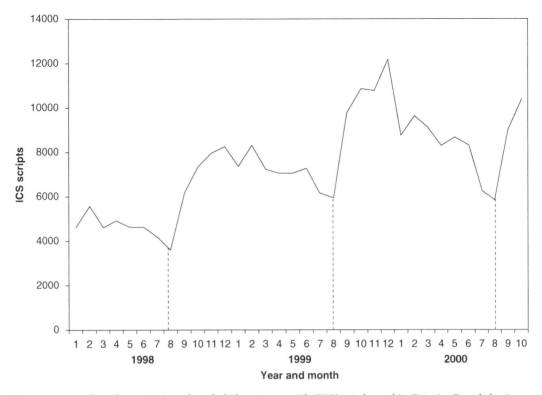

Figure 4.8 Number of prescriptions for inhaled corticosteroids (ICS) reimbursed in Ontario, Canada by Assure Health 1998–2000 by month. Reproduced with permission from reference 4

Earlier studies have also shown a strong relation of the school calendar to cycles of documented respiratory tract infections and asthma hospitalization in children,[13,21] with periods of disease exacerbation and virus detection coinciding with school attendance after vacations.

Other factors

Use of asthma control medication such as inhaled corticosteroids may influence cycles of asthma exacerbation. Filling of prescriptions for inhaled corticosteroids has an annual cycle with a low point in August and a peak in the late fall and early winter.[4,60] This cycle is shown for a 3-year period in Figure 4.8. It is possible that asthmatics may be less compliant with asthma control therapy through the summer continuing to the time after school return when

rhinovirus infections are highly prevalent and they are at greatest risk.

Increased stress has been associated with a greater risk of asthma exacerbations in children.[61] The beginning of the school year is likely to be stressful for many children and their families, and it is possible that this increases the risks posed by viral infections at that time, magnified by less use of control medication and re-exposure to allergens in the school environment.[62]

CONCLUSIONS AND IMPLICATIONS FOR DISEASE MANAGEMENT

Asthma is a disease characterized by exacerbation cycles. Some, such as the early fall peak in children in the Northern Hemisphere and others associated with the school calendar, are predictable and also occur in adults, but to a lesser extent. Given that 80% or more of asthma exacerbations in children and 50% in adults are associated with viral infections, and that periods of high prevalence of respiratory viruses are predictable, improving asthma control at these times should be a public health priority.

Short-term cycles of asthma exacerbation are associated with high levels of ambient air pollution with the risk possibly increased by certain climate patterns. The risks of exacerbation are also increased during periods of high levels of aeroallergens, again with the risk possibly compounded by climatic factors such as thunderstorms.

While reductions in levels of ambient air pollution have been addressed by most nations over the past half-century with notable success, they remain an important source of respiratory irritation and may pose particular risks to people living in highly polluted areas such as those proximal to major truck routes.

Given a low likelihood that the non-domiciliary pollution levels that individual asthma patients must endure can be modified and that aeroallergen levels and climate are beyond patient control, it would be prudent for asthma management plans to address periods such as the late summer in North America when combinations of aeroallergen and air pollution levels and climate conditions may pose a significant threat, and advise appropriate use of asthma control medications at these times.

REFERENCES

1. Unger L, Harris MC. Stepping stones in allergy. Ann Allergy 1974; 32: 214–30
2. Maimonides M. In Suessman Muntner, ed. Treatise on Asthma. Philadelphia: JB Lippincott, 1963: 1–2
3. Floyer JA. A Treatise of the Asthma, 2nd edn. Printed for R. Wilkin and W. Innys, 1717
4. Johnston NW, Johnston SL, Duncan JM, et al. The September epidemic of asthma exacerbations in children: a search for etiology. J Allergy Clin Immunol 2005; 112: 132–8

5. Crighton EJ, Mamdani MM, Upshur REG. A population based time series analysis of asthma hospitalizations in Ontario, Canada: 1988 to 2000. BMC Health Serv Res 2001; 1: 7
6. Johnston NW, Johnston SL, Norman GR, et al. The September epidemic of asthma hospitalization: school children as disease vectors. J Allergy Clin Immunol 2006; 117: 557–62
7. Bates DV, Baker-Anderson M, Sizto R. Asthma attack periodicity: a study of hospital emergency visits in Vancouver. Environ Res 1990; 51: 51–70
8. Kimes D, Levine E, Timmins S, et al. Temporal dynamics of emergency department and hospital admissions of pediatric asthmatics. Environ Res 2004; 94: 7–17
9. Silverman RA, Stevenson L, Hastings HM. Age-related seasonal patterns of emergency room visits for asthma in an urban environment. Ann Emerg Med 2003; 42: 577–86
10. Gergen PJ, Mitchell H, Lynn H. Understanding the seasonal pattern of childhood asthma: results from the National Cooperative Inner-City Asthma Study (NCICAS). J Pediatr 2002; 141: 631–6
11. Weiss KB. Seasonal trends in US hospitalizations and mortality. J Am Med Assoc 1990; 263: 2323–8
12. Fleming DM, Cross KW, Sunderland R, Ross AM. Comparison of the seasonal patterns of asthma identified in general practitioner episodes, hospital admissions and deaths. Thorax 2000; 55: 657–61
13. Storr J, Lenney W. School holidays and admissions with asthma. Arch Dis Child 1989; 64: 103–7
14. Strachan D, Hansell A, Hollowell J, et al. Collation and comparison of data on respiratory disease. Report to the Department of Health, August 1999. London: Department of Health, 1999 (http://www.sghms.ac.uk/depts/laia/COLLATE/respdata.htm) Last accessed 23 March 2002
15. Rosas I, McCartney HA, Payne RW, et al. Analysis of the relationships between environmental factors (aeroallergens, air pollution, and weather) and asthma emergency admissions to a hospital in Mexico City. Allergy 1998; 53: 394–401
16. Garty B-Z, Kosman E, Ganor E, et al. ER visits of asthmatic children, relation to air pollution, weather, and airborne allergens. Ann Allergy Asthma Immunol 1998; 81: 563–70
17. Harju T, Keistinen T, Tuuoponen T, Kivela S-L. Seasonal variation in childhood asthma hospitalizations in Finland, 1972–1992. Eur J Pediatr 1997; 156: 436–9
18. Ivey M, Simeon D, Juman S, et al. Associations between climate variables and asthma visits to accident and emergency facilities in Trinidad, West Indies. Allergol Int 2001; 50: 29–33
19. Lister S, Sheppeard V, Morgan G, et al. February asthma outbreaks in NSW: a case control study. Aust NZ J Public Health 2001; 255: 14–19

20. Kimbell-Dunn M, Pearce N, Beasley R. Seasonal variation in asthma hospitalizations and death rates in New Zealand. Respirology 2000; 5: 241–6

21. Johnston SL, Pattemore PK, Sanderson G, et al. The relationship between upper respiratory tract infections and hospital admissions for asthma: a time-trend analysis. Am J Respir Crit Care Med 1996; 154: 654–60

22. Chauhan AJ, Johnston SL. Air pollution and infection in respiratory illness. Br Med Bull 2003; 68: 95–112

23. Johnston SL, Pattemore PK, Sanderson G, et al. Community study of role of viral infections in exacerbations of asthma in 9–11 year old children. BMJ 1995; 310: 1225–8

24. Message SD, Johnston SL. Viruses in asthma. Br Med Bull 2002; 61: 29–43

25. Atkinson RW, Strachan DP. Role of outdoor aeroallergens in asthma exacerbations: epidemiological evidence. Thorax 2004; 569: 277–8

26. Ostro BD, Lipsett MJ, Wiener MB, Selner JC. Asthmatic responses to airborne acid aerosols. Am J Public Health 1991; 81: 694–702

27. Ostro BD, Lipsett MJ, Mann JK, et al. Indoor air pollution and asthma. Results from a panel study. Am J Respir Crit Care Med 1994; 149: 1400–6

28. Sunyer J, Atkinson R, Ballester F, et al. Respiratory effects of sulfur dioxide: a hierarchical multicity analysis in the APHEA 2 study. Occup Environ Med 2003; 60: e2

29. Jamason PF, Kalkstein LS, Gergen PJ. A synoptic evaluation of asthma hospital admissions in New York City. Am J Respir Crit Care Med 1997; 156: 1781–8

30. Hajat S, Haines A, Goubet SA, et al. Association of air pollution with daily general practitioner consultations for asthma and other lower respiratory conditions in London. Thorax 1999; 54: 597–605

31. Atkinson RW, Anderson HR, Strachan DP, et al. Short-term associations between outdoor air pollution and visits to accident and emergency departments in London for respiratory complaints. Eur Respir J 1999; 13: 257–65

32. Rabinovitch N, Zhang L, Murphy JR, et al. Effects of wintertime ambient air pollutants on asthma exacerbations in urban minority children with moderate to severe disease. J Allergy Clin Immunol 2004; 114: 1131–7

33. Packe GE, Ayres JG. Asthma outbreak during a thunderstorm. Lancet 1985; 2: 199–204

34. Marks GB, Colquhoun JR, Girgis ST, et al. Thunderstorm outflows preceding epidemics of asthma during spring and summer. Thorax 2001; 56: 468–71

35. Celenza A, Fothergill J, Kupek E, Shaw RJ. Thunderstorm associated asthma: a detailed analysis of environmental factors. BMJ 1996; 312: 604–7

36. Wallis DN, Webb J, Brooke D, et al. A major outbreak of asthma associated with a thunderstorm: experience of accident and emergency departments and patients' characteristics. BMJ 1996; 312: 601–4

37. Higham J, Venables K, Kupek E, et al. Asthma and thunderstorms: description of an epidemic in general practice in Britain using data from a doctor's deputising service in the UK. J Epidemiol Community Health 1997; 51: 233–8

38. Anderson W, Prescott GJ, Packham S, et al. Asthma admissions and thunderstorms: a study of pollen, fungal spores, rainfall and ozone. Q J Med 2001; 94: 429–33

39. Dales RE, Cakmak S, Judek S, et al. The role of fungal spores in thunderstorm asthma. Chest 2003; 123: 745–50

40. Dales RE, Cakmak S, Judek S, et al. Influence of outdoor aeroallergens on hospitalization for asthma in Canada. J Allergy Clin Immunol 2004; 113: 303–6

41. O'Hollaren MT, Yunginger JW, Offord KP, et al. Exposure to an aeroallergen as a possible precipitating factor in respiratory arrest in young patients with asthma. N Engl J Med 1991; 324: 359–63

42. Campbell MJ, Holgate ST, Johnston SL. Trends in asthma mortality. BMJ 1997; 315: 1012

43. Newson R, Strachan D, Emberlin AE, et al. Acute asthma epidemics, weather and pollen in England, 1987–1994. Eur Respir J 1998; 11: 694–701

44. Tan WC. Viruses in asthma exacerbations. Curr Opin Pulm Med 2004; 11: 21–6

45. Corne JM, Marshall C, Smith S, et al. Frequency, severity and duration of rhinovirus infections in asthmatic and non-asthmatic individuals: a longitudinal cohort study. Lancet 2002; 359: 831–4

46. Gern JE. Viral respiratory infection and the link to asthma. Pediatr Infect Dis J 2004; 23: S78–86

47. Lemanske RF, Busse WW. Asthma. J Allergy Clin Immunol 2003; 111: S502–19

48. Tan WC, Xiang X, Qiu D, et al. Epidemiology of respiratory viruses in patients hospitalised with near-fatal asthma, acute exacerbations of asthma or chronic obstructive pulmonary disease. Am J Med 2003; 115: 272–7

49. Teichtahl H, Buckmaster N, Pertnikovs E. The incidence of respiratory tract infection in adults requiring hospitaization for asthma. Chest 1997; 112: 591–6

50. Nicholson KG, Kent J, Ireland DC. Respiratory viruses and exacerbations of asthma in adults. BMJ 2003; 307: 982–6

51. Atmar RL, Guy E, Guntupalli KK, et al. Respiratory tract viral infections in inner-city asthmatic adults. Arch Intern Med 1998; 158: 2453–9

52. Gwaltney JM, Hendley JO, Simon G, Jordan WS. Rhinovirus infections in an industrial population. 1. The occurrence of illness. N Engl J Med 1966: 275; 1261–8

53. Arruda E, Pitkaranta A, Witek TJ, et al. Frequency and natural history of rhinovirus infections in adults during autumn. J Clin Microbiol 1997; 35: 2864–8

54. Monto AS. Epidemiology of viral respiratory infections. Am J Med 2002; 112: 4S–12S

55. Longini IM, Monto AS, Koopman JS. Statistical procedures for estimating the community probability of illness in family studies: rhinovirus and influenza. Int J Epidemiol 1984; 13: 99–106

56. Monto AS, Napier JA, Metzner HL. The Tecumseh study of respiratory illness. 1. Plan of study and observations on syndromes of acute respiratory disease. Am J Epidemiol 1971; 94: 269–79

57. Griffin MR, Coffey CS, Neuzil KM, et al. Winter viruses: influenza and respiratory syncytial virus-related morbidity in chronic lung disease. Arch Intern Med 2002; 162: 1229–36

58. Monto AS. Occurrence of respiratory virus: time, place and person. Pediatr Infect Dis J 2004; 23 (Suppl): S58–S64

59. Hendley JO, Gwaltney JM, Jordan WS. Rhinovirus infections in an industrial population. lV. Infections within families of employees during two fall peaks of respiratory illness. Am J Epidemiol 1969: 89; 184–96

60. Witt K, Knudsen E, Ditlevsen S, Hollnagel H. Academic detailing has no effect on prescribing of asthma medication in Danish general practice: a three year randomized controlled trial with 12-monthly follow-ups. Fam Pract 2004; 21: 253

61. Sandberg S, Paton JY, Ahola S. The role of acute and chronic stress in asthma attacks in children. Lancet 2000; 356: 982–7

62. Almqvist C, Wickman M, Perfetti L, et al. Worsening of asthma in children allergic to cats after indirect exposure to cat at school. Am J Respir Crit Care Med 2001; 163: 694–8

CHAPTER 5

Etiology of asthma exacerbations in children: differences from adults

James E Gern

INTRODUCTION

Asthma is difficult to define in childhood, owing to the existence of several different clinical phenotypes, as well as the shifting prevalence of these phenotypes from infancy to the school-age years and beyond. In addition to having unique clinical features, it is likely that each of these forms of childhood asthma has some distinct pathophysiological features. As a result, the types of stimuli and environmental exposures that initiate acute symptoms of wheezing and bronchospasm also vary with the age of the patient and the specific phenotype of asthma.

Most childhood asthma begins in the formative years of early childhood, which is a time of rapid development for the lungs and the immune system. During this period, environmental factors such as viral infections, pollution and allergen exposure not only influence the day-to-day occurrence of symptoms, but also have the capacity to influence the onset, course and chronicity of the disease. In this chapter, the various forms of childhood asthma are discussed, with an emphasis on the development-specific effects of viral infections, allergens and pollutants on the activity and exacerbations of asthma.

DEVELOPMENTAL CONSIDERATIONS

Children differ from adults not only in size, but also with respect to the maturity of the pulmonary and immune systems. Development in these areas occurs continuously throughout childhood, and changes are particularly marked during the first 3 years of life. Children of this age also have the highest rate of hospitalization for acute respiratory illnesses, including those associated with wheezing.[1] In fact, many children with asthma airway obstruction develop this condition before 6–7 years of age, suggesting that young children may be particularly susceptible to adverse environmental exposures during this period.[2]

Development of the lung

The process of lung development involves extensive interactions between epithelial and mesenchymal tissue beginning by the 4th week of gestation, and continues for years after birth.[3] Prenatal lung development begins with the appearance of lung buds (embryonic stage) followed by branching of the airways and blood vessels, and extension of the blood supply to the peripheral mesenchyme (canalicular stage). Differentiation of the respiratory airways and differentiation of future respiratory gas exchange (acinar) units occurs mainly in the third trimester. The final stage in differentiation is alveolar multiplication (alveolarization), which begins at term and continues for 2–3 years postnatally. This process consists of thinning of the alveolar walls and concomitant expansion of the capillary network. These two processes are mutually dependent: interference with angiogenesis will inhibit both pulmonary artery density and alveolar growth. The subdivision of the capillary walls involves co-ordinated cellular activity, including proliferation of interstitial fibroblasts, septation of existing alveoli and flattening and reduction in the numbers of alveolar epithelial cells. Following the differentiation of alveoli, the lung grows throughout childhood and this is accompanied by continuous remodeling of lung parenchyma and airways.[4] Many of the factors that regulate differentiation of alveoli and growth of airways are either induced or inhibited by acute respiratory infections.[5] This raises the possibility that viral lower respiratory infection (LRI) in early childhood could, in addition to causing acute exacerbations of asthma, also cause long-term alterations in lung architecture and physiological responses to promote asthma. Studies in animal models of virus infection[6,7] as well as long-term prospective studies of important pathogens such as respiratory syncytial virus (RSV)[8,9] are supportive of this concept, although definitive proof of causality is lacking.

Relationship of immune development to wheezing and asthma

At the time of birth, the immune system is functionally immature, and major changes in immune development occur during childhood. There has been extensive analysis of immune responses of mononuclear cells obtained at the time of birth, and these have revealed deficiencies in cytokine production, innate immunity, cellular responses and the establishment of adaptive immunity to a wide variety of pathogens (reviewed in reference 10). These deficiencies are associated with a corresponding increase in the susceptibility to a wide variety of pathogens, including bacteria, fungi and viruses. Together with the high degree of exposure of children to infected individuals at home, school and day care, this contributes to the greater number and severity of viral respiratory infections during childhood.

There are a number of mechanisms underlying the greater susceptibility to viral respiratory infections in early childhood (Table 5.1).[10–13]

Interferon (IFN) responses to mitogens and viruses are low at the time of birth, and progressively increase in the first few years. In fact, it has been demonstrated that reduced IFN-γ responses at the time of birth are associated with a greater number of symptomatic respiratory illnesses in early infancy, and this effect is especially pronounced in children who attend day care and have older siblings.[14] In addition, several studies have found evidence that specific patterns of cytokine responses at birth, including reduced phytohemagglutinin (PHA)-induced interleukin (IL)-13,[15,16] or reduced IFN-γ in response to RSV or mitogen,[16] are associated with an increased risk of subsequent wheezing. These findings suggest that wheezing may be related to overall immune maturation rather than a specific deficiency in T helper (Th)1 cytokine production.

A number of cytokine and cellular responses are impaired or delayed in early childhood and, as a result of these factors, children are more susceptible to a wide variety of bacterial and viral pathogens. In addition to having more illnesses, young children are also at greater risk of developing severe or complicated infections. For example, the severity of virus-induced respiratory symptoms is increased in early childhood in response to infection with RSV, parainfluenza, influenza and rhinoviruses. This is likely to be due to a greater propensity for these infections to involve the lower airway followed by impaired clearance of infection, along with a greater likelihood of obstruction due to anatomically smaller airways. Interestingly, the duration of susceptibility varies with the specific pathogen. The period of risk for systemic enteroviral infections extends for only a few weeks after birth,[17] while the risk for herpes simplex encephalitis is increased at least until the age of 6 years.[18]

Finally, associations between infantile wheezing and a number of genetic polymorphisms suggest additional immunological mechanisms for

Table 5.1 Deficiencies in early childhood that affect antiviral immunity[10–13]

Immune response/effector	Antiviral effects	Alteration in early childhood
Innate immunity		
Response to PAMP	Viral RNA binding to TLR-3 and TLR-7 activates innate antiviral responses	↓Type I IFN response to dsRNA
NK cells	Can lyse or induce apoptosis of virus-infected cells	↓Cytotoxicity
Neutrophils	Primary airway response to infection, antiviral effects could be mediated by reactive oxygen metabolites	↓Granulocyte storage pool
Monocytes/macrophages	Phagocytosis, production of antiviral cytokines	↓Monocyte chemotaxis
Antigen presentation	Processing of viral antigens and presentation to T cells	↓Recruitment of dendritic cells, ↓ability to activate T cells
T helper responses	Recognition of viral antigens	Delayed responses after antigen challenge, ↓help for B cell differentiation
Cytotoxic responses	Specific T cells lyse or induce apoptosis of infected cells	↓Cytotoxicity
Cytokine production	Interferons activate antiviral pathways and prime cytotoxic responses of T and NK cells	↓Production of IFN-γ, TNF-α, selected chemoattractants
Specific antibody	Prevents reinfection	↓IgA responses ↓Antibody responses to specific pathogens (e.g. measles, RSV)

dsRNA, double-stranded RNA; PAMP, pathogen-associated molecular patterns; TLR, Toll-like receptor; IFN, interferon; NK, natural killer; TNF, tumor necrosis factor; RSV, respiratory syncytial virus

this disorder. These polymorphisms include genes for chemoattractants, Th2 cytokines and receptors and other immunoregulatory genes (Table 5.2).[19–28] The precise effects of these polymorphisms on the development of antiviral responses in childhood is not well understood.

WHEEZING PHENOTYPES IN CHILDHOOD

Asthma is a syndrome rather than a single disease, and several distinct asthma phenotypes have been described in childhood. It is difficult to confidently diagnose asthma in infancy, in the sense that predicting who will and will not continue to wheeze later in childhood is an inexact

science. It is debated whether infants who wheeze primarily with respiratory infections, the so-called transient wheezers,[29] constitute a subtype of asthma. Nevertheless, this is a common syndrome that shares many features with other forms of childhood asthma, including episodic small airway obstruction, plugging of the airways with shed epithelial cells and excess mucus, and recurrent airway obstruction and wheezing. In addition, as has been demonstrated for asthma, rates of hospitalization of infants for acute virus-induced wheezing and bronchiolitis increased substantially during the period 1980–96.[30] Although virus-induced wheezing is common in infants, it is especially important in this age group to consider other causes for recurrent wheezing due to factors unrelated to the small

Table 5.2 Genetic linkages to respiratory syncytial virus-induced morbidity in infancy

Gene	Function	Associated outcome	Reference
CCR5	Receptor for chemokines (RANTES)	More severe hospitalized patients	19
IFN-γ	Antiviral responses	Severity of LRI in hospitalized infants	20
IL-4	Th2 differentiation, promotes IgE synthesis	Hospitalization	21, 22
IL-4RA	IL-4 and IL-13 receptor subunit	Hospitalization	22
IL-8	Neutrophil chemoattractant	Hospitalization	23
IL-10	Anti-inflammatory cytokines	Hospitalization	24
Surfactant protein A	Airway surfactant	Severe infection	25
Surfactant protein D	Airway surfactant	Hospitalization	26
TGFB1	Fibrosis, anti-inflammatory effects	Outpatient wheezing	27
TLR-4	Innate response to LPS	Hospitalization	28

RANTES, regulation upon activation normal T cell expressed and secreted; LPS, lipopolysaccharide; LRI, lower respiratory-tract infection

airways, such as cardiac disease, anatomic abnormalities of the large airways and immunodeficiency. In the absence of these other conditions, recurrent episodic wheezing in infancy is almost always caused by acute viral infections, and recognition of this relationship in the natural history of childhood asthma has led to speculation that viral infections may play a causative role.

Some school-aged children continue to wheeze with viruses, and very little else, and this condition has been described as wheezy bronchitis or intermittent virus-induced asthma. This condition often seems to remit in adolescence, although there may be a small subset of adults with a similar affliction. Typical atopic asthma in childhood often begins with virus-induced wheezing in infancy, but can also start later on in childhood in association with allergic sensitization. Infants with recurrent wheezing and other atopic features, such as food allergy or atopic dermatitis, or a first-degree family history of asthma, are at greatest risk of going on to develop atopic asthma.[31] Affected children can have daily symptoms, and these can be intensified by seasonal or perennial exposure to allergens. In addition to these well-recognized phenotypes, it has recently been reported that girls who experience early onset of puberty, especially in association with

excess weight during this stage of development, are at greater risk of developing asthma.[32,33] The time sequence of these events strongly suggests that sex hormones are important influences on lung physiology during puberty.

Although there is overlap in the clinical expression of wheezing and respiratory distress, these subtypes of asthma have unique risk factors and natural history, providing strong evidence that the pathophysiology of each disorder is distinct. One important distinguishing factor is age and, as illustrated above, each period of childhood is associated with a different mixture and prevalence of wheezing disorders. Although changes in lung physiology, immunological development, allergic sensitization and asthma phenotypes are in fact incremental and continuous, it is useful to think of childhood wheezing disorders in two main age groups: infancy, and children from school-age until adolescence.

CAUSES OF WHEEZING IN INFANCY

The specific pathogens that most often cause infantile wheezing are RSV, rhinoviruses (RVs), parainfluenza viruses (PIVs), metapneumovirus and influenza viruses.[34,35] RSV is the major cause of bronchiolitis during the winter months, and this pathogen accounts for about 70% of these episodes.[36] Bronchiolitis, however, represents only the most severe fraction of infections, since nearly all children are infected with this virus by age 2 years. Children aged 3–6 months are most prone to develop lower respiratory tract symptoms, suggesting that a developmental component (e.g. lung and/or immunological maturation) is an important co-factor in determining the severity of illness. Other pathogens associated with bronchiolitis are the metapneumoviruses, which cause approximately 10–15% of the non-RSV wheezing illnesses during the bronchiolitis season.[37] These viruses have a natural history that is similar to that of RSV: serological studies have shown that nearly all children are infected during the preschool years. Influenza viruses are the other major winter pathogen, and the severity of illness is strongly dependent on the prevalent serotype. Infants, along with the elderly, are clearly at greater risk of developing more severe illnesses, including LRI with wheezing. PIV infections, which are not confined to a single season, account for a significant percentage of wheezing illnesses in infants throughout the year. *Mycoplasma*, *Chlamydia* and other bacterial infections are relatively infrequent causes of recurrent wheezing, although there may be a small subset of infants who do wheeze with these pathogens.

RVs, originally identified as the most common cause of upper respiratory infection and common cold symptoms, are now recognized as an important cause of wheezing and lower respiratory symptoms in infants and children. The development of sensitive assays based on the reverse-transcription polymerase chain reaction (RT-PCR) has demonstrated that these viruses cause the majority of wheezing episodes outside of the RSV season.[34,35,38] Although the growth of most RVs is impaired at temperatures found in the alveoli (i.e. 37°C), temperatures in large and medium-sized airways are ideal for the growth of RVs, and lower airway infection has been verified after experimental inoculation of adult

volunteers.[39–41] In addition, in a small study of infants and young children with tracheostomies, RVs were more often detected in secretions from the trachea than from the nasal cavity.[42] Unlike RSV, PIVs and influenza viruses, RV pneumonia generally occurs only in immunocompromised individuals.

Non-immunological risk factors for virus-induced wheezing in infancy

Premorbid measurements of lung function indicate that children with reduced levels of lung function in infancy are at increased risk of chronic lower respiratory tract sequelae following viral infections.[29] Airway hyperresponsiveness[43] measured in early infancy is also a risk factor for asthma later on in childhood. Additional factors that predispose an infant or child to LRI and wheezing in infancy include gender, exposure to large numbers of other children at home or day care, and passive smoke exposure.

Short- and long-term effects of viral infections on lung development and asthma

Infections with respiratory viruses acutely impair lung function by directly damaging lower airway tissues, and by provoking an acute immune response with both antiviral and proinflammatory components. The epithelial cell is of primary importance during viral respiratory infections, because it serves as the host cell for viral replication, and also initiates innate and adaptive immune responses. Damage to the epithelium such as edema and shedding of dead cells, together with mucus production, can cause airway obstruction and wheezing. Virus-induced epithelial damage can also increase the permeability of the mucosal layer,[44,45] perhaps facilitating allergen contact with immune cells, and exposing neural elements to promote neurogenic inflammation. In contrast to more destructive viruses, RVs infect relatively few cells in the airway, and proinflammatory responses may be the primary mechanism for airway symptoms and lower airway dysfunction.[46] Viral infections can induce the synthesis of many of the factors that regulate airway and alveolar development and remodeling, including neutrophilic inflammation, vascular endothelial growth factor (VEGF),[47] nitric oxide (NO),[48] transforming growth factor (TGF)-β[49] and fibroblast growth factor (FGF).[50] How single or repeated bouts of virus-induced overexpression of these regulators of lung development and remodeling affect the ultimate lung structure and function is not known, but this is of interest regarding the long-term effects on the risk of asthma.

The possibility that these acute inflammatory responses, together with efforts to repair virus-induced damage to lung tissue, could have long-term consequences on lung function has been evaluated in animal models. For example, PIV infections in 3–4-week-old weanling rats can induce the development of a chronic asthma phenotype characterized by episodic, reversible airway obstruction.[7,49] To induce this response, the infection must occur in a genetically susceptible strain (the Th2-skewed Brown Norway (BN) rat as opposed to the resistant Th1-skewed F344 strain) at a critical time point in the development of the animal.[7,49] Interestingly, weanling BN rats have deficiencies in natural killer cell numbers and in their capacity to produce IFN-γ as part of the innate immune response to viral infection,[51,52] and the selective administration of IFN-γ to these animals during the acute infection inhibits the development of the chronic airway dysfunction.[53] These findings strongly support the concept that viral infections that occur in a genetically susceptible host at a critical developmental time period could promote the inception of asthma.

WHEEZING IN OLDER CHILDREN

Although infections continue to be the single most important factor related to acute exacerbations of asthma in older children, other environmental exposures assume a progressively increasing influence after 2 years of age. This trend was demonstrated in a 1-year study of hospitalizations due to asthma in Charlottesville, VA.[35] In this study, viruses were detected from nasal secretions of nearly all children less than 2 years of age. With increasing age, the percentage of children with detectable viruses gradually declined from 96% at 0–6 months of age to 50% of children aged 10–18 years. The reason for the shift in causation for acute asthma is two-fold. First, antiviral defenses are progressively strengthened during this time frame, and this is likely to be a result of maturation of innate and adaptive immune responses as well as continued growth and development of the respiratory system and the lungs. Concurrent with a lessening vulnerability to viruses is the development of respiratory allergies, which can start in the first few years of life and are associated with an increased risk of asthma.[54] Finally, other stimuli associated with bronchospasm and acute airway obstruction include bacterial sinusitis, indoor and outdoor pollutants, exercise and microbial products. The influence of these environmental factors on acute wheezing in children will be reviewed in the following sections.

Infections

The relationship between viral infections and wheezing illnesses in older children and adults has been clarified by the advent of sensitive diagnostic tests, based on the PCR, for picornaviruses such as RVs. With the advent of these more sensitive diagnostic tools, information linking common cold infections with exacerbations of asthma has come from a number of sources. Prospective studies of children with asthma have demonstrated that up to 85% of exacerbations of asthma are associated with a viral respiratory infection, compared to 40–70% of exacerbations in adults.[55,56] Although many respiratory viruses can provoke acute asthma symptoms, RVs are most often detected, especially during the spring and fall RV seasons. In fact, the spring and fall peaks in hospitalizations due to asthma closely coincide with patterns of RV isolation within the community.[57,58] Influenza and RSV are somewhat more likely to trigger acute asthma symptoms in the wintertime, but appear to account for a smaller fraction of asthma flares. RV infections are also detected in the majority of children over the age of 2 years who present to emergency departments with acute wheezing.[59,60] Together, these studies provide evidence of a strong relationship between viral infections in childhood, particularly those due to RV, and acute exacerbations of asthma.

Sinusitis and asthma

Children are at increased risk for sinus infections. Part of this risk is related to a diminished capacity to make protective antibody responses to bacteria, such as *Streptococcus pneumoniae* and *Haemophilus influenzae*, with polysaccharide coats.[10] In addition, children contract more viral upper respiratory infections, which can involve the sinuses and are also important predisposing factors to secondary bacterial infections. Finally, the anatomy of the sinuses is hampered by small outflow tracts that, when occluded, promote bacterial overgrowth in the sinuses. During childhood, the narrow diameter of these outflow tracts is accentuated.

The role of bacterial sinus infections in causing exacerbations of asthma is difficult to estimate, due to the difficulty in accurately diagnosing sinusitis in children. Moreover, common cold viruses associated with asthma exacerbations commonly involve the sinuses.[61] Acute bacterial sinusitis should be considered in children with asthma symptoms that are refractory to treatment, and especially when there has been concurrent cough and rhinitis for extended periods of time.[62] Several uncontrolled studies have demonstrated that sinus radiographs are often abnormal under these circumstances, and that treatment with antibiotics directed at likely

pathogens is often associated with clinical improvement.[63–65]

Allergens

Allergic sensitization and childhood asthma are closely linked, and it is estimated that 70–90% of children with asthma have associated allergies. The allergies most often related to asthma are dust mite, cat, *Alternaria* and, in inner-city settings, cockroach.[66] Sensitization and exposure are independent and synergistic risk factors for developing daily symptoms and exacerbations of asthma in childhood. In the Midwestern United States, it has been reported that children with *Alternaria* allergy are at greater risk for severe bronchospasm and near-fatal bouts of asthma.[67] Whether this association is due to high seasonal exposure to *Alternaria* spores or some other mechanism is unclear.

Cockroach allergy is especially common in inner-city environments, and a large multicenter co-operative study evaluated its role in acute symptoms of asthma. Children with high levels of cockroach allergen exposure and those with cockroach sensitization were frequent occurrences, but either factor alone was generally not associated with increased morbidity. Children with both sensitization and exposure to cockroach, however, were at increased risk for asthma symptoms, as well as acute care visits and hospitalizations.[68]

A different story appears to be unfolding for children exposed to cats in the home and at school. Exposure in the home or at school to small to moderate amounts of cat allergen can cause sensitization. In contrast, there is mounting evidence that exposure to larger amounts of cat allergen reduces the risk of sensitization to cat proteins and perhaps asthma.[69] While a high level of cat proteins appears to protect specifically against sensitization to cat, exposure to dogs, farm animals and endotoxin in childhood may also protect against allergies in general as well as asthma.[70] Despite the reduction in risk, children who do develop allergies to pets should avoid these animals in an effort to reduce respiratory symptoms. In fact, exposure to even low levels of cat allergens in Swedish schools has been associated with measurable increases in asthma symptoms in sensitized children.[71]

IgE-mediated food allergy is also more common in children, particularly those under the age of 3 years. Ingestion of a food allergen usually causes a constellation of symptoms, and the organ systems most commonly affected include the skin, gastrointestinal tract and respiratory tract. Although it is uncommon for a food allergen to cause adverse reactions that are limited to the respiratory tract, this does occur in a small percentage of children.[72] Consequently, food allergy should be considered when evaluating young children with frequent exacerbations or uncontrolled daily symptoms.

Pollution

There is solid evidence that a number of pollutants contribute to exacerbations of asthma, and reason to suspect that children may be especially susceptible to adverse effects of pollution. The reason for increased susceptibility may be multifactorial. First, exposures may be more intensive in children, who tend to spend more time outdoors participating in physical activity.[73] In addition, the barrier function of the airway epithelium may be suboptimal in the developing lung, and this can lead to greater penetration of pollutants into subepithelial layers.[74] There is also biochemical evidence that childhood asthma is associated with epithelial injury and stress,[75] and together with greater airway responsiveness in childhood, this could result in a reduced tolerance to environmental insults such as pollutants.

There is some evidence that certain indoor and outdoor air pollutants can cause childhood asthma. The strongest evidence is regarding environmental tobacco smoke, especially related to *in utero* exposure.[76] In addition, diesel exhaust

particles have been conclusively demonstrated to act as an adjuvant for allergic sensitization. Exposure to three other pollutants – ozone, NO_2 and particulates – has been linked to the development of asthma in some studies.[73,77]

There is conclusive evidence that acute exposure to various pollutants causes symptoms and exacerbations of asthma in children.[73,77] In model systems, pollutants such as diesel exhaust and environmental tobacco smoke can enhance allergen-induced IgE synthesis, and this may be especially important during the acquisition of new allergies during childhood. Furthermore, several forms of pollutant (e.g. tobacco smoke, NO_2) are oxidants that are capable of activating proinflammatory immune responses. In turn, there are a number of intracellular pathways that compensate for oxidant stress. A key antioxidant pathway involves the enzyme glutathione-*S*-transferase M1 (GSTM1), and there is evidence that polymorphisms of this gene can modify the pulmonary response to oxidant stress in children.[77] For example, Mexican children with a GSTM1-null genetic mutation have a greater risk for bronchoconstriction when exposed to high levels of ozone in the environment.[78] The likely explanation is that children with a reduced capacity to handle the oxidant stress are more susceptible to effects of air pollution on asthma. These findings raise the possibility that antioxidant vitamins and dietary supplements might have beneficial effects relative to lung health, and there is some evidence to support this concept. For example, supplementation with vitamins C and E prevented drops in lung function in asthmatic children exposed to high levels of ozone in Mexico City.[79] Although these results are promising, more information is needed before antioxidants can be routinely recommended for prophylaxis. Minimizing sources of pollution would help to promote lung health in childhood on a societal basis. These measures could include avoiding exposure to tobacco smoke, living away from major highways, exercising in the morning to minimize ozone exposure and societal changes to ameliorate traffic and promote the use of clean-burning fuels.[77]

Other factors

Other factors that can cause acute exacerbations of asthma in children include exercise, microbial products such as lipopolysaccharide, stress and gastroesophageal reflux. The mechanisms and effects of exercise-induced bronchospasm on asthma are likely to be similar to those in adults. An added consideration in children is that exercise, which is accompanied by deep breathing and mechanical stretching of the lung, may be an essential component in the development of healthy pulmonary physiology. Exercise is also an essential part of a healthy lifestyle to prevent obesity. In fact, it has been proposed that lack of exercise may be an important factor in the recent increase in the prevalence and severity of asthma in children, and especially children who live in inner-city environments.[80,81] With this in mind, it is essential in designing asthma treatment plans in childhood to include measures to prevent exercise-induced bronchospasm, and to actively encourage regular participation in vigorous physical activity.

It is clinically evident that stress can initiate acute asthma symptoms in children, although the mechanisms for this effect are still incompletely understood. Stress in early childhood can affect the development of the immune system, and these effects could increase the risk of developing allergy and asthma.[82] In addition to direct effects on airway physiology, a stressful environment could also reduce adherence to treatment plans. Stress can also play a role in precipitating spasm of the vocal cords, a condition that can mimic asthma, or coincide with asthma to intensify the severity of acute exacerbations.[83] Predisposing factors for vocal cord dysfunction in children include gastrointestinal reflux and allergic rhinitis, and treatment of these conditions can lead to a reduction in both vocal cord spasm and exacerbations of asthma.[84]

INTERACTIONS BETWEEN ENVIRONMENTAL FACTORS

There is great interest in determining whether there are interactive effects between environmental triggers of asthma and the unique circumstances in childhood to increase the likelihood of acute airway obstruction and respiratory symptoms (Figure 5.1). Of the various combinations of exposure, interactions between viral infections and allergy have been studied in the greatest detail. For example, in a study of children who presented to an emergency department,[60,85] detection of a respiratory virus (most commonly RV), allergen-specific IgE and eosinophilia of nasal secretions were all found to be individual risk factors for acute wheezing. Notably, viral infections and allergy (positive radioallergosorbent tests (RAST)) or allergic inflammation (eosinophilia) synergistically increased the risk of wheezing.[60] Accordingly, the risk of hospitalization among virus-infected adults is increased in patients who are both sensitized and exposed to respiratory allergens,[86] and studies of children indicate that this relationship may be even more pronounced.[87] When considered together, these findings provide strong evidence that individuals with either respiratory allergies or eosinophilic airway inflammation have an increased risk for wheezing with viral infections. Experimental models to evaluate potential mechanisms have had some conflicting results. For example, experimental inoculation with RV enhances inflammatory responses to segmental allergen challenge and the likelihood of a late phase pulmonary response after whole lung allergen challenge.[88,89] However, exposure to respiratory allergens did not enhance either the inflammatory response or the symptom severity of an experimentally induced cold.[90,91] Although additional studies are required to solve this puzzle, these findings suggest that there may be additional co-factors, related to either the host or the environment, that help to drive the synergy between colds and allergic responses.

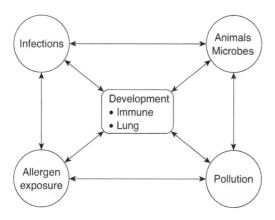

Figure 5.1 Interactions between environmental factors and development to induce exacerbations of asthma (see text)

These findings suggest that pollution, and potentially other factors, might also augment the effects of colds on childhood asthma.[92] In a 1-year study of children and adults in British Columbia, Tarlo and colleagues found that asthma exacerbations with colds were more likely to occur on days with higher levels of the outdoor pollutants sulfur dioxide and nitric oxide compared to colds without asthma exacerbations.[93] In addition, Chauhan and colleagues found evidence that school-aged children with greater personal exposure to nitrogen dioxide in the week before a viral respiratory infection had greater lower respiratory symptoms during the infection.[94] A potential mechanism of the association between pollutants and colds has been suggested by Lopez-Souza and colleagues.[95] This group of investigators evaluated the replication of rhinoviruses in well-differentiated epithelial cells in tissue culture, and found low levels of viral replication under these conditions. Replication was enhanced in poorly differentiated cell layers, and especially in those that had not yet formed tight junctions. These findings suggest that pollutants that disrupt the integrity of the epithelium could lead to greater viral replication and severity of illness and, in affected individuals, exacerbations of asthma. Additional studies will be required to test this hypothesis, and to determine whether children are more susceptible to this noxious combination.

SUMMARY AND CONCLUSIONS

Childhood is defined by developmental changes in all organ systems, and the continuous evolution of the immune and pulmonary systems is central to understanding childhood asthma and wheezing. As a result of this unique physiology, very young children and those with asthma are disproportionately affected by viral infections, allergies and pollution. Together with the effects on acute airway obstruction and respiratory symptoms, these stimuli can also have long-term effects that increase the risk of recurrent wheezing and chronic asthma. Collectively, these observations underscore the importance of gaining a better understanding of the pathogenesis of childhood asthma. In particular, the identification of critical developmental windows of susceptibility to viruses, sensitization to allergens and ill effects of pollutants would help guide efforts to treat and potentially prevent acute wheezing episodes and asthma.

ACKNOWLEDGMENTS

JEG is supported by NIH grants R01HL61879-01, P01HL70831-01 and N01-AI-25496.

REFERENCES

1. Measuring childhood asthma prevalence before and after the 1997 redesign of the National Health Interview Survey – United States. Morbid Mortal Weekly Rep 2000; 49: 908–11
2. Taussig LM, Wright AL, Holberg CJ, et al. Tucson children's respiratory study: 1980 to present. J Allergy Clin Immunol 2003; 111: 661–75
3. American Thoracic Society ad hoc Statement Committee. Mechanisms and limits of induced postnatal lung growth. Am J Respir Crit Care Med 2004; 170: 319–43

4. Xuan W, Peat JK, Toelle BG, et al. Lung function growth and its relation to airway hyperresponsiveness and recent wheeze. Results from a longitudinal population study. Am J Respir Crit Care Med 2000; 161: 1820–4

5. Gern JE, Rosenthal LA, Sorkness RL, Lemanske RF Jr. Effects of viral respiratory infections on lung development and childhood asthma. J Allergy Clin Immunol 2005; 115: 668–74

6. Castleman WL, Sorkness RL, Lemanske RF Jr, et al. Neonatal viral bronchiolitis and pneumonia induce bronchiolar hypoplasia and alveolar dysplasia in rats. Lab Invest 1988; 59: 387–96

7. Kumar A, Sorkness RL, Kaplan MR, Lemanske RF Jr. Chronic, episodic, reversible airway obstruction after viral bronchiolitis in rats. Am J Respir Crit Care Med 1997; 155: 130–4

8. Sigurs N, Bjarnason R, Sigurbergsson F, Kjellman B. Respiratory syncytial virus bronchiolitis in infancy is an important risk factor for asthma and allergy at age 7. Am J Respir Crit Care Med 2000; 161: 1501–7

9. Stein RT, Sherrill D, Morgan WJ, et al. Respiratory syncytial virus in early life and risk of wheeze and allergy by age 13 years. Lancet 1999; 354: 541–5

10. Lewis DB, Tu W. The physiologic immunodeficiency of immaturity. In Stiehm ER, Ochs HD, Winkelstein JA, eds. Immunologic Disorders in Infants and Children. Philadelphia: Elsevier, 2004: 687–760

11. Gans H, DeHovitz R, Forghani B, et al. Measles and mumps vaccination as a model to investigate the developing immune system: passive and active immunity during the first year of life. Vaccine 2003; 21: 3398–405

12. Prescott SL. Early origins of allergic disease: a review of processes and influences during early immune development. Curr Opin Allergy Clin Immunol 2003; 3: 125–32

13. West LJ. Defining critical windows in the development of the human immune system. Hum Exp Toxicol 2002; 21: 499–505

14. Copenhaver CC, Gern JE, Li Z, et al. Cytokine response patterns, exposure to viruses, and respiratory infections in the first year of life. Am J Respir Crit Care Med 2004; 170: 175–80

15. Williams TJ, Jones CA, Miles EA, et al. Fetal and neonatal IL-13 production during pregnancy and at birth and subsequent development of atopic symptoms. J Allergy Clin Immunol 2000; 105: 951–9

16. Gern JE, Brooks GD, Meyer P, et al. Bidirectional interactions between viral respiratory illness and cytokine responses in the first year of life. J Allergy Clin Immunol 2006; 117: 72–8

17. Abzug MJ. Presentation, diagnosis, and management of enterovirus infections in neonates. Paediatr Drugs 2004; 6: 1–10

18. Ito Y, Ando Y, Kimura H, et al. Polymerase chain reaction-proved herpes simplex encephalitis in children. Pediatr Infect Dis J 1998; 17: 29–32

19. Hull J, Rowlands K, Lockhart E, et al. Variants of the chemokine receptor CCR5 are associated with severe bronchiolitis caused by respiratory syncytial virus. J Infect Dis 2003; 188: 904–7

20. Gentile DA, Doyle WJ, Zeevi A, et al. Cytokine gene polymorphisms moderate illness severity in infants with respiratory syncytial virus infection. Hum Immunol 2003; 64: 338–44

21. Choi EH, Lee HJ, Yoo T, Chanock SJ. A common haplotype of interleukin-4 gene IL4 is associated with severe respiratory syncytial virus disease in Korean children. J Infect Dis 2002; 186: 1207–11

22. Hoebee B, Rietveld E, Bont L, et al. Association of severe respiratory syncytial virus bronchiolitis with interleukin-4 and interleukin-4 receptor alpha polymorphisms. J Infect Dis 2003; 187: 2–11

23. Hull J, Thomson A, Kwiatkowski D. Association of respiratory syncytial virus bronchiolitis with the interleukin 8 gene region in UK families. Thorax 2000; 55: 1023–7

24. Hoebee B, Bont L, Rietveld E, et al. Influence of promoter variants of interleukin-10, interleukin-9, and tumor necrosis factor-alpha genes on respiratory syncytial virus bronchiolitis. J Infect Dis 2004; 189: 239–47

25. Lofgren J, Ramet M, Renko M, et al. Association between surfactant protein A gene locus and severe respiratory syncytial virus infection in infants. J Infect Dis 2002; 185: 283–9

26. Lahti M, Lofgren J, Marttila R, et al. Surfactant protein D gene polymorphism associated with severe respiratory syncytial virus infection. Pediatr Res 2002; 51: 696–9

27. Hoffjan S, Ostrovnaja I, Nicolae D, et al. Genetic variation in immunoregulatory pathways and atopic phenotypes in infancy. J Allergy Clin Immunol 2003; 113: 511–18

28. Tal G, Mandelberg A, Dalal I, et al. Association between common Toll-like receptor 4 mutations and severe respiratory syncytial virus disease. J Infect Dis 2004; 189: 2057–63

29. Martinez FD, Wright AL, Taussig LM, et al. Asthma and wheezing in the first six years of life. N Engl J Med 1995; 332: 133–8

30. Shay DK, Holman RC, Newman RD, et al. Bronchiolitis-associated hospitalizations among US children, 1980–1996. J Am Med Assoc 1999; 282: 1440–6

31. Castro-Rodriguez JA, Holberg CJ, Wright AL, Martinez FD. A clinical index to define risk of asthma in young children with recurrent wheezing. Am J Respir Crit Care Med 2000; 162: 1403–6

32. Hancox RJ, Milne BJ, Poulton R, et al. Sex differences in the relation between body mass index and asthma and atopy in a birth cohort. Am J Respir Crit Care Med 2005; 171: 440–5

33. Guerra S, Wright AL, Morgan WJ, et al. Persistence of asthma symptoms during adolescence: role of obesity

and age at the onset of puberty. Am J Respir Crit Care Med 2004; 170: 78–85

34. Jartti T, Lehtinen P, Vuorinen T, et al. Respiratory picornaviruses and respiratory syncytial virus as causative agents of acute expiratory wheezing in children. Emerg Infect Dis 2004; 10: 1095–101

35. Heymann PW, Carper HT, Murphy DD, et al. Viral infections in relation to age, atopy, and season of admission among children hospitalized for wheezing. J Allergy Clin Immunol 2004; 114: 239–47

36. Wennergren G, Kristjansson S. Relationship between respiratory syncytial virus bronchiolitis and future obstructive airway diseases. Eur Respir J 2001; 18: 1044–58

37. van den Hoogen BG, de Jong JC, Groen J, et al. A newly discovered human pneumovirus isolated from young children with respiratory tract disease. Nat Med 2001; 7: 719–24

38. Lemanske RF Jr, Jackson DJ, Gangnon RE, et al. Rhinovirus illnesses during infancy predict subsequent childhood wheezing. J Allergy Clin Immunol 2005; 116: 571–7

39. Gern JE, Galagan DM, Jarjour NN, et al. Detection of rhinovirus RNA in lower airway cells during experimentally-induced infection. Am J Respir Crit Care Med 1997; 155: 1159–61

40. Papadopoulos NG, Bates PJ, Bardin PG, et al. Rhinoviruses infect the lower airways. J Infect Dis 2000; 181: 1875–84

41. Mosser AG, Vrtis R, Burchell L, et al. Quantitative and qualitative analysis of rhinovirus infection in bronchial tissues. Am J Respir Crit Care Med 2005; 171: 645–51

42. Simons E, Schroth MK, Gern JE. Analysis of tracheal secretions for rhinovirus during natural colds. Pediatr Allergy Immunol 2005; 16: 276–8

43. Palmer LJ, Rye PJ, Gibson NA, et al. Airway responsiveness in early infancy predicts asthma, lung function, and respiratory symptoms by school age. Am J Respir Crit Care Med 2001; 163: 37–42

44. Igarashi Y, Skoner DP, Doyle WJ, et al. Analysis of nasal secretions during experimental rhinovirus upper respiratory infections. J Allergy Clin Immunol 1993; 92: 722–31

45. Ohrui T, Yamaya M, Sekizawa K, et al. Effects of rhinovirus infection on hydrogen peroxide-induced alterations of barrier function in the cultured human tracheal epithelium. Am J Respir Crit Care Med 1998; 158: 241–8

46. Hendley JO. The host response, not the virus, causes the symptoms of the common cold. Clin Infect Dis 1998; 26: 847–8

47. Lee CG, Yoon HJ, Zhu Z, et al. Respiratory syncytial virus stimulation of vascular endothelial cell growth factor/vascular permeability factor. Am J Respir Cell Mol Biol 2000; 23: 662–9

48. Sanders SP. Asthma, viruses, and nitric oxide. Proc Soc Exp Biol Med 1999; 220: 123–32

49. Uhl EW, Castleman WL, Sorkness RL, et al. Parainfluenza virus-induced persistence of airway inflammation, fibrosis, and dysfunction associated with TGF-β_1 expression in Brown Norway rats. Am J Respir Crit Care Med 1996; 154: 1834–42

50. Dosanjh A, Rednam S, Martin M. Respiratory syncytial virus augments production of fibroblast growth factor basic in vitro: implications for a possible mechanism of prolonged wheezing after infection. Pediatr Allergy Immunol 2003; 14: 437–40

51. Mikus LD, Rosenthal LA, Sorkness RL, Lemanske RF Jr. Reduced interferon-gamma secretion by natural killer cells from rats susceptible to postviral chronic airway dysfunction. Am J Respir Cell Mol Biol 2001; 24: 74–82

52. Rosenthal LA, Mikus LD, Tuffaha A, et al. Attenuated innate mechanisms of interferon-gamma production in rats susceptible to postviral airway dysfunction. Am J Respir Cell Mol Biol 2004; 30: 702–9

53. Sorkness RL, Castleman WL, Kumar A, et al. Prevention of chronic postbronchiolitis airway sequelae with IFN-γ treatment in rats. Am J Respir Crit Care Med 1999; 160: 705–10

54. Lau S, Illi S, Sommerfeld C, et al. Early exposure to house-dust mite and cat allergens and development of childhood asthma: a cohort study. Multicentre Allergy Study Group. Lancet 2000; 356: 1392–7

55. Johnston SL, Pattemore PK, Sanderson G, et al. Community study of role of viral infections in exacerbations of asthma in 9–11 year old children. BMJ 1995; 310: 1225–9

56. Nicholson KG, Kent J, Ireland DC. Respiratory viruses and exacerbations of asthma in adults. BMJ 1993; 307: 982–6

57. Johnston SL, Pattemore PK, Sanderson G, et al. The relationship between upper respiratory infections and hospital admissions for asthma: a time trend analysis. Am J Respir Crit Care Med 1996; 154: 654–60

58. Johnston NW, Johnston SL, Duncan JM, et al. The September epidemic of asthma exacerbations in children: a search for etiology. J Allergy Clin Immunol 2005; 115: 132–8

59. Ingram JM, Rakes GP, Hoover GE, et al. Eosinophil cationic protein in serum and nasal washes from wheezing infants and children. J Pediatr 1995; 127: 558–64

60. Rakes GP, Arruda E, Ingram JM, et al. Rhinovirus and respiratory syncytial virus in wheezing children requiring emergency care. IgE and eosinophil analyses. Am J Respir Crit Care Med 1999; 159: 785–90

61. Gwaltney JM Jr, Phillips CD, Miller RD, Riker DK. Computed tomographic study of the common cold. N Engl J Med 1994; 330: 25–30

62. Smart BA, Slavin RG. Rhinosinusitis and pediatric asthma. Immunol Allergy Clin North Am 2005; 25: 67–82

63. Tsao CH, Chen LC, Yeh KW, Huang JL. Concomitant chronic sinusitis treatment in children with mild asthma: the effect on bronchial hyperresponsiveness. Chest 2003; 123: 757–64

64. Friedman R, Ackerman M, Wald E, et al. Asthma and bacterial sinusitis in children. J Allergy Clin Immunol 1984; 74: 185–9

65. Rachelefsky GS, Katz RM, Siegel SC. Chronic sinus disease with associated reactive airway disease in children. Pediatrics 1984; 73: 526–9

66. Litonjua AA, Carey VJ, Burge HA, et al. Exposure to cockroach allergen in the home is associated with incident doctor-diagnosed asthma and recurrent wheezing. J Allergy Clin Immunol 2001; 107: 41–7

67. O'Hollaren MT, Yunginger JW, Offard KP, et al. Exposure to an aeroallergen as a possible precipitating factor in respiratory arrest in young patients with asthma. N Engl J Med 1991; 324: 359–63

68. Rosenstreich DL, Eggleston PA, Kattan M, et al. The role of cockroach allergy and exposure to cockroach allergen in causing morbidity among inner-city children with asthma. N Engl J Med 1997; 336: 1356–63

69. Platts-Mills TAE, Vaughan JW, Blumenthal K, et al. Serum IgG and IgG4 antibodies to Fel d 1 among children exposed to 20 microg Fel d 1 at home: relevance of a nonallergic modified Th2 response. Int Arch Allergy Immunol 2001; 124: 126–9

70. Bufford JD, Gern JE. The hygiene hypothesis revisited. Immunol Allergy Clin North Am 2005; 25: 247–62

71. Perzanowski MS, Ronmark E, Nold B, et al. Relevance of allergens from cats and dogs to asthma in the northernmost province of Sweden: schools as a major site of exposure. J Allergy Clin Immunol 1999; 103: 1018–24

72. James JM, Bernhisel-Broadbent J, Sampson HA. Respiratory reactions provoked by double-blind food challenges in children. Am J Respir Crit Care Med 1994; 149: 59–64

73. Trasande L, Thurston GD. The role of air pollution in asthma and other pediatric morbidities. J Allergy Clin Immunol 2005; 115: 689–99

74. Fanucchi MV, Plopper CG. Pulmonary developmental responses to toxicants. In Roth RA, ed. Comprehensive Toxicology. New York: Pergamon, 1997: 203–20

75. Fedorov IA, Wilson SJ, Davies DE, Holgate ST. Epithelial stress and structural remodelling in childhood asthma. Thorax 2005; 60: 389–94

76. von Mutius E. Environmental factors influencing the development and progression of pediatric asthma. J Allergy Clin Immunol 2002; 109 (Suppl): S525–S532

77. Peden DB. The epidemiology and genetics of asthma risk associated with air pollution. J Allergy Clin Immunol 2005; 115: 213–19

78. Romieu I, Sienra-Monge JJ, Ramirez-Aguilar M, et al. Genetic polymorphism of GSTM1 and antioxidant supplementation influence lung function in relation to ozone exposure in asthmatic children in Mexico City. Thorax 2004; 59: 8–10

79. Romieu I, Sienra-Monge JJ, Ramirez-Aguilar M, et al. Antioxidant supplementation and lung functions among children with asthma exposed to high levels of air pollutants. Am J Respir Crit Care Med 2002; 166: 703–9

80. Motoyama EK, Brody JS, Colten HR, Warshaw JB. NHLBI workshop summary. Postnatal lung development in health and disease. Am Rev Respir Dis 1988; 137: 742–6

81. Lucas SR, Platts-Mills TA. Physical activity and exercise in asthma: relevance to etiology and treatment. J Allergy Clin Immunol 2005; 115: 928–34

82. Wright RJ, Finn P, Contreras JP, et al. Chronic caregiver stress and IgE expression, allergen-induced proliferation, and cytokine profiles in a birth cohort predisposed to atopy. J Allergy Clin Immunol 2004; 113: 1051–7

83. Selner JC, Staudenmayer H, Koepke JW, et al. Vocal cord dysfunction: the importance of psychologic factors and provocation challenge testing. J Allergy Clin Immunol 1987; 79: 726–33

84. Tilles SA. Vocal cord dysfunction in children and adolescents. Curr Allergy Asthma Rep 2003; 3: 467–72

85. Duff AL, Pomeranz ES, Gelber LE, et al. Risk factors for acute wheezing in infants and children: viruses, passive smoke, and IgE antibodies to inhalant allergens. Pediatrics 1993; 92: 535–40

86. Green RM, Cusotvic A, Sanderson G, et al. Synergism between allergens and viruses and risk of hospital admission with asthma: case–control study. BMJ 2002; 324: 763–6A

87. Murray CS, Poletti G, Kebadze T, et al. Study of modifiable risk factors for asthma exacerbations: virus infection and allergen exposure increase the risk of asthma hospital admissions in children. Thorax 2006; 61: 376–82

88. Calhoun WJ, Dick EC, Schwartz LB, Busse WW. A common cold virus, rhinovirus 16, potentiates airway inflammation after segmental antigen bronchoprovocation in allergic subjects. J Clin Invest 1994; 94: 2200–8

89. Lemanske RF Jr, Dick EC, Swenson CA, et al. Rhinovirus upper respiratory infection increases airway hyperreactivity and late asthmatic reactions. J Clin Invest 1989; 83: 1–10

90. Avila PC, Abisheganaden JA, Wong H, et al. Effects of allergic inflammation of the nasal mucosa on the severity of rhinovirus 16 cold. J Allergy Clin Immunol 2000; 105: 923–32

91. De Kluijver J, Evertse CE, Sont JK, et al. Are rhinovirus-induced airway responses in asthma aggravated by

chronic allergen exposure? Am J Respir Crit Care Med 2003; 168: 1174–80

92. Chauhan AJ, Johnston SL. Air pollution and infection in respiratory illness. Br Med Bull 2003; 68: 95–112

93. Tarlo SM, Broder I, Corey P, et al. The role of symptomatic colds in asthma exacerbations: influence of outdoor allergens and air pollutants. J Allergy Clin Immunol 2001; 108: 52–8

94. Chauhan AJ, Inskip HM, Linaker CH, et al. Personal exposure to nitrogen dioxide (NO2) and the severity of virus-induced asthma in children. Lancet 2003; 361: 1939–44

95. Lopez-Souza N, Dolganov G, Dubin R, et al. Resistance of differentiated human airway epithelium to infection by rhinovirus. Am J Physiol Lung Cell Mol Physiol 2004; 286: L373–L381

CHAPTER 6

Etiology of asthma exacerbations in adults: differences from children

Anoop J Chauhan, Simon Bourne and Sebastian L Johnston

EPIDEMIOLOGIC DIFFERENCES IN ADULT AND CHILDHOOD EXACERBATIONS

The economic impact of exacerbations is significant; expenditure for asthma costs over $9.4 billion in the USA and £2.3 billion in the UK per annum[1] and has been outlined in Chapter 3. Over half of this relates to treatment of acute exacerbations. Furthermore, in the UK for example, over 12.7 million working days are lost in adults (with a loss of productivity amounting to £1.2 billion) and school absenteeism is estimated at approximately 8.5 million school days per annum. The economic burden of exacerbations in children is more difficult to estimate but is also likely to be significant due to associated costs such as parental absenteeism from work to care for asthmatic children at home.

There are, however, noteworthy age-specific patterns of exacerbations requiring admissions to hospital. In the USA, asthma is the 11th most frequent emergency room (ER) diagnosis nationwide, and adolescents and young adults are the most frequent age groups to visit the ER for treatment.[2] Similar data from Australia, Canada and Spain report that acute asthma accounts for 1–12% of all adult ER visits.[3–5] On average, of the 1.5 million ER visits by asthma patients in 1995 in the USA, up to 30% of patients required hospital admission.[6,7]

Hospital admission rates for exacerbations for asthma in the UK showed significant differences between adults and children in the latter half of the 20th century. The largest increases in asthma admission rates occurred in children, most notably in pre-school children (0–4 age group). Admissions increased in all children up to 1988; thereafter the trends were all downward, again most obviously in younger children. Similarly, asthma admission rates in adults increased through the 1960s, declined during the 1970s, rose again from 1980 and then remained stable in the 1990s.[8] In the USA, admission rates for asthma similarly increased by 50% in adults and by over 200% in children from the 1960s to the 1980s. Rates for black patients were 50% higher in adults and 150% greater in children.

The unwanted outcome of any exacerbation is the potential for significant morbidity and mortality. Global estimates suggest that asthma accounts for about 1 in every 250 deaths, largely through the risks of life-threatening exacerbations. Many of the deaths are preventable, being due to a variety of causes from inadequate day-to-day treatment for asthma, but many relate to a delay in obtaining help during an exacerbation due to, for example, socioeconomic influences or reduced perception of the severity of an exacerbation.[9]

The age-specific asthma mortality rates from asthma in the UK show a different pattern in children and adults from the late 1950s to the

1990s. Since the early 1980s, rates among those aged under 64 had tended to decrease, whilst rates in the elderly had increased. It is more likely that there has been a small real increase in deaths over and above the increases due to minor coding changes. An irregular pattern for children is explained by variability due to the small numbers who die of asthma in this age group, but there has also been an overall decline. Asthma deaths are therefore now falling, and are currently around 1500 per year in the UK.[8] The majority of asthma deaths occur in those aged over 45, with around 40% of deaths occurring in the 75+ age group. Only a small proportion (1%) occurred in children. Similarly, in the USA death rates from asthma among the older age groups increased from the 1960s to the 1980s, with a considerable increase from 1979. For children, the evidence is less clear, but the death rate had increased for children over 5 years of age during the period from 1979 to 1982.

In many countries, asthma mortality similarly increased from the 1960s to the second half of the 1980s, but reached a plateau and has subsequently declined. This recent downward trend may reflect better management of this condition in primary care. Asthma has a low mortality rate compared with other lung diseases in adults, but mortality still occurs, typically in patients with poorly controlled disease whose condition gradually deteriorates over a period of days or even weeks. Although the admission and mortality rates overall among children and adults may appear to have stabilized in both the UK and the USA, the absolute levels of admissions and mortality still remain unacceptably high.[10]

TIME COURSE OF AN EXACERBATION IN ADULTS AND CHILDREN

Exacerbations of asthma are difficult to define but are characterized by discrete periods of increased symptoms and reduced lung function, resulting in a reduced ability to perform normal activities. Further definition is discussed in Chapter 2.

Changes that occur in symptoms and peak flow in 425 severe asthma exacerbations in adults over a 12-month period were described in the FACET study.[11] The different arms of the study included asthmatic subjects on low and high doses of budesonide with and without formoterol. A severe exacerbation was the main study endpoint (defined as the need for a course of oral corticosteroids or associated with a reduction in morning peak expiratory flow (PEF) of >30% on two consecutive days). Daily diary cards recorded PEF, symptoms and bronchodilator use over the 14 days before and after the exacerbation. Exacerbations were characterized by a gradual fall in PEF over several days, followed by more rapid changes over 2–3 days; an increase in symptoms and rescue β_2-agonist use occurred in parallel, and both the severity and time course of the changes were similar in all treatment groups (Figure 6.1). Exacerbations identified by the need for oral corticosteroids were associated with more symptoms and smaller changes in PEF than those identified on the basis of PEF criteria alone. In these adults, female sex was the main patient characteristic associated with an increased risk of having a severe exacerbation. The authors concluded that exacerbations were characterized predominantly by change in symptoms or change in PEF, but the pattern was not affected by the dose of inhaled corticosteroid or by whether the patient was taking formoterol.

The definition of exacerbations in young children is more difficult based on diary card data alone. A series of longitudinal studies of exacerbations of asthma in children have confirmed differences in exacerbations reported by subjects to those exacerbations defined by a computer algorithm.[12] The algorithm defined an exacerbation as 2 or more days with symptom scores above the median for that child (or PEF at or below the 10th centile) led by 1 day at or below the median (above the 10th centile) and followed by 2 days at or below the median (at or above the median).

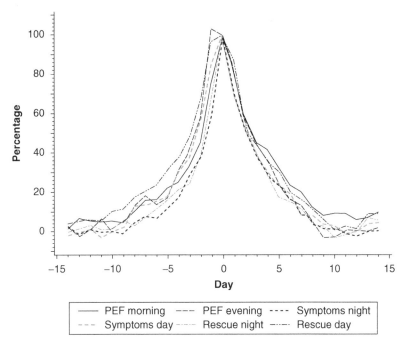

Figure 6.1 Comparison of change in morning and evening peak expiratory flow (PEF), daytime and night-time symptoms and rescue β₂-agonist use during an exacerbation of asthma in adults. Data have been standardized (day −14, 0%; maximum change, 100%) to allow comparison of changes with time between different endpoints. Reproduced with permission from reference 11

There were twice as many unreported episodes of respiratory symptoms and diminished PEF than reported exacerbations. Although the seasonal patterns of reported and unreported episodes were similar, the severity and duration of reported episodes were significantly greater than those of unreported episodes. Another study also confirmed that not every upper respiratory tract (URT) episode is followed by an exacerbation, and the propensity to develop an exacerbation also depends on other personal and environmental characteristics (Figure 6.2).[13]

In a similar study of exacerbations in 7–12-year-old asthmatic children, graphs of symptom scores and PEF measurements over a 12-month study period were examined independently by two clinicians.[14] Exacerbations were identified by symptom records without access to PEF measurements and vice versa. An upper respiratory

or PEF episode was deemed to have been present on days on which both clinicians had indicated the diagnosis. The two clinicians agreed well in their assessment of exacerbations from the daily records, with agreement in 93% of URT episodes and 94% of PEF episodes. Furthermore, when diagnosed episodes overlapped by both physicians, there was exact agreement on the date of onset for 82% of the upper respiratory episodes and 67% of the PEF episodes. It is also noteworthy that exacerbations that are reported in the community (but not requiring admission) can often show sizeable decrements in PEF rates and in some instances these are comparable to the rates of those admitted to hospital.[12]

These data therefore suggest that exacerbations are common in children and adults. Computer algorithm-defined exacerbations are more frequent but of less severity and lower duration than

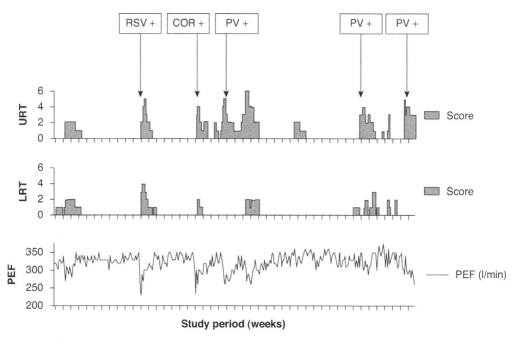

Figure 6.2 Chart of upper respiratory tract (URT) and lower respiratory tract (LRT) symptoms and peak expiratory flow (PEF) rate in relation to virus detection by reverse transcriptase-polymerase chain reaction (RT-PCR). The chart shows the temporal relation between these parameters and reported asthma exacerbations in which viruses were isolated in one child. Symptom scores are based on an arbitrary scale. Reproduced with permission from reference 13. RSV, respiratory syncytial virus; COR, coronavirus; PV, picornavirus

those reported by subjects. Compared to episodes identified by visual charts, clinicians can also consistently identify the majority of exacerbations reported by patients.

VIRUS INFECTIONS AND ASTHMA EXACERBATIONS IN ADULTS AND CHILDREN

The overwhelming evidence outlined throughout this book confirms that if adequate virus detection methods are used, viruses are detected during the great majority of asthma exacerbations. Viruses have now been implicated in asthma and satisfy many of the criteria of causality identified by Bradford Hill, namely a temporal relationship, strength of relationship, dose–response relationship, consistency, plausibility, experimental manipulation, specificity and coherence with current understanding. Some of the arguments for causality of infection in exacerbations of asthma in adults and children are presented here.

Temporal relationship and consistency

Viruses are detected in the vast majority of children (>80%) and infants (up to 100%) during wheezing illnesses. Although there are relatively fewer published studies in adults, respiratory infections are similarly associated with approximately 40–76% of exacerbations in adults.[15–17] A consistent observation in all the studies on the etiology of asthma exacerbations in children confirms rhinoviruses as the most important virus type, accounting for around 66% of infections detected.[12,13,18,19] In the studies in asthma in children, they were associated with 50% of total exacerbations.

Dose–response effect

In a study of adults admitted to the ER with asthma exacerbations, viruses were detected in sputum in 76% of these admissions. Further testing of the sputum samples included assessment for markers of cellular activation including lactate dehydrogenase (LDH) as a marker of virus-induced lower airway cell damage. LDH levels were the single strongest predictor of severity of the exacerbations measured by length of hospital stay, indicating that the degree of virus-induced lower airway cell damage was the major driver of severity of the exacerbation.[17]

The advent of sensitive molecular methods of virus detection has increasingly identified the presence of more than one virus or atypical bacterium in the same sample (co-infection) taken during acute episodes. The clinical importance of multiple infections is not known, but is likely to be related to more severe clinical episodes. In chronic obstructive pulmonary disease (COPD) simultaneous identification of bacterial and viral pathogens in sputum at the time of exacerbation is associated with enhanced airway inflammation, increased bacterial load and symptoms and a larger decrement in lung function.[20] In asthma multiple infections have been recognized but the clinical importance has not been studied in detail. In one (to-date unpublished) study, multiple infections were detected by reverse transcriptase-polymerase chain reaction (RT-PCR) in upper respiratory samples obtained from children with exacerbations of asthma and when asymptomatic. Infection was detected in 78% of exacerbation samples, and the most frequently detected organisms were picornaviruses, respiratory syncytical virus (RSV), *Mycoplasma pneumoniae* and coronaviruses (Figure 6.3).[13] Among these samples, single infections were present in 60% of exacerbation and in 17% of stable samples, dual infections in 15% and 5% and triple infections in 4% and 0% samples, respectively. An increasing number of viral infections was associated with increasing severity of URT and lower respiratory tract (LRT) symptoms and reduced peak flow in a dose–response fashion (Figure 6.4). It is likely, therefore, that co-infection between viruses may be related to clinical severity of asthma exacerbations, at least in children.

Biological plausibility and experimental manipulation

After infection, an effective antiviral immune response requires early viral clearance to reduce further inflammatory damage. The normal antiviral immune response consists of innate and specific components, requiring the co-ordinated actions of many different cell types including neutrophils, macrophages, eosinophils, dendritic cells, epithelial cells, mast cells, natural killer cells and B and T lymphocytes. Co-ordination of this response involves several cytokines and chemokines, and T lymphocytes expressing Th1 cytokines including interferon (IFN)-γ play the key role. IFN-γ has a number of potentially antiviral actions, including the activation of alveolar macrophages, and it interacts with other antiviral cytokines such as tumor necrosis factor (TNF)-α to bring about airway epithelial cell apoptosis supporting enhanced elimination of rhinovirus infection.[21]

Recent evidence suggests that adults with asthma are not at increased risk of naturally occurring rhinovirus infections compared to non-asthmatic controls, but are more susceptible to developing a clinically significant exacerbation after infection. In this study asthmatic individuals experienced LRT symptoms, and changes in peak expiratory flows were both more severe and of longer duration in the subjects than in the normal controls.[15] The reasons for this increased susceptibility in individuals with asthma are likely to be related to an amplified response of pre-existing asthmatic inflammation, a reduced ability to clear the virus effectively or probably a mixed response. Evidence for an impaired innate antiviral response in asthma has been provided from a study using primary bronchial epithelial cells from normal and asthmatic volunteers.

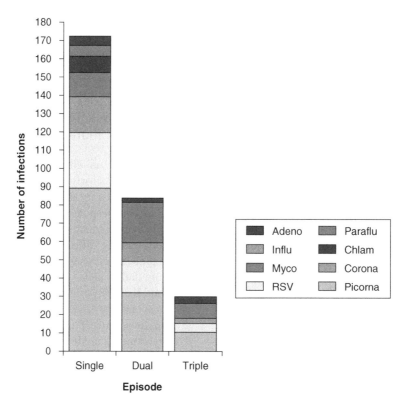

Figure 6.3 Distribution of viruses and atypical bacteria detected in 280 nasal aspirates of 7–12-year-old children during asthma exacerbations grouped by the presence of single, dual or triple infections in the same exacerbation. Adeno, adenovirus; Paraflu, parainfluenza viruses A–C; Influ, influenza viruses A and B; Chlam, *Chlamydophila pneumoniae*; Myco, *Mycoplasma pneumoniae*; Corona, coronaviruses OC43 and 229E; RSV, respiratory syncytial virus; Picorna, picornaviruses (mainly rhinovirus). Data from Chauhan AJ *et al.*, 2006, submitted for publication

Asthmatic primary bronchial epithelial cells cultured *ex vivo* and infected with rhinovirus 16 were found to have a profoundly impaired production of IFN-β and apoptosis in response to virus infection, resulting in increased virus replication.[22]

Further evidence also suggests an impaired acquired immune response to rhinovirus infections in asthma. A controlled study in asthmatic adults demonstrated an inverse correlation between induction of bronchial hyperresponsiveness after rhinovirus infection and levels of virus-induced IFN-γ in peripheral blood mononuclear cell (PBMC) cultures.[23] In another controlled *in vitro* exposure study of atopic asthmatics,

rhinovirus infection increased interleukin (IL)-4 levels (a Th2 pro-allergic response) only in subjects with asthma, and PBMCs from asthmatic subjects produced significantly lower levels of IFN-γ and IL-12 and higher levels of IL-10 than in normal controls.[24]

Asthmatic airway inflammation is characterized by an array of pathophysiological changes including the presence of T lymphocytes, eosinophils, neutrophils, mast cells and a predominantly Th2 cytokine milieu in the airways. Rhinovirus infection in both adult asthmatics and in normal subjects increased numbers of both CD4 and CD8 T cells in the bronchial mucosa, but with no difference between groups.[25]

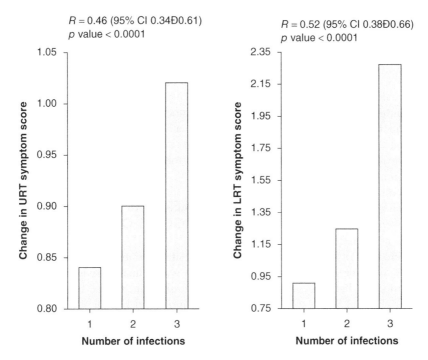

Figure 6.4 The change in daily mean upper (URT) and lower respiratory tract (LRT) symptom scores in the week after sampling in exacerbations with infection by one, two and three agents compared to exacerbations without infection. Symptom scores based on an arbitrary scale (0, absent; 1, mild; 2, moderate; 3, severe). Regression coefficient R=change in score for each successive infection. Data from Chauhan *et al.*, 2006, submitted for publication

In an experimental rhinovirus infection study of asthmatic subjects alone, sputum IFN-γ/IL-5 (relative Th1/Th2) mRNA ratios were inversely correlated with cold symptoms. The ratio was significantly higher in those who cleared virus by 2 weeks, compared with those who did not.[26] Therefore, the balance of Th1/Th2 cytokine levels in the airway is likely to influence both symptoms and virus clearance.

Specificity

Viruses other than human rhinoviruses have been implicated in asthma, although rhinoviruses are the most commonly detected pathogens in acute asthma in both adults and children. The role of RSV and the relatively recently recognized human metapneumovirus (hMPV) is discussed in Chapter 5 in this book;

hMPV is associated with up to 20% of pre-school children presenting with an acute LRT infection in which a pathogen could be detected.[27] In another study including children and adults (age range 2 months to 93 years, median 25 years), hMPV was detected in 15% of infections with a peak in isolation between February and March.[28] A third of subjects in which hMPV was detected were admitted to hospital with a range of illnesses from pneumonia to bronchiolitis. The admission rates were significantly higher among patients <5 years of age and those >50 years of age. These results provide further evidence of the importance of hMPV, particularly in young children and elderly individuals.[27] Co-infection of hMPV with human RSV confers a further 10-fold increase in risk of admission to a pediatric intensive care unit for mechanical ventilation in those admitted with bronchiolitis.[29] The importance of this virus with regard to wheezing illnesses has yet to be fully studied, but its impact is probably going to be in infants, and possibly older adults.

There is increasing (but thus far conflicting) evidence of a putative association between the atypical bacteria *Chlamydophila pneumoniae* and *Mycoplasma pneumoniae* and asthma exacerbations. These are due to the difficulties in detecting infection by serology which can now be supplemented by modern, sensitive molecular methods such as RT-PCR to detect infection. In one case–control study of 100 adults admitted with acute asthma, *M. pneumoniae* was detected by serology in 18% of asthmatics compared to only 3% of the controls.[30] There was no difference in infection between groups for *C. pneumoniae*. In children, these atypical bacteria have been detected up to seven-fold more frequently in children suffering more than four exacerbations per year[31] or associated with more prolonged exacerbations.[32] The role of these atypical bacteria has recently been reviewed.[33]

In chronic asthma, a small number of randomized placebo-controlled studies of macrolide therapy of >4 weeks' duration suggested an overall beneficial effect on symptoms and eosinophilic markers of inflammation. This suggests that infection with *C. pneumoniae* and *M. pneumoniae* in chronic stable asthma is associated with increased airway inflammation – thereby increasing asthma severity and risk of exacerbations. Of the different antibacterial drugs active against atypical bacteria, macrolides and ketolides may exert additional immunomodulatory properties. A very recent double-blind, randomized, placebo-controlled study reported a significant reduction in asthma symptom score and improvement in lung function in 278 patients treated with telithromycin for an acute exacerbation of asthma. Of these, 61% of patients had evidence of infection with *C. pneumoniae*, *M. pneumoniae* or both, but there was no relationship between bacteriological status and the response to asthma treatment. This study provides evidence of the benefit of telithromycin in adults with acute exacerbations of asthma.[34] Further studies of other related and unrelated antibiotics in this context are clearly needed.

The evidence for the specificity of many respiratory virus and atypical bacterial infections in causality of asthma exacerbations is therefore notable, but the case for causality in adults is strongest for rhinoviruses.

ALLERGENS AND OTHER TRIGGERS OF ASTHMA

Sensitization to allergens is a risk factor for chronic asthma, although the importance of any one allergen varies between countries. For example, cockroach allergen sensitization is more common in the USA than any other areas of developed countries and mite allergens are similarly common and important in Australia. Sensitization is, however, not the same as acute exposure. While there is a wealth of evidence confirming the increased risk of asthma in sensitized atopic individuals, there is increasing evidence of increased prevalence of sensitization in individuals presenting with acute asthma. It is therefore highly likely that allergen exposure can also induce exacerbations in sensitized subjects with asthma. In an experimental model, patients with late asthmatic responses demonstrate enhanced eosinophilic airway inflammation after a single allergen challenge, which is followed by an episode of increased airway hyperresponsiveness. Further repeated allergen challenge (at a level not high enough to induce an early bronchoconstrictor response, which better mimics natural, seasonal exposures) can also induce such responses. Furthermore, compared to viruses, exposure to allergens in sensitized individuals can occur seasonally or perennially, thus increasing the opportunity for high levels of exposure throughout the year. The role of allergens in childhood asthma has been discussed in the previous chapter.

In adult asthmatics, sensitization and exposure to mite-allergen is associated with increased PEF variability, reduced lung function and increased bronchial hyperresponsiveness and increased exhaled nitric oxide indicative of persistent airway inflammation.[35] Furthermore, increasing levels of mite-allergen concentrations in the home in a dose–response fashion in sensitized patients with asthma is associated with increased symptoms[36] and treatment required to control more severe asthma.[37] Given these observations, it is not surprising that exposure to a variety of allergens including mites, cats, dogs and grass is associated with an increased risk for admission or ER visit for acute asthma in children and adults.[38–40]

The association of high allergen exposure and exacerbations leading to asthma deaths is less clear, but exposure at the height of the peak mold spore season has been linked to the peak death rate in children and adults aged 5–34 years. A 200-fold increased risk of a respiratory arrest in sensitized adolescents and young adults has been similarly linked to the peak *Alternaria* spore season.[41]

Given the almost perennial exposure to both allergens and viruses in some sensitized individuals, it is likely that the synergistic effect of dual exposure in susceptible individuals increases the risk of uncontrolled asthma and exacerbations. A UK study reported a markedly increased risk of admission to hospital with acute asthma in adults with the combination of sensitization *and* current exposure to high levels of sensitizing allergens with the presence of viral infection.[42] Viral infection alone was not an independent risk for asthma admission, but, in patients both sensitized and exposed to allergens, virus infection markedly increased the risk of admission. Recent evidence further suggests a quantitative relationship between current allergen exposure and the exacerbation of asthma requiring admission to hospital (see later under Synergistic interactions).

A number of controlled exposure studies (bronchial allergen challenge and experimental rhinovirus infection) have provided further evidence of the potential synergistic effects between allergens and respiratory viral infection. In one study, adult patients were examined for bronchial hyperresponsiveness and early- and late-phase responses with ragweed antigen challenge before and after rhinovirus infection. There was a significant increase in bronchial hyperresponsiveness and, before rhinovirus infection, only one patient had a late-phase response to ragweed, compared with eight of 10 after infection.[43] These results suggest that allergens and viruses may act together to exacerbate asthma, indicating that domestic exposure to allergens acts synergistically with viruses in sensitized patients, increasing the risk of exacerbation.

Air pollution

The deaths following the early 20th century smog episodes in Europe and the USA have unequivocally confirmed the association between air pollution and respiratory disease. The historical pollutants sulfur dioxide (SO_2) and black smoke (now particulates of different-size fractions such as PM_{10} – particles with an aerodynamic diameter of 10 μm or less) and the modern gaseous pollutants nitrogen dioxide (NO_2) and ozone (O_3) from the combustion of natural gas, gasoline and diesel now pose the greatest risk of exacerbations for asthmatic subjects. The risks posed by these air pollutants are determined by seasonal outdoor concentrations, and also the personal exposure of asthmatic subjects (representing the average of the pollutant concentrations encountered in various microenvironments with weighting proportional to the time spent in each location) and interaction with other co-factors.

The evidence for air pollution suggests that it may trigger exacerbations in individuals with asthma, but there is no consistent evidence to suggest that air pollution initiates asthma in individuals with previously healthy lungs.[44] Using a variety of epidemiological approaches from case–control studies to time-series analyses, exposure to outdoor pollutants has been linked to exacerbations of respiratory symptoms by ER visits,[45,46] hospital admissions,[47,48] mortality,[49,50] increased URT and LRT symptoms[51,52] and reduced lung function.[53,54] Controlled chamber studies have also allowed investigation of airway responses provoked by inhalation of airborne pollutants that give some estimate of the propensity to cause an exacerbation. Studies in mixed populations of adult and child asthmatics have shown a variable response to air pollution across a range of exposures to different pollutants, but confirm the overall increased susceptibility of asthmatic compared to non-asthmatic subjects.[55] Examples of the association of each pollutant with asthma exacerbations are given below, but the list is not exhaustive.

A number of studies have examined the relationship between concentrations of SO_2 and daily variations in indices of health, number of deaths, hospital admissions and symptoms. Based on seven Western European cities, a $50\,\mu g/m^3$ rise in average SO_2 concentration corresponds to a 3% rise in total deaths and 2% more respiratory admissions in subjects over 65 years,[56] and a rise in 24-hour averages of black winter smoke level and SO_2 of $20\,\mu g/m^3$ would result in one additional asthma admission per day. Asthmatic patients show considerable variability in their response to SO_2 in controlled exposure studies, but, in general, they are more sensitive than normal subjects. The range of concentrations likely to provoke a doubling of airway resistance varies from above $500\,\mu g/m^3$ in adult asthmatics undergoing moderate exercise and, in the UK, outdoor concentrations of $500\,\mu g/m^3$ of SO_2 have been commonly exceeded.

The Air Pollution on Health: European Approach (APHEA) project collected data on daily pollutant levels (including O_3) from 15 European cities with a total population exceeding 25 million. The studies suggest that a rise in $50\,\mu g/m^3$ in 8-hour average O_3 concentration was associated with a 3% and 4% increase in respiratory admissions in those below and above 65 years, respectively.[57] The number of admissions specifically for asthma in those aged 15–64 years was similarly estimated as 3.5%.[58] The effects of O_3 on lung function are detectable at concentrations as low as $160\,\mu g/m^3$, but there is considerable individual variability in the responses. The O_3 level likely to trigger an exacerbation is dependent upon the total dose inhaled, integrating the intensity and duration of exposure and minute ventilation. In both normal and asthmatic adults, symptoms increase above $600\,\mu g/m^3$ of O_3. Children appear to be more sensitive to the effects of ozone, particularly if they have asthma, where the effects are seen at levels as low as $160\,\mu g/m^3$. Although the changes in forced expiratory volume (FEV_1) resolve within 24 hours after a single O_3 exposure, repeated daily exposure induces adaptation in some individuals so that the subsequent reduction in lung function becomes less marked after several days.

Epidemiological studies of the acute effects of NO_2 confirm its association with adverse outcomes. The APHEA studies reported an increase of $50\,\mu g/m^3$ in 1-hour maximum of NO_2 and O_3 was associated with a 1.3% and 2.9% increase in daily all-cause mortality,[59] and a $50\,\mu g/m^3$ increase in 24-hour average NO_2 alone was associated with an increase of 2.6% in asthma admissions,[60] often at levels well below current World Health Organization (WHO) air quality guidelines. High levels of outdoor NO_2 produced by motor vehicles are periodically experienced in urban areas (and are a good marker of vehicle-generated pollution), but the effects of NO_2 emitted indoors from unvented gas cookers seem more important. A meta-analysis of indoor NO_2 exposure studies from the UK, Europe and North America estimated an odds ratio of 1.20 for the risk for asthma-type symptoms in children for an exposure of $30\,\mu g/m^3$ of NO_2 (comparable to the increase resulting from exposure to a gas stove).[61] A further analysis of the evidence concluded that, according to age, the estimated risk is higher (1.29–1.60) in children aged 5–6 years and 6–12 years compared to infants.[62] The size of a similar collective risk in adults is not known, but one study reported the effects of daily exposure to indoor and outdoor pollution in a panel of 164 adult asthmatics (aged 18–70 years) over 3 months.[63] Significant associations were seen with indoor sources of pollution and exacerbations of asthma. The use of a gas stove was associated with shortness of breath, cough, nocturnal asthma and restrictions in activity. Controlled exposure studies suggest a small increase in bronchial hyperresponsiveness in asthmatic subjects following NO_2 exposure, but it is not a potent bronchoconstrictor as compared to SO_2, and is therefore likely to exert its effects by different mechanisms in asthma.[64]

Airborne particles have been characterized by mass (and this indirectly by size) or number concentrations per unit volume. However, particles less than 10 μm in diameter (PM_{10}) can penetrate into the thoracic airways, and to a large extent consist of finer particles smaller than a few micrometers (e.g. $PM_{2.5}$). Although the temporal and spatial variations of PM_{10} and $PM_{2.5}$ are similar, they have differences in sources of exposure and composition, and therefore health effects. There is now a wealth of evidence implicating particulate exposure and mortality from cardiovascular and respiratory diseases (especially from arid regions such as New Mexico, USA where particulate concentrations are very high), and the strength of the evidence for *fine* particulate matter is more consistent.[65] There is similarly evidence for particulate exposure and asthma morbidity, especially associations between respiratory morbidity endpoints and coarse particles in areas where no such associations with mortality were found, thus illustrating the irritative potential of fine and coarse particles. For example, an association was observed between asthma visits and PM_{10} levels, based on over 2800 ER visits in Seattle (affected by woodsmoke) over a year, and was strongest for average PM_{10} over the previous 4 days. In those under 65 years old, a 30 μg/m³ increase in 4-day average PM_{10} was associated with a 12% increase in asthma attendance.[66] An increase in asthma attendance on days with high levels of fine particulates within each season has also been observed.[67,68] Controlled exposure studies

suggest that asthmatic patients exposed to 150 μg/m³ PM_{10} (levels that can be expected in high particulate areas) show up to a 6% reduction in PEF rates.

There is now increasing evidence of a link between air pollution, asthma exacerbations and respiratory infection, and those individuals with pre-existing lung disease such as asthma are at greater risk. The majority of the studies of air pollution and infection have been conducted in children and have been described in the previous chapter, and the epidemiology and mechanisms have been reviewed elsewhere.[64,69] An overview of this range of studies of air pollutants and asthma exacerbations shows that the effects on the individual are variable and act by mechanisms other than direct bronchoconstrictor effects. The responses in individuals will depend on personal exposure, activity and probably individual and genetic susceptibility (discussed later).

Cigarette smoking

Environmental tobacco smoke (ETS) exposure, whether by active or passive (second-hand smoke; SHS) cigarette smoking, is a proven risk factor for lung cancer in adults and for recurrent respiratory illnesses,[70] asthma[71] and lung function impairment in children.[72,73] Furthermore, the risk of developing respiratory disease in children increases in direct relationship to parental smoking habits, the greatest risk being when both parents smoke. The evidence for a detrimental role of cigarette smoking and asthma exacerbations is strongest in children.

The difference between adults and children lies in the method of active and passive exposure. Young children suffer from the effects of passive smoking from adults within their household, whereas older children (adolescent) and adults are exposed to both passive and active smoke. The prevalence of adult asthmatics who smoke is 20–35%, and is surprisingly similar to smokers in the general population.[74] Furthermore, many adult asthmatics who currently smoke fail to appreciate the detrimental effects of ETS on asthma control. In one study of asthmatic adults presenting to ERs with an exacerbation of asthma, 50% of current smokers believed that smoking made their asthma symptoms worse but only 4% stated that smoking was responsible for their current exacerbation.[75]

In adults, ER visits and hospital admissions as a result of asthma occur more frequently amongst cigarette smokers with asthma,[76] especially following days with high levels of outdoor pollution;[77] there is evidence that current smoking is a risk factor for near-fatal and fatal asthma.[78] In another study, adult asthmatics exposed to ETS were compared to asthmatics not exposed.[79] Asthmatics exposed to ETS had significantly more ER visits for asthma, hospital admissions for acute asthma, more exacerbations at home and increased use of bronchodilators, and they had more ER visits and absences from work as a result of uncontrolled asthma.

Evidence for the role of passive ETS or SHS exposure in triggering and exacerbating asthma in adults (compared to poor asthma symptom control) is, however, surprisingly limited. A study of some 11 000 adults participating in the US National Health and Nutrition Survey (NHANES III) found impairment of lung function with exposure in women, especially those with asthma,[80] and another study confirmed that exposure to SHS was associated with a lowered FEV_1 and forced vital capacity (FVC).[81] A controlled exposure study reported significant declines in FEV_1 and FVC in both men and women after an acute exposure to passive ETS.[82] A recent population-based case–control study from Finland has also provided evidence that adult-onset asthma is significantly increased by recent exposure to SHS at work and at home.[83]

Stress

Stress has been defined as a process in which environmental demands far exceed the adaptive capacity of an individual, resulting in psychological stress and biological changes that place a person at risk of disease. Stress and other psychological factors have long been hypothesized to be associated with asthma symptoms and in some individuals may cause a reduction in lung function.[84,85] In children the relationship between stress and asthma was described as *asthma nervosa* in the early part of the past century. Some asthmatic patients experience asthma exacerbations in response to acute stress, such as watching emotionally charged films[86] or listening to stressful interactions.[87] Children and adults have different adaptive mechanisms and stressors and there are consequently different effects on asthma control and exacerbations. In adults and children severe asthma is significantly associated with psychological pressures, in particular depression.[88,89]

In one study of older children the presence of severe life events both on their own and in conjunction with high levels of chronic stress significantly increased the risk of new asthma exacerbations. Major life events alone increased the risk of exacerbations for 4 weeks following an initial delay of 2 weeks. When severe life events occurred in combination with chronic stress the risk of acute asthma events rose sharply and almost immediately within the first 2 weeks. The risk therefore of acute asthma exacerbations in children is enhanced and starts earlier if the child's life situation is characterized by multiple chronic stressors.[90] Similar links with psychological stressors has been identified in adults. One study identified that 50% of 32 asthmatic subjects followed serially over 140 days had significant associations between pulmonary function and psychological variables.[91]

The mechanisms of the relationship of stress, socioeconomic status (SES) and asthmatic airway inflammation have been studied. Adolescents from a low SES in one study had greater stress experience and lower overall beliefs about control over their health but ironically increased levels of IL-5 and IFN-γ, and lower levels of early morning cortisol, than those from higher SES.[92] The exacerbation alone is unlikely to invoke a psychological stressor response in asthmatics, as one study in 74 adults reported no significant adrenal cortical suppression on presentation with acute asthma to the ER.[93] In another study, children with asthma who simultaneously experienced acute and chronic stress exhibited a five-fold reduction in glucocorticoid receptor mRNA and a ten-fold reduction in β_2-adrenergic receptor mRNA relative to children with asthma without comparable stressor exposure, suggesting that stressful experience diminishes expression of the glucocorticoid and β_2-adrenergic receptor genes in children with asthma.[94]

Food

There have been frequent case reports demonstrating that asthma exacerbations can be triggered by foods, and that this reaction can be controlled by an alteration in diet. Respiratory symptoms due to an IgE-mediated food allergic reaction can occur if the food is not routinely ingested, resulting in anaphylaxis, which may be accompanied by severe asthma. If the food is routinely ingested it may present with chronic asthma that is often associated with atopic dermatitis. In infants and young children, symptoms may take the form of classical asthma but there may be intermittent exacerbations of dyspnea, tachypnea and occasionally fever.[95]

A large proportion of adults with asthma perceive that diet plays an important part in their asthma control. In a recent survey of 135 adult asthmatics attending an allergy clinic, 73% reported perceived food-induced asthma, and 61% had tried to modify their diet in order to improve their asthma control.[96] In another study, 17% of adults with asthma reported food intolerance, and were also more likely to be atopic.[97] Most cases of food-induced asthma are observed in infancy and are then often related to cow's milk hypersensitivity, egg, wheat flour and peanuts. Despite the perceived importance of foods in asthma, double-blind, placebo-controlled food challenges in controlled environments are the 'gold standard' for the diagnosis of adverse reactions to foods and

food additives. Such evidence has shown that less than 1% of patients may have objective evidence of food-induced asthma.[98] The overall prevalence of food allergy and acute asthma is probably around 4–6% in children, but less than 1% in adult patients.

Aspirin

Aspirin-induced asthma (AIA) is more prevalent than was previously thought, with estimates of 21% in adults and 5% in children.[99] Many also have nasal polyposis, and sensitivity to aspirin or non-steroidal anti-inflammatory drugs (NSAIDs) as part of the clinical triad with asthma. AIA tends to present in the third or fourth decade in adults not necessarily known to be sensitive to aspirin or NSAIDs. Acute exacerbations of asthma can occur after inadvertent exposure, are often slow in onset but can progress rapidly after 30 minutes to 2 hours and are accompanied by ocular and rhinitic symptoms; occasionally, anaphylaxis, urticaria and angioedema can occur. The clinical manifestations depend on the increased activity of active arachidonic acid metabolites derived through the action of 5-lipoxygenase enzymes. A definitive diagnosis often requires pulmonary function assessment following an aspirin challenge under controlled circumstances. NSAID avoidance (occasionally desensitization) in addition to leukotriene modifiers and standard asthma therapy are the key to treatment.

Pregnancy

Pregnancy has a variable effect on the course of asthma and the 'rule of thirds' applies, with 35% experiencing a worsening of asthma during pregnancy, improvement in 28% and unchanged in 33%,[100] although the best predictor of asthma morbidity is likely to be asthma severity before pregnancy.[101] There is an unequal distribution of asthma exacerbations in pregnancy (with exacerbations occurring in 20–30% of pregnant asthmatic subjects), although the mechanisms for this are not clear. In one study of 504 pregnant asthmatic subjects, asthma exacerbations occurred most frequently between weeks 17 and 24 of the gestation.[102] Another study of 146 patients revealed a peak incidence of severe exacerbations between weeks 14 and 24, and mild exacerbations between weeks 25 and 32.[103] It is possible that many women may reduce or stop taking their medication (in the belief they may harm the fetus) shortly after becoming pregnant, accounting for some of the early exacerbations.

Gastroesophageal reflux

Gastroesophageal reflux disease (GORD) is a potential trigger of asthma; antireflux therapy may be helpful in select patients with poorly controlled asthma including recurrent exacerbations. Several studies have correlated esophageal acid events with asthma symptoms, supporting the hypothesis that GORD may be a trigger for asthma, often in the absence of significant reflux symptoms.[104] A variety of mechanisms are likely to operate but increased vagal tone following acid-stimulated esophageal receptors, microaspiration of gastric acid in the upper airway and increased minute ventilation after acid exposure are the most plausible explanations. Standard antireflux therapy is likely to improve outcome in 20–70% of adult asthmatics.[105,106] A systematic review that included 396 patients reported that nine of the total 12 studies demonstrated significant improvements in at least one outcome such as wheezing, lung function or overall symptoms, but the effects were not consistent across the studies.[107]

Exercise

Exercise is a common trigger for bronchoconstriction leading to an exacerbation in patients with asthma. Exercise-induced asthma is present in probably up to 80% of patients with poorly controlled asthma but with different levels of severity. The mechanisms are not known but probably relate to the underlying severity of bronchial hyperresponsiveness triggered by inhalation of

cold, dry air during exercise with increased minute ventilation. Bronchoconstriction occurs after 5 minutes, peaks at 15 minutes and usually resolves by 60 minutes. This early-phase response is not invariably followed by a late-phase response after several hours (as is more commonly observed in an allergen challenge model), thus potentially aggravating the severity and duration of the exacerbation. Treating the airway inflammation specifically by leukotriene modifiers and long-acting β_2-agonists can reduce the severity of bronchoconstriction.

Synergistic interactions

A review of the etiology of asthma exacerbations in adults and children confirms the wide variety of environmental, personal and infective triggers that increase upper and lower airway symptoms and reduce lung function. Some of this evidence has already been discussed earlier in this chapter. There is evidence that air pollution, virus infections, allergens and stress can act synergistically in asthma exacerbations and a brief review is presented here. The increased risk of hospital admission for acute asthma in sensitized adults exposed to allergens with the presence of viral infection has been described earlier. Another recent study in children confirmed that asthma exacerbations were associated with the combination of both sensitization and current high exposure to sensitizing allergen and the presence of naturally occurring virus infection. Their combined effect was much greater than the individual effects.[108]

The relationship between allergen-triggered epidemics of asthma with ambient air pollution has been most widely reported from Barcelona in the 1980s with the unloading of soy beans in the harbor. It is noteworthy that soy beans were unloaded on 123 days between 1985 and 1987, of which only 13 days were associated with asthma epidemics. Furthermore, the levels of NO_2 and SO_2 were higher on these 13 days compared to the rest of the 123 days, thus suggesting air pollution may have played a synergistic role in the epidemics.[109] Other discrete epidemics of asthma (causing an excess of hospital admissions and primary care visits) in relation to thunderstorms have also been described in Birmingham, UK,[110] in London, UK[111] and Melbourne, Australia.[112] It is postulated that the dispersal of pollen grains after aqueous contact following the thunderstorm released smaller and more potent allergens that were small enough to enter the airways and exacerbate asthma. Although the disruption of grass pollens after thunderstorms may be the likeliest cause, air pollution may potentiate the attacks of asthma; a controlled study demonstrated *in vitro* that exhaust carbon particles derived from a stationary diesel engine bound avidly to the major grass pollen allergen *lol p1* representing a possible mechanism by which allergens could become concentrated in polluted air and thus trigger attacks of asthma in atopic individuals.[113]

Other studies also suggest that air pollution exposure either alone or in combination with other pollutants may alter the early and late asthmatic response to inhaled allergen. Exposure of ten adult asthmatic subjects to the higher concentration of NO_2 led to greater reductions in lung function in both the early and late asthmatic responses compared to air-exposed subjects.[114] In another study, ten mild asthmatic subjects exposed to air, NO_2 or SO_2, or both gases together, were followed by allergen challenge. The decreases in PD_{20} FEV_1 (the dose of allergen required to produce a 20% fall in FEV_1) after exposure to each agent alone were not significant, but the decrease after exposure to the combination was significant.[115] The findings from these studies suggest that air pollution at concentrations encountered in the home environment can potentiate the specific airway response of patients with asthma to inhaled allergen.

Several studies have also sought to determine whether a chronic stressful life event (such as final examinations in high-school students) enhances the airway inflammatory response to antigen. In one study psychological stress and airway inflammation following antigen challenge was evaluated during both a low- and a high-stress phase (final examination week) in 20 subjects with mild asthma. Anxiety and depression scores were significantly higher during the examination period, and markers of eosinophilic airway inflammation at 6 and 24 hours after antigen challenge were significantly increased during the high-stress phase.[116]

Our own observations also provide some evidence of a synergistic link between upper respiratory virus infections, personal NO_2 air pollutant exposure and the severity of asthma exacerbations. Asthma exacerbations were analyzed in relation to high versus low NO_2 exposures in the week prior to an upper respiratory viral infection in a cohort of asthmatic children followed for a year. There were significant increases in the severity of asthma symptoms, with 60% increased severity for all virus and >200% for RSV infections for high compared with low NO_2 exposure. The highest category of NO_2 exposure was also associated with more severe falls in PEF with virus infection. These effects were observed at levels within current air-quality standards.[13] The schematic role of the different trigger factors leading to an asthma exacerbation is given in Figure 6.5.

GENETIC SUSCEPTIBILITY TO ENVIRONMENTALLY TRIGGERED EXACERBATIONS

Gene–environment interactions are important in influencing the vulnerability of asthmatic individuals to environmental triggers. Both airway and alveolar epithelial cells are lined by fluids containing protective antioxidants, for example the glutathione *S*-transferase superfamily (GSFM1, GSTT1 and GSTP1). The GST enzymes have an important role in neutralizing reactive oxygen species, thus preventing oxidative stress. There are common variants of the four GST genes, of which some are associated with asthma. For example, in one study the GSTP1 genotype increased both the risk and the severity of respiratory infection in school-age

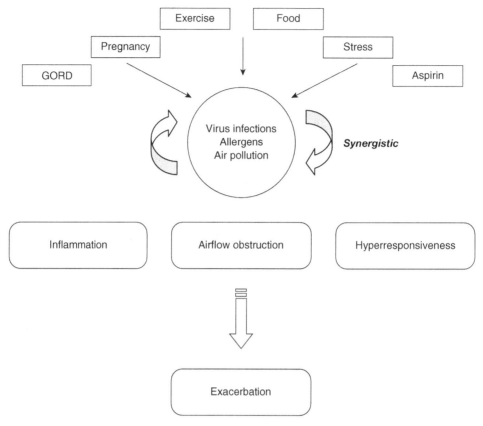

Figure 6.5 The synergistic role of trigger factors in asthmatic airway inflammation, airflow obstruction, bronchial hyperresponsiveness and exacerbations. GORD, gastroesophageal reflux disease

children, and another study has shown that GSTM1-deficient asthmatic children in Mexico City were more susceptible to small airway damage after O_3 exposure.[117]

GSTM1-deficient subjects also have a larger increase in IgE and histamine in nasal lavage fluid after challenge with diesel exhaust particles or allergen than children with a functional GSTM1 genotype. Other studies have also demonstrated that the '308 promoter' polymorphism of TNF-α increases the sensitivity of the airways to the bronchoconstrictor response to inhaled SO_2[118] and O_3.[119] In addition, supplementation of their diet with vitamin C (250 mg/day) and vitamin E is able to compensate for this genetic susceptibility. As the

ability of diesel exhaust particles to trigger allergic responses is repeatable and reproducible within individuals these findings support the view that genetic factors are important in determining individual sensitivity to air pollution and possibly infection, and the antioxidant status of the diet and the clinical manifestations of air pollutant injury in asthma are mediated through this mechanism.

SUMMARY

Exacerbations of asthma are common in children and adults with broadly similar etiologies (Table 6.1). The majority of exacerbations are

Table 6.1 The etiology of asthma exacerbations in adults and children

Factor	Adults	Children
Any virus	+++	+++
RSV	+	+++
Rhinovirus	+++	+++
hMPV	+	++
Coronavirus	++	++
Chlamydophila pneumoniae	++	+
Mycoplasma pneumoniae	++	+
Allergens	++	++
Air pollution	++	+++
Cigarette smoking	++	+++
Stress	++	++
Foods	+	++
Aspirin	+	+
Pregnancy	+	−
GORD	+	−
Exercise	+	+

RSV, respiratory syncytial virus; hMPV, human metapneumovirus; GORD, gastroesophageal reflux disease
'+', The putative strength of evidence implicating the factor in the pathogenesis and ability to trigger an exacerbation of asthma either in isolation or in interaction with other co-factors

characterized by upper respiratory viral infections, of which rhinoviruses are the most important in both children and adults. The abilities of environmental, personal and infective factors in triggering exacerbations are likely to be related to the severity of underlying airway inflammation, genetic susceptibility, an impaired innate immune response in asthma and a synergistic interaction between factors.

REFERENCES

1. Smart BA. Statistical Abstract of the United States 1996. Washington, DC: United States Bureau of the Census, 1996
2. Burt CW, Knapp DE. Ambulatory care visits for asthma in United States, 1993–1994. Adv Data 1996; 277: 1–3
3. Krahn MD, Berka C, Langlois P, et al. Direct and indirect costs of asthma in Canada 1990. Can Med Assoc J 1996; 154: 821–31
4. Mellis CM, Peat JK, Bauman AE, Woolcock AJ. The cost of asthma in New South Wales. Med J Aust 1991; 155: 522–8
5. Otero Gonzalez I, Blanco Aparicio M, Montero Martinez C. Características epidemiológicas de las exacerbaciones por EPOC y asma en un hospital general. Arch Bronconeumol 2002; 38: 256–62
6. Centers for Disease Control and Prevention C. Asthma mortality and hospitalization among children and adults, United States 1980–1993. Morbid Mortal Weekly Rep 1996; 45: 350–3
7. Weber EJ, Silverman RA, Callaham ML, et al. A prospective multicenter study of factors associated with hospital admission among adults with acute asthma. Am J Med 2002; 113: 371–8
8. AIA. Asthma Morbidity and Mortality Report: Lung and Asthma Information Agency. UK, 2006. Online access at http://www.laia.ac.uk/index.htm
9. Masoli M, Fabian D, Holt S, Beasley R. The Global Burden of Asthma: Executive Summary of the GINA Dissemination Committee Report: Global Initiative for Asthma (GINA) Program, 2005
10. Sly RM. Continuing decreases in asthma mortality in the United States. Ann Allergy Asthma Immunol 2004; 92: 313–18
11. Tattersfield AE, Postma DS, Barnes PJ, et al. Exacerbations of asthma: a descriptive study of 425 severe exacerbations. The FACET International Study Group. Am J Respir Crit Care Med 1999; 160: 594–9
12. Johnston SL, Pattemore PK, Sanderson G, et al. Community study of role of viral infections in exacerbations of asthma in 9–11 year old children [see comments]. BMJ 1995; 310: 1225–8
13. Chauhan AJ, Inskip HM, Linaker CH, et al. Personal exposure to nitrogen dioxide (NO_2) and the severity of virus-induced asthma in children. Lancet 2003; 361: 1939–44
14. Linaker CH, Coggon D, Holgate ST, et al. Personal exposure to nitrogen dioxide and risk of airflow obstruction in asthmatic children with upper respiratory infection. Thorax 2000; 55: 930–3
15. Corne JM, Marshall C, Smith S, et al. Frequency, severity, and duration of rhinovirus infections in asthmatic and nonasthmatic individuals: a longitudinal cohort study. Lancet 2002; 359: 831–4
16. Grissell TV, Powell H, Shafren DR, et al. Interleukin-10 gene expression in acute virus-induced asthma. Am J Respir Crit Care Med 2005; 172: 433–9
17. Wark PA, Johnston SL, Moric I, et al. Neutrophil degranulation and cell lysis is associated with clinical severity in virus-induced asthma. Eur Respir J 2002; 19: 68–75
18. Rakes GP, Arruda E, Ingram JM, et al. Rhinovirus and respiratory syncytial virus in wheezing children

requiring emergency care. IgE and eosinophil analyses. Am J Respir Crit Care Med 1999; 159: 785–90

19. Freymuth F, Vabret A, Brouard J, et al. Detection of viral, Chlamydia pneumoniae and Mycoplasma pneumoniae infections in exacerbations of asthma in children. J Clin Virol 1999; 13: 131–9

20. Wilkinson TMA, Hurst JR, Perera WR, et al. Effect of interactions between lower airway bacterial and rhinoviral infection in exacerbations of COPD. Chest 2006; 129: 317–24

21. Trautmann A, Schmid-Grendelmeier P, Kruger K, et al. T cells and eosinophils cooperate in the induction of bronchial epithelial cell apoptosis in asthma. J Allergy Clin Immunol 2002; 109: 329–37

22. Wark PA, Johnston SL, Bucchieri F, et al. Asthmatic bronchial epithelial cells have a deficient innate immune response to infection with rhinovirus. J Exp Med 2005; 201: 937–47

23. Brooks GD, Buchta KA, Swenson CA, et al. Rhinovirus-induced interferon-gamma and airway responsiveness in asthma. Am J Respir Crit Care Med 2003; 168: 1091–4

24. Papadopoulos NG, Stanciu LA, Papi A, et al. A defective type 1 response to rhinovirus in atopic asthma. Thorax 2002; 57: 328–32

25. Fraenkel DJ, Bardin PG, Sanderson G, et al. Lower airways inflammation during rhinovirus colds in normal and in asthmatic subjects. Am J Respir Crit Care Med 1995; 151: 879–86

26. Gern JE, Vrtis R, Grindle KA, et al. Relationship of upper and lower airway cytokines to outcome of experimental rhinovirus infection. Am J Respir Crit Care Med 2000; 162: 2226–31

27. Kahn JS. Human metapneumovirus: a newly emerging respiratory pathogen. Curr Opin Infect Dis 2003; 16: 255–8

28. Bastien N, Ward D, Van Caeseele P, et al. Human metapneumovirus infection in the Canadian population. J Clin Microbiol 2003; 41: 4642–6

29. Semple MG, Cowell A, Dove W, et al. Dual infection of infants by human metapneumovirus and human respiratory syncytial virus is strongly associated with severe bronchiolitis. J Infect Dis 2005; 191: 382–6

30. Lieberman D, Printz S, Ben-Yaakov M, et al. Atypical pathogen infection in adults with acute exacerbation of bronchial asthma. Am J Respir Crit Care Med 2003; 167: 406–10

31. Cunningham AF, Johnston SL, Julious SA, et al. Chronic Chlamydia pneumoniae infection and asthma exacerbations in children. Eur Respir J 1998; 11: 345–9

32. Thumerelle C, Deschildre A, Bouquillon C, et al. Role of viruses and atypical bacteria in exacerbations of asthma in hospitalized children: a prospective study in the Nord-Pas de Calais region (France). Pediatr Pulmonol 2003; 35: 75–82

33. Johnston SL, Martin RJ. Chlamydophila pneumoniae and Mycoplasma pneumoniae: a role in asthma pathogenesis? Am J Respir Crit Care Med 2005; 172: 1078–90

34. Johnston SL, Blasi F, Black PN, et al., TELICAST-Investigators. The effect of telithromycin in acute exacerbations of asthma. N Engl J Med 2006; 354: 1589–600

35. Custovic A, Taggart SC, Francis HC, et al. Exposure to house dust mite allergens and the clinical activity of asthma. J Allergy Clin Immunol 1996; 98: 64–72

36. Vervloet D, Charpin D, Haddi E, et al. Medication requirements and house dust mite exposure in mite-sensitive asthmatics. Allergy 1991; 46: 554–8

37. Tunnicliffe WS, Fletcher TJ, Hammond K, et al. Sensitivity and exposure to indoor allergens in adults with differing asthma severity. Eur Respir J 1999; 13: 654–9

38. Gelber LE, Seltzer LH, Bouzoukis JK, et al. Sensitization and exposure to indoor allergens as risk factors for asthma among patients presenting to hospital. Am Rev Respir Dis 1993; 147: 573–8

39. Nelson RPJ, DiNicolo R, Fernandez-Caldas E, et al. Allergen-specific IgE levels and mite allergen exposure in children with acute asthma first seen in an emergency department and in nonasthmatic control subjects. J Allergy Clin Immunol 1996; 98: 258–63

40. Rosas I, McCartney HA, Payne RW, et al. Analysis of the relationships between environmental factors (aeroallergens, air pollution, and weather) and asthma emergency admissions to a hospital in Mexico City. Allergy 1998; 53: 394–401

41. O'Hollaren MT, Yunginger JW, Offord KP, et al. Exposure to an aeroallergen as a possible precipitating factor in respiratory arrest in young patients with asthma. N Engl J Med 1991; 324: 359–63

42. Green RM, Custovic A, Sanderson G, et al. Synergism between allergens and viruses and risk of hospital admission with asthma: case–control study. BMJ 2002; 324: 763–7

43. Lemanske RF Jr, Dick EC, Swenson CA, et al. Rhinovirus upper respiratory infection increases airway hyperreactivity and late asthmatic reactions. J Clin Invest 1989; 83: 1–10

44. Van der Zee SC, Hoek G, Boezen HM, et al. Acute effects of urban air pollution on respiratory health of children with and without chronic respiratory symptoms. Occup Environ Med 1999; 56: 802–12

45. Buchdahl R, Parker A, Stebbings T, Babiker A. Association between air pollution and acute childhood wheezy episodes: prospective observational study [see comments]. BMJ 1996; 312: 661–5

46. Kesten S, Szalai J, Dzyngel B. Air quality and the frequency of emergency room visits for asthma. Ann Allergy Asthma Immunol 1995; 74: 269–73

47. Bates DV, Sizto R. Air pollution and hospital admissions in Southern Ontario: the acid summer haze effect. Environ Res 1987; 43: 317–31

48. Ponka A, Virtanen M. Chronic bronchitis, emphysema, and low-level air pollution in Helsinki, 1987–1989. Environ Res 1994; 65: 207–17

49. Anderson HR, Limb ES, Bland JM, et al. Health effects of an air pollution episode in London, December 1991. Thorax 1995; 50: 1188–93

50. Saldiva PH, Lichtenfels AJ, Paiva PS, et al. Association between air pollution and mortality due to respiratory diseases in children in Sao Paulo, Brazil: a preliminary report. Environ Res 1994; 65: 218–25

51. Braun-Fahrlander C, Ackermann-Liebrich U, Schwartz J, et al. Air pollution and respiratory symptoms in preschool children. Am Rev Respir Dis 1992; 145: 42–7

52. Mukala K, Pekkanen J, Tiittanen P, et al. Seasonal exposure to NO2 and respiratory symptoms in preschool children. J Exposure Anal Environ Epidemiol 1996; 6: 197–210

53. Frischer T, Studnicka M, Beer E, Neumann M. The effects of ambient NO$_2$ on lung function in primary schoolchildren. Environ Res 1993; 62: 179–88

54. Scarlett JF, Abbott KJ, Peacock JL, et al. Acute effects of summer air pollution on respiratory function in primary school children in southern England. Thorax 1996; 51: 1109–14

55. Advisory Group on the Med Aspects of Air Pollution Episodes. Oxides of Nitrogen (3rd Report). London: Department of Health, 1993: 29–49

56. Katsouyanni K, Touloumi G, Spix C, et al. Short-term effects of ambient sulphur dioxide and particulate matter on mortality in 12 European cities: results from time series data from the APHEA project. Air Pollution and Health: a European Approach. Br Med J 1997; 314: 1658–63

57. Spix C, Anderson HR, Schwartz J, et al. Short-term effects of air pollution on hospital admissions of respiratory diseases in Europe: a quantitative summary of APHEA study results. Air Pollution and Health: a European Approach. Arch Environ Health 1998; 53: 54–64

58. Ponka A, Virtanen M. Asthma and ambient air pollution in Helsinki. J Epidemiol Commun Health 1996; 50: s59–62

59. Touloumi G, Katsouyanni K, Zmirou D, et al. Short-term effects of ambient oxidant exposure on mortality: a combined analysis within the APHEA project. Air Pollution and Health: a European Approach. Am J Epidemiol 1997; 146: 177–85

60. Sunyer J, Spix C, Quenel P, et al. Urban air pollution and emergency admissions for asthma in four European cities: the APHEA Project. Thorax 1997; 52: 760–5

61. Hasselblad V, Eddy DM, Kotchmar DJ. Synthesis of environmental evidence: nitrogen dioxide epidemiology studies. J Air Waste Manage Assoc 1992; 42: 662–71

62. Li Y, Powers TE, Roth HD. Random-effects linear regression meta-analysis models with application to the nitrogen dioxide health effects studies. J Air Waste Manage Assoc 1994; 44: 261–70

63. Ostro BD, Lipsett M, Mann JK, et al. Indoor air pollution and asthma. Am J Respir Crit Care Med 1994; 149: 1400–6

64. Chauhan AJ, Krishna MT, Frew AJ, Holgate ST. Exposure to nitrogen dioxide (NO$_2$) and respiratory disease risk. Rev Environ Health 1998; 13: 73–90

65. Dockery DW, Pope ACd, Xu X, et al. An association between air pollution and mortality in six U.S. cities [see comments]. N Engl J Med 1993; 329: 1753–9

66. Schwartz J, Slater D, Larson TV, et al. Particulate air pollution and hospital emergency room visits for asthma in Seattle. Am Rev Respir Dis 1993; 147: 826–31

67. Rennick GJ, Jarman FC. Are children with asthma affected by smog? Med J Aust 1992; 156: 837–41

68. Delfino RJ, Becklake MR, Hanley JA. The relationship of urgent hospital admissions for respiratory illnesses to photochemical air pollution levels in Montreal. Environ Res 1994; 67: 1–19

69. Chauhan AJ, Johnston SL. Air pollution and infection in respiratory illness. Br Med Bull 2003; 68: 95–112

70. Beeber SJ. Parental smoking and childhood asthma. J Pediatr Health Care 1996; 10: 58–62

71. Soussan D, Liard R, Zureik M, et al. Treatment compliance, passive smoking, and asthma control: a three year cohort study. Arch Dis Child 2003; 88: 229–33

72. Chilmonczyk BA, Salmun LM, Megathlin KN, et al. Association between exposure to environmental tobacco smoke and exacerbations of asthma in children. N Engl J Med 1993; 328: 1665–9

73. Lewis S, Richards D, Bynner J, et al. Prospective study of risk factors for early and persistent wheezing in childhood. Eur Respir J 1995; 8: 349–56

74. Chalmers GW, Macleod KJ, Little SA, et al. Influence of cigarette smoking on inhaled corticosteroid treatment in mild asthma. Thorax 2002; 57: 226–30

75. Silverman RA, Boudreaux ED, Woodruff PG, et al. Cigarette smoking among asthmatic adults presenting to 64 emergency departments. Chest 2003; 123: 1472–9

76. Thomson NC, Chaudhuri R, Livingston E. Asthma and cigarette smoking. Eur Respir J 2004; 24: 822–33

77. Cassino C, Ito K, Bader I, et al. Cigarette smoking and ozone-associated emergency department use for asthma by adults in New York City. Am J Respir Crit Care Med 1999; 159: 1773–9

78. Mitchell I, Tough SC, Semple LK, et al. Near-fatal asthma: a population-based study of risk factors. Chest 2002; 121: 1407–13

79. Jindal S, Gupta D, Singh A. Indices of morbidity and control of asthma in adult patients exposed to environmental tobacco smoke. Chest 1994; 106: 746–9

80. Eisner MD. Environmental tobacco smoke exposure and pulmonary function among adults in NHANES III: impact on the general population and adults with

current asthma. Environ Health Perspect 2002; 110: 765–70

81. Chen R, Tunstall-Pedoe H, Tavendale R. Environmental tobacco smoke and lung function in employees who never smoked: the Scottish MONICA study. Occup Environ Med 2001; 58: 563–8

82. Smith CJ, Bombick DW, Ryan BA, et al. Pulmonary function in nonsmokers following exposure to sidestream cigarette smoke. Toxicol Pathol 2001; 29: 260–4

83. Jaakkola MS, Piipari R, Jaakkola N, Jaakkola J. Environmental tobacco smoke and adult-onset asthma: a population-based incident case–control study. Am J Public Health 2003; 93: 2055–60

84. Isenberg SA, Lehrer PM, Hochron SM. The effects of suggestion and emotional arousal on pulmonary function in asthma: a review and a hypothesis regarding vagal mediation. Psychosom Med 1992; 54: 192–216

85. Lehrer PM, Isenberg S, Hochron SM. Asthma and emotion: a review. J Asthma 1993; 30: 5–21

86. Beggs PJ, Curson PH. An integrated environmental asthma model. Arch Environ Health 1995; 50: 87–94

87. Kolbe J, Garrett J, Vamos M, Rea HH. Influences on trends in asthma morbidity and mortality: the New Zealand experience. Chest 1994; 106: 211S–15S

88. Busse WW, Kiecolt-Glaser JK, Coe C, et al. NHLBI Workshop summary: stress and asthma. Am J Crit Care Med 1995; 151: 249–52

89. Miller BD. Depression and asthma: a potentially lethal mixture. J Allergy Clin Immunol 1987; 80: 481–6

90. Sandberg S, Paton JY, Ahola S, et al. The role of acute and chronic stress in asthma attacks in children [see comment]. Lancet 2000; 356: 982–7

91. Schmaling KB, McKnight PE, Afari N. A prospective study of the relationship of mood and stress to pulmonary function among patients with asthma. J Asthma 2002; 39: 501–10

92. Chen E, Fisher EB, Bacharier LB, Strunk RC. Socioeconomic status, stress, and immune markers in adolescents with asthma. Psychosom Med 2003; 65: 984–92

93. Cydulka RK, Emerman CL. Adrenal function and physiologic stress during acute asthma exacerbation. Ann Emerg Med 1998; 31: 558–61

94. Miller GE, Chen E. Life stress and diminished expression of genes encoding glucocorticoid receptor and β_2-adrenergic receptor in children with asthma. Proc Natl Acad Sci USA 2006; 103: 5496–501

95. Hill DJ, Firer MA, Shelton MJ, Hosking CS. Manifestations of milk allergy in asthmatic children. J Paediatr 1986; 109: 270–6

96. Dawson KP, Ford RPK, Mogridge N. Childhood asthma: what do parents add or avoid in their children's diets? NZ Med J 1990; 103: 239–40

97. Woods RK, Abramson M, Raven JM, et al. Reported food intolerance and respiratory symptoms in young adults. Eur Respir J 1998; 11: 151–5

98. Bock SA, Aitkens FM. Patterns of food hypersensitivity during sixteen years of double-blind placebo controlled food challenges. J Paediatr 1990; 117: 561–7

99. Jenkins C, Costello J, Hodge L. Systematic review of prevalence of aspirin induced asthma and its implications for clinical practice. BMJ 2004; 328: 434–41

100. Schatz M. Asthma and pregnancy. Lancet 1999; 353: 1202–4

101. Namazy JA, Schatz M. Pregnancy and asthma: recent developments. Curr Opin Pulm Med 2005; 11: 56–60

102. Stenius-Aarniala BS, Hedman J, Teramo KA. Acute asthma during pregnancy. Thorax 1996; 51: 411–14

103. Murphy VE, Gibson PG, Talbot PI, Clifton VL. Severe asthma exacerbations during pregnancy. Obstet Gynecol 2005; 106: 1046–54

104. Harding SM, Guzzo MR, Richter JE. 24-hr esophageal pH testing in asthmatics: respiratory symptom correlation with esophageal acid events. Chest 1999; 115: 654–9

105. Harding SM, Richter JE, Guzzo MR, et al. Asthma and gastroesophageal, reflux: acid suppressive therapy improves asthma outcome. Am J Med 1996; 100: 395–405

106. Kiljander TO, Salomaa ER, Hietanen EK, Terho EO. Gastroesophageal reflux in asthmatics: a double-blind, placebo-controlled crossover study with omeprazole. Chest 1999; 116: 1257–64

107. Coughlan JL, Gibson PG, Henry RL. Medical treatment for reflux oesophagitis does not consistently improve asthma control: a systematic review. Thorax 2001; 56: 198–204

108. Murray CS, Poletti G, Kebadze T, et al. A study of modifiable risk factors for asthma exacerbations: virus infection and allergen exposure synergistically increase risk of asthma hospitalization in children. Thorax 2006; 61: 376–82

109. Castellsague J, Sunyer J, Salz M, et al. Effect of air pollution in asthma epidemics caused by soya bean dust [Abstract]. Eur Respir J 1992; 15: 413S

110. Packe GE, Ayres JG. Asthma outbreak during a thunderstorm. Lancet 1985; 2: 199–204

111. Higham J, Venables K, Kopek E, Bajekal M. Asthma and thunderstorms: description of an epidemic in general practice in Britain using data from a doctors' deputising service in the UK. J Epidemiol Community Health 1997; 51: 233–8

112. Bellomo R, Gigliotti P, Treloar A, et al. Two consecutive thunderstorm associated epidemics of asthma in the city of Melbourne. The possible role of rye grass pollen. Med J Aust 1992; 156: 834–7

113. Knox RB, Suphioglu C, Taylor P, et al. Major grass pollen allergen Lol p 1 binds to diesel exhaust

particles: implications for asthma and air pollution. Clin Exp Allergy 1997; 27: 246–51

114. Tunnicliffe WS, Burge PS, Ayres JG. Effect of domestic concentrations of nitrogen dioxide on airway responses to inhaled allergen in asthmatic patients. Lancet 1994; 344: 1733–6

115. Devalia JL, Rusznak C, Herdman MJ, et al. Effect of nitrogen dioxide and sulphur dioxide on airway response of mild asthmatic patients to allergen inhalation. Lancet 1994; 344: 1668–71

116. Liu LY, Coe CL, Swenson CA, et al. School examinations enhance airway inflammation to antigen challenge. Am J Respir Crit Care Med 2002; 165: 1062–7

117. Romieu I, Sienra-Monge JJ, Ramirez-Aguilar M, et al. Genetic polymorphism of GSTM1 and antioxidant supplementation influence lung function in relation to ozone exposure in asthmatic children in Mexico City. Thorax 2004; 59: 8–10

118. Winterton DL, Kaufman J, Keener CV, et al. Genetic polymorphisms as biomarkers of sensitivity to inhaled sulfur dioxide in subjects with asthma. Ann Allergy Asthma Immunol 2001; 86: 232–8

119. Bergamaschi E, De Palma G, Mozzoni P, et al. Polymorphism of quinone-metabolizing enzymes and susceptibility to ozone-induced acute effects. Am J Crit Care Med 2001; 163: 1426–31

CHAPTER 7

Modes of transmission of respiratory viral infections

M Patricia Fabian, James J McDevitt and Donald K Milton

RELATIONSHIP BETWEEN VIRAL RESPIRATORY DISEASES AND ASTHMA

Respiratory viruses are one of the most common causes of infectious disease and have a wide range of health effects, from mild symptoms to life-threatening diseases.[1] Most respiratory viruses spread rapidly through communities via person-to-person transmission, particularly in crowded indoor environments such as schools. The cost of viral infections includes decreased productivity and time lost from work or school, visits to health-care providers and purchase of pharmaceuticals.[2] A recent report estimated that 500 million episodes of viral respiratory infections (VRI) occur annually in the USA resulting in $16.8 billion in direct costs and $7.6 billion in indirect costs for employed individuals.[3] Data from a 1996 survey conducted by the Centres for Disease Control (CDC) reported that respiratory infections resulted in 148 million days of restricted activity, nearly 20 million days of missed work, 22 million days of missed school and 45 million bedridden days.[4]

The association between infection with respiratory viruses and asthma exacerbation in children and adult populations has been reviewed by multiple authors[5–9] and is considered elsewhere in this volume. Infections with the viral pathogens shown in Table 7.1 have been associated with increased morbidity and mortality due to exacerbation of asthma and may be the most important triggers of asthma and wheezing in children. Respiratory viral infections caused by parainfluenza,[10,11] influenza,[10,11] human rhinovirus,[10–13] human metapneumovirus,[14,15] adenovirus[16] and coronavirus[10,11] have been shown to be associated with asthma exacerbations. Respiratory syncytial virus (RSV) infection may cause exacerbations among persons with pre-existing asthma and may also increase the risk of developing asthma for children in whom early life infection is severe and involves bronchiolitis.[17,18] Human metapneumovirus may also be associated with bronchiolitis.[12] Given that asthma prevalence has increased in recent decades[19,20] and that more than 75% of asthma exacerbations in both adults and children are associated with respiratory viral infections,[5,11] understanding modes of virus transmission is important not only for prevention of severe viral illnesses such as influenza, but also for reduction of asthma-related morbidity and mortality associated with viral infections.

MODES OF TRANSMISSION

The primary mode of transmission of respiratory viruses has often been debated. Transmission routes are often difficult to identify definitively because many factors are involved, including variable survival on surfaces and in

Table 7.1 Viruses associated with asthma exacerbations and their characteristics

Name	Family	Envelope	Size (nm)
Respiratory syncytial virus	Paramyxoviridae	Yes	120–300
Parainfluenza	Paramyxoviridae	Yes	150–300
Influenza	Orthomyxoviridae	Yes	80–120
Rhinovirus	Picornaviridae	No	27
Human metapneumovirus	Paramyxoviridae	Yes	150–300
Adenovirus	Adenoviridae	No	65–80
Coronavirus	Coronaviridae	Yes	80–120

Adapted from reference 9

air, dependent on characteristics of the virus and environmental conditions, aerosol generation, host susceptibility and regional expression of receptors,[21,22] and because multiple routes may be important for some viruses.

There are no known environmental reservoirs where common respiratory viruses survive for months or years. Therefore, the transmission of viral infection begins with shedding of infectious virus by an infected person. Respiratory viruses are shed primarily in nasal and oral secretions or by generation of virus-containing droplets from respiratory tract fluids. However, some respiratory viruses may also be shed in urine and feces; it appears that in certain instances SARS Co-V was transmitted by aerosolized fecal material.[23,24] The routes of transmission for respiratory viruses include a continuum from direct contact to transmission by airborne droplet nuclei and contact with contaminated objects. Direct contact between mucosal surfaces and viral deposition onto the oral, nasal or ocular mucosa by a direct hit with a large droplet (> 10–100 μm diameter), released with sufficient momentum to reach the susceptible host, may be considered one end of this continuum. These routes require close proximity; large-droplet spray can be considered an extension of direct contact. However, droplets of respiratory fluid evaporate quickly, lose most of their mass within seconds and produce droplet nuclei.[25] The resulting droplet nuclei do not have sufficient momentum to be carried directly from the infected to the susceptible host. They are true aerosols, wafted on air currents, and can be a

vehicle of contact between a source and susceptible host at both short and longer distances – depending on survival of the virus and dilution by ventilation. Respiratory viruses may also be transmitted via hand-to-hand contact and intermediate contact with inanimate objects (fomites) prior to autoinoculation by the fingers of the susceptible host placed on the upper respiratory or ocular mucosa, again dependent on survival of the virus on the contaminated surface.

Discrimination between the various modes of transmission has been difficult for several reasons. First, the concentration of infectious particles in air required to transmit infection is very low – thus it can be very difficult to detect them and prove that the particles exist.[25] Second, the nature of human source aerosols and their dissemination has not been well understood or widely appreciated. Recent advances in measuring and analyzing aerosols generated by the human respiratory tract may lead to a clearer understanding of the role of airborne transmission in respiratory infections.

Most previous work on human source aerosols focused on generation of aerosols from the upper respiratory mucosa[25] and used techniques generally insensitive to particles less than 1.0 μm in diameter. Early studies found that as many as 40 000 droplets are generated during a sneeze, about one order of magnitude more than coughing and two to four orders more than when talking loudly.[26] Most of the particles detected were less than 4 μm.[27,28] Very few particles were thought to be liberated during quiet breathing,[25] and there were few data to suggest interindividual differences in generation of aerosols during coughing, sneezing or talking. Thus, the 'disseminator' or 'super-spreader' phenomenon was difficult to explain as it was not clearly associated with disease severity, especially for certain viral infections where the patient was contagious prior to clinical illness (e.g. measles). Edwards and colleagues,[29] however, have recently shown that large numbers of particles are generated by the human respiratory system during quiet mouth breathing. Using laser light scattering to detect particles of ≥ 150 nm, they observed a bimodal distribution of production rates. Six of 11 volunteers consistently exhaled an average of >500 particles per liter over 6 hours, up to 3230 particles per liter, during quiet breathing. The remaining five volunteers produced from 14 to 71 particles per liter. Integrated over time, the 'high-producers' liberated 5000–32 000 particles per minute, greater numbers than those reported in the early studies of coughing and sneezing. A major factor in the detection of these large numbers of particles may be the use of instruments sensitive to smaller particles than could be detected in the early studies; most of the particles observed were $<1.0\,\mu m$ in diameter. The mechanism by which these submicron droplet nuclei are generated is not known. Microdroplets formed by bursting films of respiratory fluid during inhalation are a possible mechanism for generation of these human-source nanoparticles. Further research is needed to identify mechanisms of generation, to characterize particle production during nose breathing and to determine whether the phenomenon of particle high-producers can account for the occurrence of super-spreaders of certain respiratory infections such as SARS, measles and influenza.

Riley and O'Grady[25] characterized airborne exposure to pathogens as occurring in two distinct modes: either organisms in 'dust', using the word in the sense that Wells had[30] to mean large particles with high settling velocities resuspended from environmental reservoirs, or organisms carried in droplet nuclei, resulting from the desiccation of larger droplets to produce aerosol particles that remained suspended for many minutes to hours. For tuberculosis, experimental studies in animals exposed to artificial aerosols demonstrated that only small aerosol particles able to reach the distal air spaces were capable of transmitting infection. This is a consequence of the unique suitability of the alveolus and the alveolar macrophage as susceptible environments for growth of *Mycobacterium tuberculosis*. Thus, tuberculosis may be classified as an obligate airborne transmitted infection. Many respiratory viruses can initiate infection in other tissues including upper respiratory mucosa so that larger particles ('dust', large droplets or resuspended organisms attached to skin scales) and sometimes fomites are capable of transmitting infection, e.g. human rhinovirus and RSV. Viruses in this category can use any of these routes depending on the environment, and many respiratory viral infections may be classified as opportunistic airborne transmitted infections when there is evidence of transmission by droplet nuclei. Certain respiratory viruses, such as some strains of adenoviruses,[31] may not be capable of efficiently initiating infection and disease except in the lower respiratory tract, and may therefore be considered obligate airborne transmitted infections.

Once expelled from an infected source, the potential for subsequent infections in other individuals is a function of the removal of the virus from the environment due to physical decay of the aerosol and biological decay of the virus in the aerosol or on surfaces. The size of the virus-laden aerosol greatly influences the fate of the particle in air. Smaller particles can remain suspended in the air for long periods of time, and thereby increase the probability of being inhaled and causing infection. The size of an aerosol is typically described by the particles' aerodynamic equivalent diameter (AED). The AED of a particle is the diameter of a unit density sphere ($1\,g/cm^3$) which has the same settling velocity as that particle. The terminal

Table 7.2 Settling velocities calculated for particles in still air

Particle aerodynamic diameter*	Settling velocity (cm/s)	Settling time, 2-meter
1	0.003	18.5 hours
2.5	0.019	3.0 hours
5	0.075	44 minutes
10	0.3	11 minutes
100	30	6.7 seconds

*Unit density sphere in still air

settling velocity, the resultant vector of the force of gravity and drag forces, is higher for droplets with large AEDs and results in short residence times in the air. Droplet nuclei have very low settling velocities and small AEDs and can remain airborne for long periods of time. Settling velocities for some aerosol particles in still air are shown in Table 7.2.[32] Large droplets (>10 μm) typically settle out of the air very quickly, limiting their impact to people in close proximity to the generator.[28] However, depending on environmental conditions (e.g. temperature and relative humidity) larger particles can quickly evaporate to become droplet nuclei (<5 μm) that can stay suspended in the air for long periods of time.[33,34] Wells suggested that particles as large as 100 μm could evaporate to become droplet nuclei,[35] although 15–20 μm is a more probable upper limit on the size for this phenomenon. A large starting volume may result in relatively large numbers of virions per droplet nucleus compared with the number of virions contained in the exhaled nanoparticles described above. Whether a greater infection risk is generated by a smaller number of intermittently exhaled particles containing large numbers of virions per particle or a larger number of constantly exhaled nanoparticles containing fewer virions per particle is likely to depend on the infectiousness of the virus and its ability to survive evaporation and concentration of other solutes in the droplet nucleus.

Thus, infectiousness of the resulting aerosol is likely to vary depending on the virus and environmental conditions.

The relative humidity of the air plays a part in changing the size of aerosolized particles. The relationship between relative humidity and particle size is complex, owing to the dynamic nature of liquid aerosols. Particles produced from the saturated environment of the respiratory tract will lose moisture and shrink in size when expired into the ambient air. Similarly, when hydroscopic particles are inhaled from ambient air they will increase in size due to the addition of moisture from the respiratory tract. As a result, infectious aerosols are likely to exhibit dynamic particle sizes and their deposition characteristics may not be accurately predicted by their behavior in room air.

Upon exhalation large droplets will quickly settle and therefore will have little opportunity for transport from the source of generation. Reception of large droplets will therefore be limited to persons very close to the generator[28] or be subject to indirect transmission through fomites. Persons in this so-called 'near field' may potentially be exposed to the droplet by direct deposition into the upper respiratory tract or ocular membranes. Persons in the near field may also inhale the droplet prior to its settling, as well as being subject to physical contact with the droplet on their person with subsequent autoinoculation. Owing to their short residence time in air, large droplets are not subject to ventilation factors such as dilution, transport and removal, which play an important role in determining the fate of fine particles in air. Droplets which settle out of the air may become re-entrained when subject to sweeping or high-velocity air streams, but may have limited capacity for establishing infection due to loss of viability on surfaces.

The 'near field' may also contain higher concentrations of exhaled droplet nuclei. The infectious aerosol particle concentration in the near field will be most concentrated since droplets' nuclei have not had an opportunity to be diluted by ventilation. If the rate of generation of infectious droplet nuclei is low, air is poorly mixed, the biological decay of infectiousness is rapid and ventilation does not carry the aerosol into other occupied spaces, then risk of infection may be largely confined to the near field, giving rise to an impression that prolonged face-to-face exposure is required for transmission. It is important to recognize that this observation may not be a reliable indicator of the mode of transmission. Application of computational fluid dynamics may allow more accurate identification of risks of infection based on patterns of non-uniform air mixing and convection around room occupants, allowing discrimination between deposition on exposed mucosal surfaces and inhalation.[36]

It is also important to consider the dose required to initiate infection. A person with a tidal volume of 10 liters per minute will 'sample' more than $14 \, m^3$ of air per day. If there is one infectious dose in that large volume of air, the probability that a person breathing that air volume would not receive an infectious dose is described by a Poisson distribution and is $e^{-1} = 0.37$ (i.e. the probability of infection would be $1 - e^{-1} = 0.63$), assuming that infection is ultimately initiated by a single particle as seems to be the case for tuberculosis and measles.[25,37] Thus, one can appreciate the difficulty in detecting that small dose by the usual small-volume sampling devices. This also implies that lowering the concentration of infectious particles via ventilation is a difficult task requiring vast and usually impractical amounts of dilution ventilation. This realization led to the interest in use of upper-room germicidal ultraviolet (UVC) lights for continuous sterilization of large volumes of air.[38,39] The well-known decline in both respiratory infections and asthma exacerbations during the summer (Figure 7.1) could be an indication that a large portion of the respiratory infection burden is driven by airborne transmission, mitigated in summer months by large amounts of ventilation via open windows.[25] However, because this trough in infection and exacerbation is coincident with school vacations, it cannot be considered strong evidence for the route of transmission.[40]

Virus stability in the environment plays an important role in transmission with respect to biological decay. Virus survival in the environment is dependent on factors such as virus type, temperature, relative humidity, ultraviolet radiation and deposition surface. Non-enveloped viruses are much more resistant to environmental degradation than enveloped viruses.[41] The lipid layer on enveloped viruses is easily destroyed, thus inactivating the virus since it cannot bind to target cells. Relative humidity of the air plays a part both in changing the size of aerosolized particles and in influencing the viability of particles in the air. Low relative humidity was believed to contribute to an outbreak of measles in a physician's office.[42] In controlled laboratory experiments airborne influenza A and vaccinia viruses were found to survive best at low relative humidity (17–25%),[43] rotavirus SA11 at medium relative humidity (50±5%),[44] human coronavirus at medium relative humidity (50%)[45] and rhinovirus at high relative humidity (80±5%).[46] At optimal relative humidity, all viruses remained culturable for over 24 hours, the rotavirus remaining viable for over 9 days. Once deposited, the deposition surface type plays an important role in virus survival. RSV has been shown to survive for up to 6 hours on smooth countertops, but survives for periods of only 20–30 minutes on cloth gowns or paper tissue.[47] On hard non-porous environmental surfaces influenza viruses A and B have been found to survive and remain infectious for 24–48 hours, on cloth, paper and tissues for less than 8–12 hours and on hands after transfer from environmental surfaces for around 5 minutes.[48] Parainfluenza virus was shown to survive for at least 7 days in an open plastic dish at room temperature.[49] Viruses are also subject to inactivation by ultraviolet radiation[50,51] and possibly visible light.[52] Jensen showed that germicidal ultraviolet radiation (254 nm) inactivated more than 99.9% of vaccinia and other viruses with exposure periods of less than 1 second;[53] unfortunately, the dose delivered cannot be accurately determined from these data. The

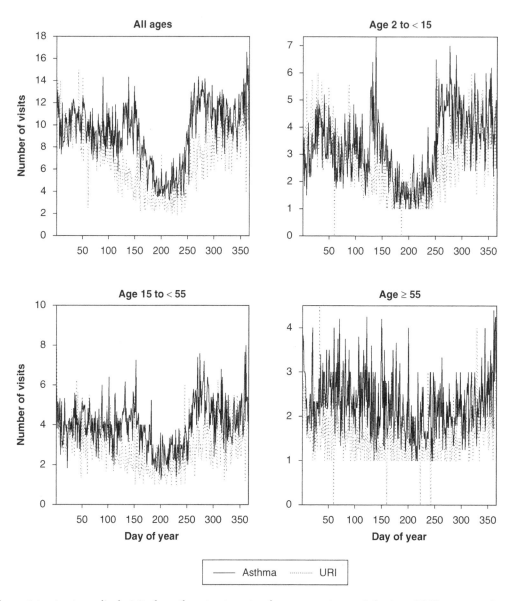

Figure 7.1 Acute medical visits for asthma treatment and upper respiratory infections (URI) among asthmatics with at least one acute asthma intervention during the period 1 January 1999 and 30 June 2004 at the Fallon Community Health Plan, Worcester, MA, by age group

various environmental factors act together and the resultant outcome will determine the probability of survival.

Viruses deposited in the respiratory tract must adhere to cell surfaces and enter susceptible cells to initiate infection. Most virus attachment and entry is mediated by binding to specific receptor and/or co-receptor molecules located on the cell surface.[54] Therefore, virus particles must be deposited in regions with corresponding receptors to establish infection. If appropriate receptors are not present at the site of deposition, they may be encountered during clearance from the site of deposition. Thus, if a virus particle is inhaled and deposited within the respiratory tract, infection may not occur if the appropriate cell type and receptor is not present at the sight of deposition or along the avenue of clearance. In addition, the virus must be able to evade the host immune systems successfully. Hall and Douglas showed that the site of inoculation of respiratory syncytial virus played a role in the establishment of infection. Inoculation of RSV solutions into the eye and nose caused infection, while inoculation of the mouth did not.[55] A study by Mills et al.[56] suggested that there was more efficient infection of RSV when nebulized virus was administered via an intranasal route. Human rhinovirus (HRV) can infect cells of both the upper and lower airways.[57] Thus, the portal of entry, dose and site of deposition (form of inocula) play a role in the initiation of infection.

EVIDENCE FOR TRANSMISSION OF THREE SPECIFIC INFECTIOUS AGENTS

The three most studied viruses in explaining modes of transmission are RSV, rhinovirus and influenza. The first of these appears to be primarily direct contact-transmitted; the second is likely to have mixed modes and is the subject of a longstanding controversy regarding its predominant modes of transmission; and the last is reasonably well established as being transmitted by airborne droplet nuclei. Following is a summary of the evidence for transmission of these three infectious agents.

Respiratory syncytial virus

RSV infection causes acute respiratory illness in patients of all ages and produces bronchiolitis in infants.[7] The majority of the studies of RSV transmission have focused on nosocomial infection in infants. RSV is widely believed to be transmitted by contact. This conclusion is supported by studies showing that RSV can survive for up to 6 hours on fomites,[47] that the eyes and nose are sensitive routes for RSV infection[58] and that the use of gloves and gowns was effective in preventing infection in the presence of increased compliance. A hand-washing and education campaign targeted at staff and parents reduced hospital-acquired RSV infection in children, from 4.2% to 0.6%.[59] Other authors have also shown that the use of protective equipment decreased the rate of RSV infections.[60–62] Gala et al. found that hospital-acquired RSV infection increased from 5% (staff) and 6% (children) to 34% (staff) and 43% (children) after nurses stopped using goggles.[60]

Hall and Douglas[58] studied the transmission of RSV from infected infants to caregivers who were categorized as 'cuddlers' in direct contact with infants (five of seven infected), 'touchers' in contact with RSV-contaminated surfaces but not directly with the infants (four of ten infected) and 'sitters' without direct or indirect contact via room surfaces who sat 6 feet from infants (none of 14 infected). This study strongly suggests that direct and indirect contact were the primary modes of transmission. Unfortunately, no information was reported about the room layout, ventilation rates or air mixing patterns, and no air monitoring was performed. Thus, we cannot conclusively eliminate the possibility that a combination of low rates of infectious particle generation and uneven ventilation and air mixing skewed the results. There are some data regarding RSV aerosols in children's hospital rooms. Aintablian et al. detected the presence of RSV by air sampling and polymerase chain reaction (PCR) analysis in 63% of rooms containing children with RSV infection.[63] Nucleic acid from RSV was detected as far as 21 feet from patient beds. Although the presence of nucleic acid does not necessarily prove the existence of infectious virus, it does indicate the possibility of airborne transmission of RSV. Since viable virus monitoring was not performed as part of this study, no correlation studies between positive

PCR results and airborne infection were possible. This raises the possibility that residual transmission in the studies of personal protective equipment may have been due to airborne transmission. However, the weight of the evidence favors direct contact and fomites as the primary mode of transmission.

Human rhinovirus

There are two groups that have intensively studied the modes of HRV transmission and they reached opposite conclusions. Their work was recently reviewed by Goldmann[64] and re-evaluated in light of new mathematical models for estimating the risk of airborne infection.[65] The group from Virginia reported that direct contact and fomites were the primary modes of transmission, while the group from Wisconsin reported that HRV was primarily transmitted via droplets or airborne droplet nuclei.

One point of contention has been survival of HRV on hands. Ansari et al. found that HRV could survive on hands for at least 20 minutes,[66] consistent with the earlier data from the Virginia group that HRV could be isolated from the hands of 39% of study subjects with cold symptoms, and that volunteers whose hands were intentionally contaminated with HRV could become infected after self-inoculation of their eyes or nose.[67] Later, blinded, controlled experiments found that regularly treating fingers with iodine decreased transmission.[68] The most often cited experiments carried out by the Virginia group[69] involved intranasally infected students used to expose three groups of susceptible students via direct contact, large droplets and droplet nuclei:

(1) Direct contact: infected donors contaminated their hands with nasal secretions which the recipients then rubbed with their hands. The recipients then rubbed their eyes and put their fingers in their noses. Both donors and recipients wore masks during contact.

(2) Large droplets: one donor and four recipients sat around a table. The donor sang, coughed and sneezed for 15 minutes. Both donor and recipients wore gloves during the experiment.

(3) Droplet nuclei: one donor and one or two recipients were housed together for 3 days in a large room separated by a wire mesh to limit contact and large-droplet transmission.

In the direct hand contact/self-inoculation group 11 of 15 recipients became infected; in the large droplet group one of 12 recipients became infected and in the droplet nuclei group none of 10 recipients were infected. The authors concluded that transmission was mainly via the contact route, with large droplets playing a small role and droplet nuclei not playing a role at all. A recent analysis by Myatt et al.[65] found that the power to detect infection in the small-particle aerosol experiment was very low, particularly if the infectious particle generation rate was low; thus airborne infection could not be rejected.

The Wisconsin group performed a similarly convincing series of experiments with very different results. They also used students intranasally infected with HRV. They found that very long duration of exposures (hundreds of hours) in poorly ventilated rooms was required to reliably transmit infection.[70] They therefore considered that the Virginia group had not exposed subjects for long enough to rule out airborne transmissions, consistent with the recent mathematical model. They then performed a series of experiments in which 24 donors and 36 recipients played 12-hour poker games.[71] Half the recipients were restrained from touching their faces using an arm brace or shield. They found that the attack rates were 56% and 67% in restrained and unrestrained volunteers, respectively, and concluded that airborne transmission was the only way to account for similar attack rates in the groups. Another group of 12 susceptible student recipients played cards in a separate room with chips and cards heavily contaminated with secretions from the first experiments. The recipients were encouraged to touch their face and put their fingers in their noses. None of the recipients became ill, supporting their initial conclusion that airborne transmission dominates HRV transmission. These results with fomites and those from direct contact and fomites by the Virginia group are difficult to reconcile. One suggestion is that the Virginia group exposed volunteers to fresher, still wet secretions[64] 'by volunteers who essentially blew their noses into their hands' immediately before contact. One peculiar result from the Wisconsin group, however, was the finding that virucidal facial tissues were effective in preventing transmission of HRV infection.[72] In this experiment, face covering during coughing, sneezing, as well as nose blowing was strictly enforced during the intervention with the virucidal tissues. These measures were not enforced during the control periods when cloth handkerchiefs were used. It is difficult to understand why the virucidal properties of the cloth or tissue would matter here. It seems more likely that the enforced face covering was the effective element. Given that this intervention would have decreased large droplet spray and droplet nuclei from coughs and sneezes, but not have had much effect on microdroplets and their submicron droplet nuclei generated during quiet breathing, this experiment may suggest that the latter, recently described phenomenon is not significantly involved in transmission of HRV. Future studies with greater attention to ventilation rates, exposure times, relative humidity and other factors involved in biological decay in air and on surfaces, and realistic exposure to fomites and hands of infected donors, will be required to define the relative importance of contact and airborne modes of HRV transmission. At present it seems prudent to assume that both modes play a role.

Human influenza virus

Both epidemiology and animal models suggest that influenza is primarily transmitted via the airborne route, although the fomite and direct contact routes remain possible, minor transmission pathways.[1,64,73] It has been suggested that young children are the main transmitters in households[74] and that vaccination of school-age children may prevent morbidity and mortality in the elderly.[75]

The epidemiological literature relevant to the mode of influenza transmission consists largely of outbreak reports. The most often cited is an apparently airborne transmitted outbreak of influenza reported by Moser et al.[76] among passengers of an airplane grounded for 4.5 hours with its ventilation system shut off. One passenger became ill within 15 minutes of boarding. Of 54 other passengers, 25 of 29 who remained on board throughout the delay and seven of 25 who deplaned for part of the delay became infected with influenza. The source had not been in close contact with most of the passengers, so that airborne droplet nuclei appeared to be the most plausible explanation. Drinka et al. found, during influenza surveillance of a multi-building nursing home, that one building with higher ventilation rates and higher square footage per resident had lower influenza A attack rates than other buildings.[77] However, further studies did not confirm this trend,[78] and they concluded that an outlier in the initial study had driven the initial reported association.[79] The nursing home report, however, was not based on a study designed to test the effectiveness of ventilation, and the very high ventilation rates that would be expected to be necessary for control of influenza[25,80] were not used. Only one intervention study specifically designed to control droplet-nuclei transmission of influenza has been reported. That study[81] was conducted during two waves of acute febrile respiratory illness between July 1957 and March 1958 at the Livermore, California Veterans Administration Hospital. Baseline serology was obtained in July 1957 and serum was drawn again in November 1957 after the first wave and a third time in March 1957 after a second wave of acute respiratory illness. Upper-room UVC was in use to

Table 7.3 Influenza serology of acute respiratory illness at Livermore Veterans Hospital 1957–58. Adapted from reference 81

	Upper-room UVC		No UVC	
Time interval	Positive	Negative	Positive	Negative
July–November 15	2	10	3	60
November 16–March	0	4	39	28

prevent tuberculosis transmission in one wing of the hospital, but not in another. Patients were restricted to the hospital so that their only source of infection was virus brought in by infectious staff and visitors. Over the course of both waves of illness, 18% of staff and 19% of patients in the wing without UVC developed a four-fold rise in influenza titers. However, only 2% of patients in the wing with upper-room UVC seroconverted. As shown in Table 7.3, the first wave of illness was mostly not due to influenza, but UVC protected against this unknown illness as well. During the second wave, both influenza and non-influenza-related acute respiratory illness were lower in the wing with upper-room UVC. Riley and O'Grady[25] pointed out that this experiment, however strongly it seemed to support droplet nuclei as the primary mode of influenza transmission, was properly considered as only one experimental data point. At the time of this writing, almost 45 years later, with rising concern about emergent avian influenza, it is unfortunate that this experiment has never been repeated.

Experimental human infection via aerosol was achieved by Alford et al.,[82] who exposed subjects to low doses of influenza virus carried in airborne particles 1–3 μm in diameter. They were able to infect four out of 23 volunteers (17%). A larger body of animal experimental data demonstrated infection transmission by droplet nuclei both from experimental aerosols, and in animal-to-animal transmission experiments. Loosli et al. performed a series of experiments infecting mice using influenza aerosolized via an atomizer.[83–85] Edward et al. infected mice via experimental influenza aerosols[86] and showed that airborne influenza exposed to UVC was not capable of initiating infection, while 100% of the mice exposed to airborne influenza that was not treated with UVC either died or developed significant disease.[87] Animal-to-animal transmission experiments have shown the importance of droplet nuclei in both ferrets and mice. In one experiment, influenza A transmission from sick to healthy ferrets was achieved through different-shaped ducts (straight, S or U shape). The ducts were mechanically ventilated and the ferrets separated by a length of duct considered sufficient to eliminate large droplet or other large particle transmission. Ferrets became sick in all experiments, supporting the hypothesis that influenza was transmitted via droplet nuclei.[88] Schulman and Kilbourne[89] developed a mouse model for influenza and found an inverse correlation between air exchange and infection rate regardless of whether mice were able to mingle in one cage or were separated by two layers of wire mesh, indicating that droplet nuclei were the vehicle of transmission. In subsequent experiments,[90,91] Schulman showed that influenza virus strains which were equally infectious when administered by experimental aerosols were not equally transmissible from mouse to mouse, and that the ability to detect influenza in exhaust air from the cage of infected mice correlated with the transmissibility of the virus strain. Strains related to a pandemic influenza virus were more transmissible via droplet nuclei, suggesting that mutations promoting transmission via droplet nuclei are key steps in the evolution of pandemic influenza. These human and animal data suggest that, although influenza has been shown to survive for minutes to a few hours on fomites,[48] it is unlikely that direct contact and fomites play an important role in transmission of influenza.

CONCLUSIONS

Respiratory viruses are transmitted by a variety of mechanisms: some primarily via small-particle, droplet nuclei, aerosols and others primarily by direct contact and/or fomites. Some, and particularly rhinovirus, may be entirely opportunistic, using all available modes. Recent advances in detection of human exhaled breath particles and computational fluid dynamic modeling of particle dispersion in indoor air may lead to a better understanding of the role of 'near field' exposures and ability to determine when face-to-face exposure implies large droplets and when it indicates short-lived organisms in droplet nuclei. These advances may lead to improved ability to design public health interventions to prevent transmission.

REFERENCES

1. Barker J, Stevens D, Bloomfield SF. Spread and prevention of some common viral infections in community facilities and domestic homes. J Appl Microbiol 2001; 91: 7–21

2. Bertino JS. Cost burden of viral respiratory infections: issues for formulary decision makers. Am J Med 2002; 112 (Suppl 6A): 42S–49S

3. Fendrick A, Monto A, Sarnes M, Nightengale B. The economic burden of viral respiratory infection in the United States [abstract]. Value Health 2001; 4: 412

4. Adams P, Hendershot G, Marano M. Current estimates from the national health interview survey, 1996. National center for health statistics. Vital Health Stat 1999; 10: 1–203

5. Johnston SL. Mechanisms of asthma exacerbation. Clin Exp Allergy 1998; 28 (Suppl 5): 181–6; discussion 203–5

6. Cohen L, Castro M. The role of viral respiratory infections in the pathogenesis and exacerbation of asthma. Semin Respir Infect 2003; 18: 3–8

7. Lemanske RF Jr. Viruses and asthma: inception, exacerbation, and possible prevention. J Pediatr 2003; 142 (Suppl): S3–7; discussion S7–8

8. Schwarze J, Johnston SL. Unravelling synergistic immune interactions between respiratory virus infections and allergic airway inflammation. Clin Exp Allergy 2004; 34: 1153–5

9. MacDowell AL, Bacharier LB. Infectious triggers of asthma. Immunol Allergy Clin North Am 2005; 25: 45–66

10. Nicholson KG, Kent J, Ireland DC. Respiratory viruses and exacerbations of asthma in adults. BMJ 1993; 307: 982–6

11. Johnston SL, Pattemore PK, Sanderson G, et al. Community study of role of viral infections in exacerbations of asthma in 9–11 year old children. BMJ 1995; 310: 1225–9

12. Rawlinson WD, Waliuzzaman Z, Carter IW, et al. Asthma exacerbations in children associated with rhinovirus but not human metapneumovirus infection. J Infect Dis 2003; 187: 1314–18

13. Johnston NW, Johnston SL, Duncan JM, et al. The September epidemic of asthma exacerbations in children: a search for etiology. J Allergy Clin Immunol 2005; 115: 132–8

14. Williams JV, Harris PA, Tollefson SJ, et al. Human metapneumovirus and lower respiratory tract disease in otherwise healthy infants and children. N Engl J Med 2004; 350: 443–50

15. Bosis S, Esposito S, Niesters HG, et al. Impact of human metapneumovirus in childhood: comparison with respiratory syncytial virus and influenza viruses. J Med Virol 2005; 75: 101–4

16. Tan WC, Xiang X, Qiu D, et al. Epidemiology of respiratory viruses in patients hospitalized with near-fatal asthma, acute exacerbations of asthma, or chronic obstructive pulmonary disease. Am J Med 2003; 115: 272–7

17. Hall CB. Nosocomial respiratory syncytial virus infections: The 'cold war' has not ended. Clin Infect Dis 2000; 31: 590–6

18. Hall CB. Respiratory syncytial virus and parainfluenza virus. N Engl J Med 2001; 344: 1917–28

19. Evans RD, Mullally DI, Wilson RW, et al. National trends in the morbidity and mortality of asthma in the US. Prevalence, hospitalization and death from asthma over two decades: 1965–1984. Chest 1987; 91 (Suppl): 65S–74S

20. Woolcock AJ, Peat JK, Evidence for the increase in asthma worldwide. Ciba Found Symp 1997; 206: 122–34; discussion 134–9, 157–9

21. Cole EC, Cook CE. Characterization of infectious aerosols in health care facilities: an aid to effective engineering controls and preventive strategies. Am J Infect Control 1998; 26: 453–64

22. Roy CJ, Milton DK. Airborne transmission of communicable infection – the elusive pathway. N Engl J Med 2004; 350: 1710–12

23. Yu IT, Li Y, Wong TW, et al. Evidence of airborne transmission of the severe acute respiratory syndrome virus. N Engl J Med 2004; 350: 1731–9

24. Li Y, Duan S, Yu IT, Wong TW. Multi-zone modeling of probable SARS virus transmission by airflow between flats in block E, Amoy Gardens. Indoor Air 2005; 15: 96–111

25. Riley RL, O'Grady F. Airborne Infection: Transmission and Control. New York: Macmillan, 1961

26. Cox CS. The Aerobiological Pathway of Micro-organisms. Chichester: Wiley, 1987

27. Duguid J. The size and duration of air-carriage of respiratory droplets and droplet-nuclei. J Hyg 1946; 44: 471–9

28. Gerone P, Couch R, Keefer G, et al. Assessment of experimental and natural viral aerosols. Bacteriol Rev 1966; 30: 576–88

29. Edwards DA, Man JC, Brand P, et al. Inhaling to mitigate exhaled bioaerosols. Proc Natl Acad Sci USA 2004; 101: 17383–8

30. Wells WF. Airborne Contagion and Air Hygiene: an Ecological Study of Droplet Infection. Cambridge, MA: Harvard University Press, 1955

31. Couch RB, Cate TR, Douglas RG Jr, et al. Effect of route of inoculation on experimental respiratory viral disease in volunteers and evidence for airborne transmission. Bacteriol Rev 1996; 30: 517–29

32. Hinds WC. Aerosol Technology: Properties, Behavior, and Measurement of Airborne Particles. New York: John Wiley & Sons, 1999

33. Owen MK, Ensor DS, Sparks LE. Airborne particle sizes and sources found in indoor air. Atmospheric Environ 1992; 26A: 2149–62

34. Sattar SA, Ijaz MK. Airborne viruses. In: Wilkes P, Stenzenbach LD, eds. Manual of Environmental Microbiology. Washington, DC: ASM Press, 2002: 682–92

35. Wells WF. On air-borne infection. Study ii. Am J Hyg 1934; 20: 611–18

36. Murakami S. Analysis and design of micro-climate around the human body with respiration by cfd. Indoor Air 2004; 14: 144–56

37. Riley EC, Murphy G, Riley RL. Airborne spread of measles in a suburban elementary school. Am J Epidemiol 1978; 107: 421–32

38. Riley RL, Nardell EA. Clearing the air. The theory and application of ultraviolet air disinfection. Am Rev Respir Dis 1989; 139: 1286–94

39. Nardell EA, Keegan J, Cheney SA, Etkind SC. Airborne infection. Theoretical limits of protection achievable by building ventilation. Am Rev Respir Dis 1991; 144: 302–6

40. Johnston SL, Pattemore PK, Sanderson G, et al. The relationship between upper respiratory infections and hospital admissions for asthma: a time-trend analysis. Am J Respir Crit Care Med 1996; 154: 654–60

41. Schurmann W, Eggers HJ. Antiviral activity of an alcoholic hand disinfectant. Comparison of the in vitro suspension test with in vivo experiments on hands, and on individual fingertips. Antiviral Res 1983; 3: 25–41

42. Remington PL, Hall WN, Davis IH, et al. Airborne transmission of measles in a physician's office. J Am Med Assoc 1985; 253: 1574–7

43. Harper GJ. Airborne micro-organisms: survival tests with four viruses. J Hyg 1961; 59: 479–86

44. Sattar SA, Ijaz MK, Johnson-Lussenburg CM, Springthorpe VS. Effect of relative humidity on the airborne survival of rotavirus sa11. Appl Environ Microbiol 1984; 47: 879–81

45. Ijaz MK, Brunner AH, Sattar SA, et al. Survival characteristics of airborne human coronavirus 229e. J Gen Virol 1985; 66: 2743–8

46. Karim YG, Ijaz MK, Sattar SA, Johnson-Lussenburg CM. Effect of relative humidity on the airborne survival of rhinovirus-14. Can J Microbiol 1985; 31: 1058–61

47. Hall CB, Douglas RG Jr, Geiman JM. Possible transmission by fomites of respiratory syncytial virus. J Infect Dis 1980; 141: 98–102

48. Bean B, Moore B, Peterson L, et al. Survival of influenza viruses on environmental surfaces. J Infect Dis 1982; 146: 47–51

49. Parkinson AJ, Muchmore HG, Scott EN, Scott LV. Survival of human parainfluenza viruses in the south polar environment. Appl Environ Microbiol 1983; 46: 901–5

50. Nuanualsuwan S, Mariam T, Himathongkham S, Cliver DO. Ultraviolet inactivation of feline calicivirus, human enteric viruses and coliphages. Photochem Photobiol 2002; 76: 406–10

51. Nuanualsuwan S, Cliver DO. Capsid functions of inactivated human picornaviruses and feline calicivirus. Appl Environ Microbiol 2003; 69: 350–7

52. Roberts P, Hope A. Virus inactivation by high intensity broad spectrum pulsed light. J Virol Methods 2003; 110: 61–5

53. Jensen MM. Inactivation of airborne viruses by ultraviolet irradiation. Appl Microbiol 1964; 12: 418–20

54. Flint SJ, Enquist LW, Racaniello VR, Skalka AM. Attachment and entry. In Principles of Virology. Washington, DC: ASM Press, 2004: 126–75

55. Hall CB, Douglas RG Jr. Nosocomial respiratory syncytial viral infections. Should gowns and masks be used? Am J Dis Child 1981; 135: 512–15

56. Mills JT, Van Kirk JE, Wright PF, Chanock RM. Experimental respiratory syncytial virus infection of adults. Possible mechanisms of resistance to infection and illness. J Immunol 1971; 107: 123–30

57. Gern JE, Galagan DM, Jarjour NN, et al. Detection of rhinovirus RNA in lower airway cells during experimentally induced infection. Am J Respir Crit Care Med 1997; 155: 1159–61

58   Hall CB, Douglas RG Jr. Modes of transmission of respiratory syncytial virus. J Pediatr 1981; 99: 100–3

59.   Isaacs D, Dickson H, O'Callaghan C, et al. Hand-washing and cohorting in prevention of hospital acquired infections with respiratory syncytial virus. Arch Dis Child 1991; 66: 227–31

60.   Gala CL, Hall CB, Schnabel KC, et al. The use of eye–nose goggles to control nosocomial respiratory syncytial virus infection. J Am Med Assoc 1986; 256: 2706–8

61.   Madge P, Paton JY, McColl JH, Mackie PL. Prospective controlled study of four infection-control procedures to prevent nosocomial infection with respiratory syncytial virus. Lancet 1992; 340: 1079–83

62.   Karanfil LV, Conlon M, Lykens K, et al. Reducing the rate of nosocomially transmitted respiratory syncytial virus. Am J Infect Control 1999; 27: 91–6

63.   Aintablian N, Walpita P, Sawyer MH. Detection of bordetella pertussis and respiratory synctial virus in air samples from hospital rooms. Infect Control Hosp Epidemiol 1998; 19: 918–23

64.   Goldmann DA. Transmission of viral respiratory infections in the home. Pediatr Infect Dis J 2000; 19 (Suppl): S97–102

65.   Myatt TA, Johnston SL, Zuo Z, et al. Detection of airborne rhinovirus and its relation to outdoor air supply in office environments. Am J Respir Crit Care Med 2004; 169: 1187–90

66.   Ansari SA, Springthorpe VS, Sattar SA, et al. Potential role of hands in the spread of respiratory viral infections: studies with human parainfluenza virus 3 and rhinovirus 14. J Clin Microbiol 1991; 29: 2115–19

67.   Hendley JO, Wenzel RP, Gwaltney JM Jr. Transmission of rhinovirus colds by self-inoculation. N Engl J Med 1973; 288: 1361–4

68.   Hendley JO, Gwaltney JM Jr. Mechanisms of transmission of rhinovirus infections. Epidemiol Rev 1988; 10: 243–58

69.   Gwaltney JM Jr, Moskalski PB, Hendley JO. Hand-to-hand transmission of rhinovirus colds. Ann Intern Med 1978; 88: 463–7

70.   Meschievitz CK, Schultz SB, Dick EC. A model for obtaining predictable natural transmission of rhinoviruses in human volunteers. J Infect Dis 1984; 150: 195–201

71.   Dick EC, Jennings LC, Mink KA, et al. Aerosol transmission of rhinovirus colds. J Infect Dis 1987; 156: 442–8

72.   Dick EC, Hossain SU, Mink KA, et al. Interruption of transmission of rhinovirus colds among human volunteers using virucidal paper handkerchiefs. J Infect Dis 1986; 153: 352–6

73.   Riley RL. Airborne infection. Am J Med 1974: 57: 466–75

74.   Viboud C, Boelle PY, Cauchemez S, et al. Risk factors of influenza transmission in households. Br J Gen Pract 2004; 54: 684–9

75.   Reichert TA, Sugaya N, Fedson DS, et al. The Japanese experience with vaccinating schoolchildren against influenza. N Engl J Med 2001; 344: 889–96

76.   Moser MR, Bender TR, Margolis HS, et al. An outbreak of influenza aboard a commercial airliner. Am J Epidemiol 1979; 110: 1–6

77.   Drinka PJ, Krause P, Schilling M, et al. Report of an outbreak: nursing home architecture and influenza-a attack rates. J Am Geriatr Soc 1996; 44: 910–13

78.   Drinka PJ, Krause P, Nest L, et al. Delays in the application of outbreak control prophylaxis for influenza a in a nursing home. Infect Control Hosp Epidemiol 2002; 23: 600–3

79.   Drinka PJ, Krause P, Nest L, Tyndall D. Report of an outbreak: nursing home architecture and influenza-a attack rates: update. J Am Geriatr Soc 2004; 52: 847–8

80.   Rudnick SN, Milton DK. Risk of indoor airborne infection transmission estimated from carbon dioxide concentration. Indoor Air 2003; 13: 237–45

81.   McLean RL. The effect of ultraviolet radiation upon the transmission of epidemic influenza in long-term hospital patients. Am Rev Respir Dis 1961; 83: 36–8

82.   Alford RH, Kasel JA, Gerone PJ, Knight V. Human influenza resulting from aerosol inhalation. Proc Soc Exp Biol Med 1996; 122: 800–4

83.   Loosli CG, Lemon HM, Robertson OH, Appel E. Experimental air-borne influenza infection. I. Influence of humidity on survival of virus in air. Proc Soc Exp Biol 1943; 53: 205–6

84.   Loosli CG, Hamre D, Berlin BS. Air-borne influenza virus a infections in immunized animals. Trans Assoc Am Physicians 1953; 66: 222–30

85.   Loosli CG, Hertweck MS, Hockwald RS. Airborne influenza pr8-a virus infections in actively immunized mice. Arch Environ Health 1970; 21: 332–46

86.   Edward D, Elford W, Laidlaw P. Studies of air-borne virus infections. I. Experimental technique and preliminary observations on influenza and infectious ectromelia. J Hyg (Lond) 1943; 43: 1–10

87.   Edward D, Elford W, Laidlaw P. Studies of air-borne virus infections. II. The killing of virus aerosols by ultra-violet radiation. J Hyg (Lond) 1943; 43: 11–15

88.   Andrewes CH, Glover RE. Spread of infection from the respiratory tract of the ferret. I. Transmission of influenza a virus. Br J Exp Pathol 1941; 22: 91–7

89.   Schulman JL, Kilbourne ED. Airborne transmission of influenza virus infection in mice. Nature 1962; 195: 1129–30

90.   Schulman JL. Experimental transmission of influenza virus infection in mice. IV. Relationship of transmissibility of different strains of virus and recovery of airborne virus in the environment of infector mice. J Exp Med 1967; 125: 479–88

91.   Schulman JL. The use of an animal model to study transmission of influenza virus infection. Am J Public Health Nations Health 1968; 58: 2092–6

PART II

Pathophysiology

CHAPTER 8

Mechanisms of
asthma exacerbation

Anh L Innes and John V Fahy

INTRODUCTION

The clinical characteristics of an asthma exacerbation include symptoms of dyspnea, chest tightness and mucus hypersecretion. These characteristics represent the clinical expression of airway inflammation and changes in airway structural cells that are quite complex and not fully understood. Surprisingly few mechanistically oriented studies in human asthma have attempted to unravel this complexity. From available data, it is clear that intense airway inflammation is characteristic of asthma exacerbation and that changes occur in structural airway cells such as smooth muscle cells, mucous cells and cells in the bronchial microvasculature. The net effect of this pathology is airflow obstruction occurring not just because of concentric smooth muscle contraction, but also because of edema of the airway wall and mucous plugging of the airway lumen.

The smooth muscle contraction, bronchial edema and mucus hypersecretion that contribute to significant airflow obstruction during acute asthma exacerbations occur in the context of pre-existing airway remodeling.[1,2] This remodeling primes the airway for the exacerbation response. Thus, although airway hyperresponsiveness in asthma usually refers to responses of airway smooth muscle, it also extends to hyperresponsiveness of vascular endothelial cells and of airway mucous cells.

Together, structural changes in muscle, blood vessels and mucous cells render the asthmatic airway vulnerable to exaggerated responses to environmental stimulation. It is this priming of the airway by remodeling that renders asthmatics sensitive to the exacerbation response (Figure 8.1). Examination of endobronchial biopsies from asthmatics with and without airflow obstruction demonstrates that airway remodeling occurs in asthmatics with normal or mild airflow obstruction. This finding helps explain the occurrence of asthma exacerbations (sometimes severe and even life-threatening) in asthmatics with normal airflow between exacerbations. Remodeling can thus be silent to tests of airflow, and the most prominent clinical manifestation of airway remodeling in asthma may be susceptibility to asthma exacerbation.

If structural changes in the asthmatic airway render asthmatics susceptible to exacerbation responses, then triggers must exist to activate these responses. These triggers are usually environmental, although non-compliance with medication can also contribute, as can asthmatic reactions to medications such as non-steroidal anti-inflammatory medications. Examples of environmental stimuli are viruses, air pollutants and aeroallergens. One paradigm for the pathogenesis of asthma exacerbation is a two-phase process, as follows. Phase 1 is the activation of ciliated airway epithelial cells by environmental stimuli, degranulation of mast

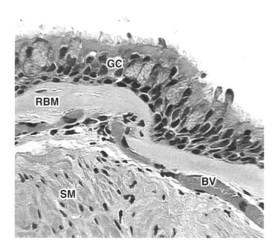

Figure 8.1 Airway pathology in asthma is depicted in this photomicrograph of a section from an endobronchial biopsy taken during bronchoscopy from a subject with mild chronic asthma. Goblet cell (GC) hyperplasia, reticular basement membrane (RBM) fibrosis, smooth muscle (SM) hypertrophy and blood vessel (BV) engorgement are shown. (Hematoxylin and eosin stain.) See also Color Plate I

cells or basophils within the epithelial layer, and recruitment of eosinophils and neutrophils to the airway from the vascular space. Phase 2 is inflammation-induced activation of structural cells such as muscle cells, mucous cells and vascular cells. Activation of these structural cells causes airflow obstruction.

In this chapter, we review mechanisms of asthma exacerbation by first discussing the role of the airway epithelium, then we discuss the role of mast cells, basophils and leukocytes. Finally, we discuss three of the most important causes of airflow limitation in acute exacerbation: airway smooth muscle contraction, airway edema and airway mucus hypersecretion.

AIRWAY EPITHELIUM

Airway epithelial cells line the airways, secrete mucus and provide barrier protection and a system of mucociliary clearance necessary for proper host defense.[3–5] Abnormalities in airway epithelial cell function have long been suspected to play a pathophysiological role in asthma exacerbations. Desquamation of airway epithelial cells, possibly due to the action of inflammatory mediators such as eosinophil granule proteins, is considered one mechanism of epithelial injury during acute asthma exacerbations.[6–8] Indeed, the loss of airway epithelium in asthma has been hypothesized to result in the loss of an epithelium-derived relaxing factor, inducing airway narrowing and airway hyperreactivity.[9,10] Experimental evidence to support the existence of these relaxing factors comes from animal models where endogenous mediators such as prostaglindin E_2 and nitric oxide induce relaxation of tracheas containing epithelium. In contrast, tracheas denuded of epithelium, when stimulated with histamine, acetylcholine or endotoxin, exhibit increased contractile responses.[11,12] The exact role of epithelium-derived relaxing factors is not yet defined, however, and the desquamation of epithelial cells in acute asthma exacerbation is not a consistent finding.[7,13–15] This is hardly surprising, because the older concept of the epithelium as a simple physical barrier between the host and the environment, the loss of which is detrimental to the host, is changing. Instead, current concepts for the role of epithelial cells posit more sophisticated host defense functions, including modulation of local immune responses and limitation of inflammatory processes by degrading or inhibiting proinflammatory mediators and proteins.[5,16] In this scenario, epithelial cells do not simply 'give up' when subjected to environmental stimuli. Rather, these cells are well equipped to 'fight back', with cytoprotective as well as proinflammatory responses. For example, activation of protease-activated receptor 2 (PAR-2) on epithelial cells may represent a mechanism for prostanoid-dependent cytoprotection in the airways.[17] In addition, airway clara cells secrete clara cell secretory protein (CCSP), one of the most abundant

Table 8.1 Epithelium-derived cytokines. Adapted from reference 5

| Colony stimulating factors | Pleiotropic cytokines | Growth factors | Receptor antagonists | Chemoattractant cytokines | | |
				Lymphocyte chemoattractant factor	C-x-C/α chemokines	C-C/β chemokines
GM-CSF	IL-6	TGF-α	Type 1 TNFR	IL-16	GRO-α	RANTES
G-CSF	IL-11	TGF-β	icIL-1Ra Type 1		GRO-γ	MCP-1
M-CSF	IL-1	SCF			IL-8	MCP-4
CSF-1	IL-10 TNFα	bFGF				Eotaxin-1, 2, 3

secreted proteins of the airway lining fluid and a potent inhibitor of allergic airway inflammation.[18,19] Finally, other protective responses of the epithelium include the secretion of interleukin (IL)-10 and transforming growth factor (TGF)-β, cytokines that inhibit many inflammatory responses.[20,21] These inflammation-limiting responses do not always predominate, however, and the epithelium can respond to stimulation by producing biologically active mediators that promote airway inflammation. These mediators include cytokines and chemokines that promote inflammatory cell accumulation and activation (Table 8.1) as well as lipid and peptide mediators (e.g. arachidonic acid metabolites), endothelin-1 and reactive oxygen species.[22]

The mechanisms responsible for epithelial cell activation during asthma exacerbations will differ according to the stimuli for the exacerbation. The provoking stimuli range from medication non-compliance, resulting in loss of asthma control, to acute exacerbations, resulting from exposure to environmental insults as diverse as viral infection, aeroallergens, air pollutants and inhaled recreational drugs. Exposure to environmental tobacco smoke provokes exacerbations of asthma, and asthmatic children of smoking parents have more frequent exacerbations and more severe symptoms.[23–25]

Rhinovirus (RV), the most common viral infection of the respiratory tract, is the virus most frequently implicated in asthma exacerbations. Asthmatics are at increased risk for lower respiratory tract symptoms when infected with RV,[26] and they are at increased risk for infection-induced reductions in airflow.[27] The mechanism of virus-induced airflow obstruction in asthma may be virus-induced activation of airway epithelial cells with upregulation of chemokines and proinflammatory cytokines such as IL-6, IL-8, granulocyte–macrophage colony-stimulating factor and IL-16.[28,29] Analysis of airway secretions from infected asthmatics shows increases in IL-8,[30,31] IL-10[32] and IL-6. Increases in IL-6 in airway secretions from asthmatics in acute exacerbation are particularly striking,[33–35] although it is not clear from clinical studies that the mechanism of this increase is always virus-associated. The specific role of IL-6 in acute asthma is also not clear. IL-6 is a pleiotropic cytokine with a wide range of biological activities. It helps regulate immune reactivity, the acute-phase response, inflammation and hematopoiesis.[36] IL-6 can also bind to the soluble IL-6 receptor and induce proliferation of T cells expressing the cognate receptor gp130.[37]

Seasonal allergens, specifically mold spores, have been implicated in exacerbations and even sudden death attributed to asthma.[4,38,39] A synergistic interaction between respiratory viral infection and allergen exposure has been suggested by data both in experimental RV infection[40] as well as in children[41] and adults[42] hospitalized for asthma exacerbation, an effect which may be explained by the augmentation of proinflammatory responses in the airways. The risk for hospitalization is increased with the combination of sensitization, current exposure to allergens and the presence of viral infection. A possible mechanism for this synergism suggested by experimental RV-16 infection is the persistently enhanced airway inflammation which has been noted after local antigen challenge in allergic subjects. Thus, viruses and allergens may act synergistically to induce asthma exacerbations in some instances. In addition, there are examples of other environmental stimuli acting in concert, leading to exacerbation. For example, exposure to diesel engine emissions increases susceptibility to respiratory syncytial virus (RSV) infection in a mouse model,[43] and high exposure to nitrogen dioxide in children prior to a respiratory viral infection is associated with increased severity of the resulting asthma exacerbation.[44]

The airway epithelium is a complex structure with multiple resident cell types, and the complexity in asthma is increased by the presence of significant numbers of non-resident cells such as mast cells and basophils. Activation of mast cells and basophils in the epithelial layer by inhaled environmental stimuli may be particularly important in the pathogenesis of asthma exacerbations, as outlined below.

ROLE OF MAST CELLS AND BASOPHILS

The airways of patients who die from asthma are infiltrated with basophils and mast cells,[45,46] and airway secretions from asthmatics in exacerbation show increased concentrations of mast cell- and basophil-associated mediators such as tryptase and histamine.[47] Mast cells and basophils are IgE-effector cells, and IgE-mediated type 1 hypersensitivity reactions cause acute bronchospasm in allergic asthmatic subjects exposed to aeroallergen.[48,49] The specific mechanism is that allergen molecules crosslink adjacent Fab components of IgE on mast cells and basophils causing secretion of preformed mediators such as histamine, tumor necrosis factor (TNF)α, tryptase and chymase, as well as newly generated mediators such as cytokines and eicosanoids.[47] There is ample evidence from the laboratory to demonstrate that aeroallergen challenge causes significant airflow narrowing and that the response is a two-phase phenomenon. Specifically, the early phase is acute airflow obstruction occurring immediately after aeroallergen inhalation. This early obstruction to airflow resolves spontaneously within 2 hours, but it is followed by the late-phase response, a decrease in airflow which occurs 2–8 hours after aeroallergen inhalation. The resolution of the late phase can take several hours. IgE-effector cells are implicated in the pathophysiology of both early- and late-phase responses, as evidenced by attenuation of both responses in asthmatics pretreated with omalizumab (a monoclonal antibody directed against IgE) prior to allergen challenge.[50,51] The late-phase response is thought to be a consequence of allergen-induced inflammation and vascular leak, and the efficacy of omalizumab in attenuation of this response suggests that omalizumab has anti-inflammatory effects. This suggestion has been borne out in studies which demonstrate a marked reduction in airway eosinophilia in asthmatics treated with omalizumab.[52] Even so, it has been surprising to see the efficacy of omalizumab in preventing asthma exacerbations. Treatment of asthmatics with omalizumab results in a 50% reduction in the frequency of asthma exacerbation,[53–55] strong evidence for an important role for IgE and its effector cells in the pathophysiology of asthma exacerbation.[56]

CELLULAR INFLAMMATION

Asthma exacerbations are characterized by recruitment and activation of inflammatory cells to the airway. These cells include eosinophils, neutrophils and T cells. For example, examination of inflammatory cells in airway secretions collected from patients in asthma exacerbation and in airway tissue in fatal asthma shows accumulation of eosinophils and neutrophils.[33,57–60] In fatal asthma, specific patterns of leukocyte accumulation in the airway submucosa have been associated with specific cellular phenotypes.[59] Rapid-onset fatal asthma is associated with a predominance of submucosal neutrophils, whereas slow-onset fatal asthma is associated with predominance of submucosal eosinophils.[59] These findings raise the possibility that the mechanisms of cellular inflammation in fatal asthma exacerbations differ depending on the time course of the exacerbation, which may in turn depend on the specific precipitants of the exacerbation.[61,62]

The role of T cells in asthma is well established, and a central role for CD4+ T cells as orchestrators of inflammation and remodeling in asthma is widely accepted.[63] In acute severe asthma, it has been found that T cells are activated. Specifically, peripheral blood T cells have upregulation of activation markers such as interleukin-2 receptor (IL-2R), class 2 histocompatibility antigen (HLA-DR) and very late activation antigen (VLA-1).[64] In addition, CD8+/perforin+ T cells are prominent in the airways of patients who die of acute asthma. In particular, perforin helps to eradicate virus, but it will also damage host tissues,[65] contributing to the airway pathology of fatal asthma.

Differences have been found in how eosinophil and neutrophil numbers change during treatment of severe asthma exacerbations.[58] Whereas eosinophil numbers in airway secretions decrease quickly and almost completely during treatment, neutrophil numbers actually increase, at least initially. This difference is probably explained by the differential effects of corticosteroids on neutrophils and eosinophils. Corticosteroids are used to treat acute severe asthma, and steroids have been shown to promote apoptosis of eosinophils but inhibit apoptosis of neutrophils *in vitro*.[66] Of course, the numbers of neutrophils may not be the only important variable, because steroids may stabilize neutrophil activation or modify the response of airway structural cells to the actions of neutrophil products.

The mechanism of recruitment of inflammatory cells to the airway during asthma exacerbation probably involves the upregulation of chemokines and cytokines. As discussed above, airway epithelial cells or IgE-effector cells in the airway epithelium can be activated by inhaled triggers, and this activation process can result in release of multiple proinflammatory mediators that can cause leukocyte accumulation in the airway. IL-5, IL-8, TNFα, platelet activating factor and IL-1β are but a few of the chemoattractant mediators capable of this action.

Neutrophils and eosinophils secrete multiple soluble mediators that can perturb airway function, and these include proteases, cationic proteins, lipid mediators and cytokines. As discussed elsewhere in this chapter, the biological consequences of excess concentrations of these proteins include smooth muscle contraction, increased vascular permeability and mucous cell degranulation. Among these mediators, TNFα is deserving of special mention. The concentrations of TNFα are increased in serum from patients with acute asthma,[67–69] and this can have multiple consequences ranging from airway infiltration of neutrophils and eosinophils, activation of airway smooth muscle, activation of myofibroblasts and changes in vascular permeability.[70] Inhibition of TNFα in an experimental model of asthma abrogates allergen-induced airway responses.[71] More importantly, inhibition of TNFα in patients with refractory asthma significantly improves lung function and bronchial hyperresponsiveness.[72] It is not unreasonable to hope that further clinical trials will demonstrate that TNFα inhibition may help prevent and treat exacerbations of asthma.

AIRWAY SMOOTH MUSCLE

Airway smooth muscle is hypertrophied and hyperplastic in cases of fatal asthma.[14,73–75] Hyperplasia seems to dominate over hypertrophy as the dominant abnormality of airway smooth muscle in asthma,[76] with the number of smooth muscle cells increased 2–3-fold above normal.[73,77,78] Studies of airway smooth muscle cells in culture have identified several potential mitogens, which include growth factors whose receptors have intrinsic tyrosine kinase activity (platelet-derived growth factor (PDGF), insulin-like growth factor (IGF)-I, epidermal growth factor (EGF), fibroblast growth factor (FGF)), inflammatory mediators (leukotriene D4, thromboxane), cytokines (IL-Iβ) and serine proteases (thrombin, tryptase).

Mathematical models suggest that simply increasing the volume of smooth muscle in the airway without an increase in contractility can lead to airway hyperresponsiveness through local mechanical effects.[79–81] Some data have also demonstrated that even a 40% increase in muscle volume can lead to a dramatic increase in responsiveness to constrictor agonists.[79–81]

Contraction of airway smooth muscle undoubtedly contributes to the mechanism of airflow obstruction in asthma exacerbations. Of the inflammatory mediators released by epithelial cells, IgE effector cells and leukocytes, those most active on smooth muscle are tryptase, histamine, LTC4 and LTD4. Indeed, in the laboratory the early bronchoconstrictor response to inhaled allergen is significantly attenuated by leukotriene receptor antagonists,[82] and the combination of antihistamines and antileukotrienes is more effective than antileukotrienes alone.[83]

The effects of smooth muscle shortening in asthmatic airways are greatly amplified in airways which are edematous and which have luminal occlusion with mucus. This is conceptually very important because of the implications for treatment of exacerbation, and is discussed in more detail below.

AIRWAY MICROVASCULATURE

The number and size of bronchial blood vessels is increased in asthma,[84] and these vessels have a role in regulating airway caliber. Increases in blood vessels and vascular volume will result in swelling of the mucosa and narrowing of the airway lumen,[85] and increased vascular permeability will result in plasma protein extravasation into the airway wall and lumen. Many inflammatory mediators cause vasodilatation and increased permeability at the post-capillary venule.[86–88] In experimental models, mediators such as histamine, substance P, bradykinin, LTC4, LTD4 and platelet-activating factor (PAF) increase airway microvascular permeability.[89,90] In humans, allergen challenge[91] and ozone exposure cause a rise in airway lavage protein levels, providing evidence that these exposures cause an increase in bronchovascular permeability and that this increase may be implicated in the changes in non-specific hyperresponsiveness induced by these exposures. Histamine also causes a reversible and reproducible plasma leakage in the human nasal airway.[92]

Increased bronchovascular permeability will result in plasma exudation, and the exuded plasma can contribute to airway narrowing in asthma exacerbation in several ways. Acute severe asthma is associated with increased concentrations of plasma proteins such as albumin in airway secretions.[93] Plasma proteins will combine with mucins to alter the physical properties of the mucin gel matrix. For example, the mixture of albumin and mucin yields a very viscous material[94] which will ultimately worsen mucus clearance – a major problem in asthma exacerbations. Second, the surface tension-lowering properties of surfactant help maintain the patency of distal airways, and plasma proteins such as fibrin can inactivate surfactant. Interestingly, fibrin has been immunolocalized on the distal airway epithelium of a patient who died from fatal asthma.[95] Third, bronchial edema will increase mucosal and submucosal thickness, alter the mechanical properties of the airway wall and decouple the airway wall from its parenchymal attachments.[86] Edematous airways may cause airway narrowing simply by displacing airway mass toward the lumen. Even more important than this displacement is the amplification of the effects of smooth muscle contraction. The airway epithelium normally rests on an unfolded basement membrane, but contraction of airway smooth muscle results in ridges that protrude into the lumen. These ridges are formed by epithelial projections, with intervening spaces that fill with fluid if there is plasma exudation.[86] This filling will decrease the cross-sectional area of the lumen, affecting the dynamics of airflow.

Taken together, there is convincing evidence that increased bronchovascular permeability with leakage of plasma proteins into the airway wall and lumen contributes to the mechanism of airflow obstruction in asthma. Although there is good evidence that β-agonists decrease bronchovascular permeability in animal models and cell culture systems,[96,97] the evidence for this effect in humans *in vivo* is not strong. Specific therapies targeting vascular remodeling and vascular leakage in asthma are likely to be helpful in the treatment and prevention of exacerbations.

MUCOUS CELLS

Excessive sputum production is a common symptom of acute asthma exacerbations.[98] In

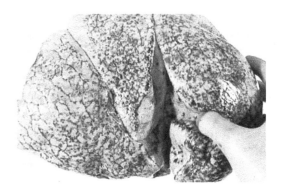

Figure 8.2 Lungs at autopsy in fatal asthma, demonstrating severe hyperinflation and resistance to deflation

addition, mucous plugging of the airway is a consistent finding in autopsy studies in fatal asthma,[7,99] resulting in severe hyperinflation and resistance to deflation of the lungs even when removed from the chest (Figure 8.2). For example, in the 1960s, Dunnill provided graphic descriptions in 20 cases of fatal asthma. For a typical case of fatal asthma he noted that '...the cut surface of the lung showed a striking picture with numerous grey, glistening, mucous plugs scattered throughout the airway passages'. He summarized that 'pathologically the outstanding feature of the asthmatic lung lies in the failure of clearance of the bronchial secretions'.[100] Others have confirmed this summary, and it is only a small minority of asthma deaths that are not associated with airway mucus impaction.[99,101] It is thus hard to over-emphasize the importance of mucus hypersecretion in the pathophysiology of asthma exacerbations. The combination of airway narrowing from concentric smooth muscle contraction and luminal obstruction with mucous plugs is particularly dangerous and marks asthma as unique among airway diseases in its propensity for sudden and sometimes fatal exacerbations.

The sources of mucin glycoproteins in the airway are goblet cells in the surface epithelium and mucous cells in submucosal glands. Goblet cells and glands are both likely to increase their secretory function during asthma exacerbations. For glands, it has been shown that their enlargement is characteristic of more severe forms of asthma,[73] and for goblet cells it has been shown that luminal mucins can be traced to a goblet cell origin.[102,103] The mechanism of airway mucous cell hyperplasia must be separated from mechanisms of mucous cell degranulation. Recently discovered mediators of mucous cell metaplasia include IL-13, ligands for the EGF receptor and a calcium-activated chloride channel (CLCA1).[104] Mucous cell degranulation is calcium-mediated and can be rapidly triggered by a wide variety of physiological agents, including cytokines/chemokines, bacterial exoproducts, nucleotides, neurotransmitters and proteases.[105] Specific mucin secretagogues that may be particularly important in asthma exacerbation include neutrophil elastase, chymase, leukotrienes, eosinophil cationic protein and nucleotides.[104,106] All of these secretagogues may be implicated in the pathophysiology of mucus hypersecretion in asthma exacerbation, since the cells that secrete them are known to accumulate in acute severe asthma. Neutrophil elastase may be an especially important secretagogue in acute exacerbations of asthma, since free elastase activity is detectable in airway secretions during exacerbations.[33,107]

Direct evidence for the importance of mucus hypersecretion in acute asthma exacerbation comes from animal models. In mice sensitized and challenged with ovalbumin, it is possible to induce death by asphyxiation, and autopsy reveals complete luminal occlusion with mucins.[108] Leukotrienes are important mediators of mucous cell degranulation in this instance, because the effect is blocked by zileuton, a specific inhibitor of 5-lipoxygenase.[109] The effect of allergen challenge in airway mucous cells has also been studied in an experiment in human asthma.[110] Interestingly, although aerosolized allergen challenge caused significant eosinophilic inflammation, it was not associated with goblet cell degranulation.[110]

Thus, in humans there appear to be mechanisms preventing goblet cell degranulation following allergen exposure, at least most of the time. The occurrence of goblet cell degranulation in fatal asthma may represent a unique, and as yet incompletely understood, circumstance where this protection is overridden. A better understanding of mechanisms inhibiting goblet cell degranulation is needed, because knowledge of such mechanisms would advance the understanding of mucus hypersecretion in acute asthma.

The mucus that occludes the lumen in asthma exacerbation is quite a complex biological material, and analysis of mucous plugs in fatal asthma shows that they comprise a mixture of mucins, plasma proteins and products of cell death.[99] Important plasma proteins include albumin and fibrinogen, and important products of cell death include DNA and actin. The relative concentration of mucin, plasma proteins, DNA and actin will have consequences for the physical properties of the mucus. For example, the 'rubbery' consistency of asthmatic mucus is probably a consequence of the relatively high concentrations of mucins and albumin compared to mucus from diseases such as cystic fibrosis, where concentration of DNA is high[111] but the relative amount of plasma protein is low.

The accumulation of the mucin component of mucus in the airway lumen in asthma exacerbation is a combined consequence of increased mucin and decreased mucociliary clearance.[112] Mucociliary clearance relies upon normal functioning of cilia on epithelial cells and optimal rheological properties of airway mucus. The cephalad movement of mucus and airway secretions propelled by the co-ordinated, rhythmic beating of epithelial cilia is sometimes referred to as the mucociliary escalator. This escalator relies not only on ciliary movement but also on the optimal rheological properties of mucus. Elasticity is necessary for cilia to transmit kinetic energy to the mucous layer to propel it forward, but high elastic recoil would impede the mucociliary escalator by the resistance to extrusion from goblet cells as well as the resistance to propulsion by epithelial cilia.[113] A rheological balance between elasticity and viscosity is therefore necessary, and this balance is perturbed in airway diseases such as asthma, when mucus is produced which is abnormal both in volume and in composition.

The clearance of airway mucus depends upon its proper hydration. Normally, airway mucus exists in two layers, the gel (formed principally of secreted mucins) and the sol – a watery layer on which the gel sits, and in which epithelial cilia can beat freely.[112] Optimal maintenance of the sol requires a process of active ion transport, regulated by ion channels such as cystic fibrosis transmembrane conductance regulator (CFTR). Purinergic receptors expressed by airway epithelia are hypothesized to have roles in the autocrine regulation of the sol volume. Functional data suggest that ATP mediates acute responses via P2Y2 receptor stimulation,[114] and that ATP metabolism provides a source of adenosine for stimulation of the A2b adenosine receptor.[115] Dehydration of the sol because of the loss of sol homeostasis is considered an important mechanism of mucus stasis in cystic fibrosis,[116] and this mechanism could conceivably also operate in acute asthma. Administration of hypertonic saline by aerosol can rehydrate the sol, and inhaled hypertonic saline improves mucociliary clearance[117] and lung function[118] in patients with cystic fibrosis. Hypertonic saline is associated with bronchospasm in asthmatics; therefore, its use in acute asthma is problematic. However, these data demonstrate that improvement in mucociliary clearance using treatment strategies focused on mucus and mucociliary clearance is a viable strategy for improving airflow in diseases associated with mucus hypersecretion.

It is not just fatal asthma exacerbations that provide evidence for mucous plugs in the airways of asthmatics in exacerbation. Clinically, it is not uncommon to find segmental collapse

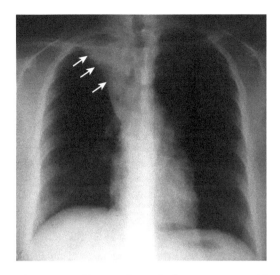

Figure 8.3 Chest radiograph from a 20-year-old woman admitted to the intensive care unit for management of acute severe asthma. The chest radiograph shows collapse of the right upper lobe (arrows) secondary to mucus impaction. The abnormality resolved completely within 24 hours of treatment with mechanical ventilation, corticosteroids and bronchodilators

of lung lobes because of luminal occlusion (Figure 8.3), and lavage in these situations yields mucous plugs that have formed airway casts (Figure 8.4). These findings emphasize that asthma exacerbations involve a process of luminal occlusion as well as airway narrowing from smooth muscle contraction. This explains why β-agonists are not sufficient therapy for asthma exacerbations and why new treatment modalities are needed to degrade mucous plugs and promote their clearance.

SUMMARY

Asthma exacerbations represent an extreme of loss of asthma control and as such can be viewed as a 'storm' of airway activity, in which several components of normal airway

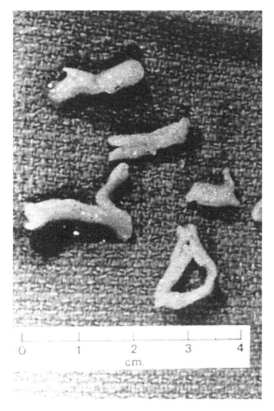

Figure 8.4 Airway casts recovered from broncho-alveolar lavage from an asthmatic subject in acute exacerbation. From reference 119

homeostasis are perturbed, leading to airflow obstruction. Airway smooth muscle contraction, mucous cell degranulation and bronchial edema all contribute to airflow obstruction during asthma exacerbations. Severe asthma exacerbations can lead to fatal or near-fatal asthma, and these situations can be considered a 'perfect storm' in which a combination of factors arise at once and lead to catastrophic airway obstruction. Understanding the contributors to these 'storm conditions' in acute asthma as well as the mechanisms that normally dispel these conditions is the key to better management and prevention of asthma exacerbations.

REFERENCES

1. Woodruff PG, Fahy JV. Airway remodeling in asthma. Semin Respir Crit Care Med 2002; 23: 361–7
2. Vignola AM, Chiappara G, Chanez P, et al. Growth factors in asthma. Monaldi Arch Chest Dis 1997; 52: 159–69
3. Davies RJ, Devalia JL. Epithelial cells. Br Med Bull 1992; 48: 85–96
4. Campbell AM. Bronchial epithelial cells in asthma. Allergy 1997; 52: 483–9
5. Polito AJ, Proud D. Epithelial cells as regulators of airway inflammation. J Allergy Clin Immunol 1998; 102: 714–18
6. Cardell BS, Pearson RSB. Death in asthmatics. Thorax 1959; 14: 341–52
7. Houston JC, De Navasquez S, Trounce JR. A clinical and pathological study of fatal cases of status asthmaticus. Thorax 1953; 8: 207–13
8. Azzawi M, Johnston PW, Majumdar S, et al. T lymphocytes and activated eosinophils in airway mucosa in fatal asthma and cystic fibrosis. Am Rev Respir Dis 1992; 145: 1477–82
9. Aizawa H, Miyazaki N, Shigematsu N, et al. A possible role of airway epithelium in modulating hyperresponsiveness. Br J Pharmacol 1988; 93: 139–45
10. Vanhoutte PM. Epithelium-derived relaxing factor(s) and bronchial reactivity. J Allergy Clin Immunol 1989; 83: 855–61
11. Folkerts G, Nijkamp FP. Virus-indued airway hyperresponsiveness: role of inflammatory cells and mediators. Am J Respir Crit Care Med 1995; 151: 1666–74
12. Sparrow MP, Omari TI, Mitchell HW. The epithelial barrier and airway responsiveness. Can J Physiol Pharmacol 1995; 73: 180–90
13. Ordoñez C, Ferrando R, Hyde DM, et al. Epithelial desquamation in asthma: artifact or pathology? Am J Resp Crit Care Med 2000; 162: 2324–9
14. Carroll N, Elliot J, Morton A, et al. The structure of large and small airways in nonfatal and fatal asthma. Am Rev Respir Dis 1993; 147: 405–10
15. Lozewicz S, Wells C, Gomez E, et al. Morphological integrity of the bronchial epithelium in mild asthma. Thorax 1990; 45: 12–15
16. Fahy JV. Remodeling of the airway epithelium in asthma. Am J Respir Crit Care Med 2001; 164: S46–51
17. Cocks TM, Fong B, Chow JM, et al. A protective role for protease-activated receptors in the airways. Nature 1999; 398: 156–60
18. Wang SZ, Rosenberger CL, Espindola TM, et al. CCSP modulates airway dysfunction and host responses in an Ova-challenged mouse model. Am J Physiol Lung Cell Mol Physiol 2001; 281: L1303–11

19. Chen Y, Zhao YH, Wu R. Differential regulation of airway mucin gene expression and mucin secretion by extracellular nucleotide triphosphates. Am J Respir Cell Mol Biol 2001; 25: 409–17

20. Aubert JD, Dalal BI, Bai TR, et al. Transforming growth factor beta 1 gene expression in human airways. Thorax 1994; 49: 225–32

21. Bonfield TL, Konstan MW, Burfeind P, et al. Normal bronchial epithelial cells constitutively produce the anti-inflammatory cytokine interleukin-10, which is downregulated in cystic fibrosis. Am J Respir Cell Mol Biol 1995; 13: 257–61

22. Behera AK, Kumar M, Matsuse H, et al. Respiratory syncytial virus induces the expression of 5-lipoxygenase and endothelin-1 in bronchial epithelial cells. Biochem Biophys Res Commun 1998; 251: 704–9

23. Chilmonczyk BA, Salmun LM, Megathlin KN, et al. Association between exposure to environmental tobacco smoke and exacerbations of asthma in children. N Engl J Med 1993; 328: 1665–9

24. Evans D, Levison MJ, Feldman CH, et al. The impact of passive smoking on emergency room visits of urban children with asthma. Am Rev Respir Dis 1987; 135: 567–72

25. Murray AB, Morrison BJ. The effect of cigarette smoke from the mother on bronchial responsiveness and severity of symptoms in children with asthma. J Allergy Clin Immunol 1986; 77: 575–81

26. Corne JM, Marshall C, Smith S, et al. Frequency, severity, and duration of rhinovirus infections in asthmatic and non-asthmatic individuals: a longitudinal cohort study. Lancet 2002; 359: 831–4

27. Grunberg K, Timmers MC, de Klerk EP, et al. Experimental rhinovirus 16 infection causes variable airway obstruction in subjects with atopic asthma. Am J Respir Crit Care Med 1999; 160: 1375–80

28. Papadopoulos NG, Bates PJ, Bardin PG, et al. Rhinoviruses infect the lower airways. J Infect Dis 2000; 181: 1875–84

29. Subauste MC, Jacoby DB, Richards SM, et al. Infection of a human respiratory epithelial cell line with rhinovirus. Induction of cytokine release and modulation of susceptibility to infection by cytokine exposure. J Clin Invest 1995; 96: 549–57

30. Gern JE, Martin MS, Anklam KA, et al. Relationships among specific viral pathogens, virus-induced interleukin-8, and respiratory symptoms in infancy. Pediatr Allergy Immunol 2002; 13: 386–93

31. Gern JE, Vrtis R, Grindle KA, et al. Relationship of upper and lower airway cytokines to outcome of experimental rhinovirus infection. Am J Respir Crit Care Med 2000; 162: 2226–31

32. Grissell TV, Powell H, Shafren DR, et al. Interleukin-10 gene expression in acute virus-induced asthma. Am J Respir Crit Care Med 2005; 172: 433–9

33. Fahy JV, Kim KW, Liu J, et al. Prominent neutrophilic inflammation in sputum from subjects with asthma exacerbation. J Allergy Clin Immunol 1995; 95: 843–52

34. Tillie-Leblond I, Pugin J, Marquette CH, et al. Balance between proinflammatory cytokines and their inhibitors in bronchial lavage from patients with status asthmaticus. Am J Respir Crit Care Med 1999; 159: 487–94

35. Broide DH, Lotz M, Cuomo AJ, et al. Cytokines in symptomatic asthma airways. J Allergy Clin Immunol 1992; 89: 958–67

36. Hirano T, Akira S, Taga T, et al. Biological and clinical aspects of interleukin 6. Immunol Today 1990; 11: 443–9

37. Doganci A, Sauer K, Karwot R, et al. Pathological role of IL-6 in the experimental allergic bronchial asthma in mice. Clin Rev Allergy Immunol 2005; 28: 257–70

38. O'Hollaren MT, Yunginger JW, Offord KP, et al. Exposure to an aeroallergen as a possible precipitating factor in respiratory arrest in young patients with asthma. N Engl J Med 1991; 324: 359–63

39. Weiss KB, Wagener DK. Geographic variations in US asthma mortality: small-area analyses of excess mortality, 1981–1985. Am J Epidemiol 1990; 132: S107–15

40. Calhoun WJ, Dick EC, Schwartz LB, et al. A common cold virus, rhinovirus 16, potentiates airway inflammation after segmental antigen bronchoprovocation in allergic subjects. J Clin Invest 1994; 94: 2200–8

41. Murray CS, Poletti G, Kebadze T, et al. A study of modifiable risk factors for asthma exacerbations: virus infection and allergen exposure increase the risk of asthma hospitalization in children. Thorax 2006; 61: 376–82

42. Green RM, Custovic A, Sanderson G, et al. Synergism between allergens and viruses and risk of hospital admission with asthma: case–control study. BMJ 2002; 324: 763

43. Harrod KS, Jaramillo RJ, Rosenberger CL, et al. Increased susceptibility to RSV infection by exposure to inhaled diesel engine emissions. Am J Respir Cell Mol Biol 2003; 28: 451–63

44. Chauhan AJ, Inskip HM, Linaker CH, et al. Personal exposure to nitrogen dioxide (NO_2) and the severity of virus-induced asthma in children. Lancet 2003; 361: 1939–44

45. Kepley CL, McFeeley PJ, Oliver JM, et al. Immunohistochemical detection of human basophils in postmortem cases of fatal asthma. Am J Respir Crit Care Med 2001; 164: 1053–8

46. Koshino T, Teshima S, Fukushima N, et al. Identification of basophils by immunohistochemistry in the airways of post-mortem cases of fatal asthma. Clin Exp Allergy 1993; 23: 919–25

47. Hart PH. Regulation of the inflammatory response in asthma by mast cell products. Immunol Cell Biol 2001; 79: 149–53

48. Marks GB. Environmental factors and gene–environment interactions in the aetiology of asthma. Clin Exp Pharmacol Physiol 2006; 33: 285–9

49. Cockcroft DW, Murdock KY, Kirby J, et al. Prediction of airway responsiveness to allergen from skin sensitivity to allergen and airway responsiveness to histamine. Am Rev Respir Dis 1987; 135: 264–7

50. Fahy JV, Cockcroft DW, Boulet LP, et al. Effect of aerosolized anti-IgE (E25) on airway responses to inhaled allergen in asthmatic subjects. Am J Resp Crit Care Med 1998; 157: A410

51. Boulet LP, Chapman KR, Cote J, et al. Inhibitory effects of an anti-IgE antibody E25 on allergen-induced early asthmatic response. Am J Respir Crit Care Med 1997; 155: 1835–40

52. Djukanovic R, Wilson SJ, Kraft M, et al. Effects of treatment with anti-immunoglobulin E antibody omalizumab on airway inflammation in allergic asthma. Am J Respir Crit Care Med 2004; 170: 583–93

53. Busse W, Corren J, Quentin Lanier B, et al. Omalizumab, anti-IgE recombinant humanized monoclonal antibody, for the treatment of severe allergic asthma. J Allergy Clin Immunol 2001; 108: 184–90

54. Soler M, Matz J, Townley R, et al. The anti-IgE antibody omalizumab reduces exacerbations and steroid requirement in allergic asthmatics. Eur Respir J 2001; 18: 254–61

55. Milgrom H, Fick RB, Su JQ, et al. Treatment of allergic asthma with monoclonal anti-IgE antibody. N Engl J Med 1999; 341: 1966–73

56. Seymour ML, Gilby N, Bardin PG, et al. Rhinovirus infection increases 5-lipoxygenase and cyclooxygenase-2 in bronchial biopsy specimens from nonatopic subjects. J Infect Dis 2002; 185: 540–4

57. Lamblin C, Gosset P, Tillie-Leblond I, et al. Bronchial neutrophilia in patients with non-infectious status asthmaticus. Am J Respir Crit Care Med 1998; 157: 394–402

58. Ordoñez CO, Shaughnessy TE, Matthay MA, et al. Increased neutrophil numbers and IL-8 levels in airway secretions in acute severe asthma. Am J Respir Crit Care Med 2000; 161: 15–20

59. Sur S, Crotty TB, Kephart GM, et al. Sudden-onset fatal asthma. A distinct entity with few eosinophils and relatively more neutrophils in the airway submucosa? Am Rev Respir Dis 1993; 148: 713–19

60. Carroll N, Lehmann E, Barret J, et al. Variability of airway structure and inflammation in normal subjects and in cases of nonfatal and fatal asthma. Pathol Res Pract 1996; 192: 238–48

61. Metzger WJ, Richerson HB, Worden K, et al. Bronchoalveolar lavage of allergic asthmatic patients following allergen bronchoprovocation. Chest 1986; 89: 477–83

62. Hunt LW, Gleich GJ, Ohnishi T, et al. Endotoxin contamination causes neutrophilia following pulmonary allergen challenge. Am J Respir Crit Care Med 1994; 149: 1471–5

63. Tillie-Leblond I, Gosset P, Tonnel AB. Inflammatory events in severe acute asthma. Allergy 2005; 60: 23–9

64. Corrigan CJ, Hartnell A, Kay AB. T lymphocyte activation in acute severe asthma. Lancet 1988; 1: 1129–32

65. O'Sullivan S, Cormican L, Faul JL, et al. Activated, cytotoxic CD8(+) T lymphocytes contribute to the pathology of asthma death. Am J Respir Crit Care Med 2001; 164: 560–4

66. Nittoh T, Fujimori H, Kozumi Y, et al. Effects of glucocorticoids on apoptosis of infiltrated eosinophils and neutrophils in rats. Eur J Pharmacol 1998; 354: 73–81

67. Thomas PS. Tumour necrosis factor-alpha: the role of this multifunctional cytokine in asthma. Immunol Cell Biol 2001; 79: 132–40

68. Koizumi A, Hashimoto S, Kobayashi T, et al. Elevation of serum soluble vascular cell adhesion molecule-1 (sVCAM-1) levels in bronchial asthma. Clin Exp Immunol 1995; 101: 468–73

69. Kobayashi T, Hashimoto S, Imai K, et al. Elevation of serum soluble intercellular adhesion molecule-1 (sICAM-1) and sE-selectin levels in bronchial asthma. Clin Exp Immunol 1994; 96: 110–15

70. Erzurum SC. Inhibition of tumor necrosis factor alpha for refractory asthma. N Engl J Med 2006; 354: 754–8

71. Kim J, McKinley L, Natarajan S, et al. Anti-tumor necrosis factor-alpha antibody treatment reduces pulmonary inflammation and methacholine hyper-responsiveness in a murine asthma model induced by house dust. Clin Exp Allergy 2006; 36: 122–32

72. Berry MA, Hargadon B, Shelley M, et al. Evidence of a role of tumor necrosis factor alpha in refractory asthma. N Engl J Med 2006; 354: 697–708

73. Dunnill MS, Massarella GR, Anderson JA. A comparison of the quantitative anatomy of the bronchi in normal subjects, in status asthmaticus, in chronic bronchitis, and in emphysema. Thorax 1969; 24: 176–9

74. Ebina M, Takahashi T, Chiba T, et al. Cellular hypertrophy and hyperplasia of airway smooth muscles underlying bronchial asthma. Am Rev Respir Dis 1993; 148: 720–6

75. Roche WR. Inflammatory and structural changes in the small airways in bronchial asthma. Am J Resp Crit Care Med 1998; 157: S191–4

76. Knox AJ. Airway remodeling in asthma – role of airway smooth muscle. Clin Sci 1994; 86: 647–52

77. Heard BE, Hossain S. Hyperplasia of bronchial muscle in asthma. J Pathol 1973; 110: 319–31

78. Hossain S. Quantitative measurement of bronchial muscle in men with asthma. Am Rev Respir Dis 1973; 107: 99–109

79. James AL, Pare PD, Hogg JC. The mechanics of airway narrowing in asthma. Am Rev Respir Dis 1989; 139: 242–6

80. Lambert RK, Wiggs BR, Kuwano K, et al. Functional significance of increased airway smooth muscle in asthma and COPD. J Appl Physiol 1993; 74: 2771–81

81. Macklem PT. A theoretical analysis of the effect of airway smooth muscle load on airway narrowing. Am J Respir Crit Care Med 1996; 153: 83–9

82. Diamant Z, Grootendorst DC, Veselic-Charvat M, et al. The effect of montelukast (MK-0476), a cysteinyl leukotriene receptor antagonist, on allergen-induced airway responses and sputum cell counts in asthma. Clin Exp Allergy 1999; 29: 42–51

83. Roquet A, Dahlen B, Kumlin M, et al. Combined antagonism of leukotrienes and histamine produces predominant inhibition of allergen-induced early and late phase airway obstruction in asthmatics. Am J Respir Crit Care Med 1997; 155: 1856–63

84. Li X, Wilson JW. Increased vascularity of the bronchial mucosa in mild asthma. Am J Resp Crit Care Med 1997; 156: 229–33

85. Mitzner W, Wagner E, Brown RH. Is asthma a vascular disorder? Chest 1995; 107: 97S-102S

86. Yager D, Kamm RD, Drazen JM. Airway wall liquid. Sources and role as an amplifier of bronchoconstriction. Chest 1995; 107: 105S-110S

87. Laitinen LA, Laitinen A, Widdicombe JG. Effects of inflammatory and other mediators on airway vascular beds. Am Rev Respir Dis 1987; 135: S67–S70

88. McDonald DM. Neurogenic inflammation in the respiratory tract: actions of sensory nerve mediators on blood vessels and epithelium in the airway mucosa. Am Rev Respir Dis 1987; 136: S65–S72

89. Erjefalt I, Persson CG. Inflammatory passage of plasma macromolecules into airway wall and lumen. Pulm Pharmacol 1989; 2: 93–102

90. Rogers DF, Boschetto P, Barnes PJ. Plasma exudation. Correlation between Evans blue dye and radiolabeled albumin in guinea pig airways in vivo. J Pharmacol Methods 1989; 21: 309–15

91. Fick RB Jr, Metzger WJ, Richerson HB, et al. Increased bronchovascular permeability after allergen exposure in sensitive asthmatics. J Appl Physiol 1987; 63: 1147–55

92. Svensson C, Baumgarten CR, Pipkorn U, et al. Reversibility and reproducibility of histamine induced plasma leakage in nasal airways. Thorax 1989; 44: 13–18

93. Lemjabbar H, Gosset P, Lamblin C, et al. Contribution of 92 kDa gelatinase/type IV collagenase in bronchial inflammation during status asthmaticus. Am J Respir Crit Care Med 1999; 159: 1298–307

94. List SJ, Findlay BP, Fornster GG, et al. Enhancement of the viscosity of mucin by serum albumin. Biochem J 1978; 175: 565–71

95. Wagers SS, Norton RJ, Rinaldi LM, et al. Extravascular fibrin, plasminogen activator, plasminogen activator inhibitors, and airway hyperresponsiveness. J Clin Invest 2004; 114: 104–11

96. O'Donnell SR, Persson CG. Beta-adrenoceptor mediated inhibition by terbutaline of histamine effects on vascular permeability. Br J Pharmacol 1978; 62: 321–4

97. Persson CG, Erjefalt I, Andersson P. Leakage of macromolecules from guinea-pig tracheobronchial microcirculation. Effects of allergen, leukotrienes, tachykinins, and anti-asthma drugs. Acta Physiol Scand 1986; 127: 95–105

98. Turner-Warwick M, Openshaw P. Sputum in asthma. Postgrad Med J 1987; 63 (Suppl 1): 79–82

99. Kuyper LM, Pare PD, Hogg JC, et al. Characterization of airway plugging in fatal asthma. Am J Med 2003; 115: 6–11

100. Dunnill MS. The pathology of asthma with special reference to changes in the bronchial mucosa. J Clin Pathol 1960; 13: 27–33

101. Reid LM. The presence or absence of bronchial mucus in fatal asthma. J Allergy Clin Immunol 1987; 80: 415–16

102. Aikawa T, Shimura S, Sasaki H, et al. Marked goblet cell hyperplasia with mucus accumulation in the airways of patients who died of severe acute asthma attack. Chest 1992; 101: 916–21

103. Shimura S, Andoh Y, Haraguchi M, et al. Continuity of airway goblet cells and intraluminal mucus in the airways of patients with bronchial asthma. Eur Respir J 1996; 9: 1395–401

104. Fahy JV. Goblet cell and mucin gene abnormalities in asthma. Chest 2002; 122: 320S–6S

105. Perez-Vilar J, Olsen JC, Chua M, et al. pH-dependent intraluminal organization of mucin granules in live human mucous/goblet cells. J Biol Chem 2005; 280: 16868–81

106. Kim KC, Lee BC. P2 purinoceptor regulation of mucin release by airway goblet cells in primary culture. Br J Pharmacol 1991; 103: 1053–6

107. Nadel JA, Takeyama K. Mechanisms of hypersecretion in acute asthma, proposed cause of death, and novel therapy. Pediatric Pulmonol 1999; 18: 54–5

108. Ohkawara Y, Lei XF, Stampfli MR, et al. Cytokine and eosinophil responses in the lung, peripheral blood, and bone marrow compartments in a murine model of allergen-induced airways inflammation. Am J Respir Cell Mol Biol 1997; 16: 510–20

109. Henderson WR Jr, Lewis DB, Albert RK, et al. The importance of leukotrienes in airway inflammation in a mouse model of asthma. J Exp Med 1996; 184: 1483–94

110. Hays SR, Fahy JV. The role of mucus in fatal asthma. Am J Med 2003; 115: 68–9

111. Brandt T, Breitenstein S, von der Hardt H, et al. DNA concentration and length in sputum of patients with cystic fibrosis during inhalation with recombinant human DNase. Thorax 1995; 50: 880–2

112. Fahy JV. Airway mucus and the mucociliary system. In Middleton E, Reed CE, Ellis EF, et al., eds. Allergy Principles and Practice. St Louis, MO: Mosby, 1998: 520–31

113. King M, Rubin BK. Pharmacological approaches to discovery and development of new mucolytic agents. Adv Drug Deliv Rev 2002; 54: 1475–90

114. Hwang TH, Schwiebert EM, Guggino WB. Apical and basolateral ATP stimulates tracheal epithelial chloride secretion via multiple purinergic receptors. Am J Physiol 1996; 270: C1611–23

115. Stutts MJ, Fitz JG, Paradiso AM, et al. Multiple modes of regulation of airway epithelial chloride secretion by extracellular ATP. Am J Physiol 1994; 267: C1442–51

116. Ratjen F. Restoring airway surface liquid in cystic fibrosis. N Engl J Med 2006; 354: 291–3

117. Donaldson SH, Bennett WD, Zeman KL, et al. Mucus clearance and lung function in cystic fibrosis with hypertonic saline. N Engl J Med 2006; 354: 241–50

118. Elkins MR, Robinson M, Rose BR, et al. A controlled trial of long-term inhaled hypertonic saline in patients with cystic fibrosis. N Engl J Med 2006; 354: 229–40

119. Lang DM, Simon RA, Mathison DA, et al. Safety and possible efficacy of fiberoptic bronchoscopy with lavage in the management of refractory asthma with mucous impaction. Ann Allergy 1991; 67: 324–30

CHAPTER 9

Virus induction of neurogenic inflammation and airway responsiveness

Giovanni Piedimonte

INTRODUCTION

Local stimulation of vagal polymodal nociceptive afferent nerves (C-fibers) in the respiratory tract results in a series of co-ordinated biological responses aimed at expelling the noxious agents and starting the inflammatory and immune responses. This constellation of events is referred to as neurogenic inflammation and is due to the local release of peptide neurotransmitters stored in terminal varicosities of these nerves.

The first part of this chapter focuses on the receptors and enzymes involved in the regulation of the biological responses to inflammatory neuropeptides in the respiratory tract, their distribution, function and biological effects.

The second part focuses on the effects of viral respiratory infections on sensory innervation of the airways at different developmental stages and explores the pathophysiological manifestations of these effects, such as changes in vascular permeability and bronchial responsiveness occurring during and after the infection. Also reviewed are the interactions between the sensorineural pathways and different effector cell types involved in immune and inflammatory responses, such as lymphocytes, monocytes and mast cells, and the critical role of neurotrophic factors in the co-ordination and modulation of these interactions. A new model deriving from these data is discussed that could explain some

of the unique phenotypic features of asthma in childhood.

In the last part, specific attention is directed towards the possible therapeutic strategies aimed at controlling neurogenic inflammatory responses.

INFLAMMATORY NEUROPEPTIDES

Peptides

Mammalian tachykinins include substance P (SP), neurokinin A (NKA), neurokinin B (NKB), and the N-terminal extended forms of NKA (neuropeptide K, NPK; neuropeptide γ, NPγ). Their agonist activity is associated with the shared carboxy terminal domain (Phe-X-Gly-Leu-Met-NH$_2$), whereas the amino terminal domains confer binding selectivity for different receptor subtypes.[1] Two distinct preprotachykinin (PPT) genes control the synthesis of tachykinin peptides.[2] While NKB is the only product from the PPT-B gene, the PPT-A gene directs the synthesis of several different peptides. As a result of alternative RNA splicing, three different mRNA transcripts are produced from the PPT-A gene: the αPPT-A mRNA can encode only SP, whereas the βPPT-A and γPPT-A mRNAs can encode both SP and NKA. Post-translational processing of the βPPT-A mRNA product can yield NKA or NPK, while γPPT-A mRNA can yield NKA or NPγ.[3,4] Thus, by virtue of the alternative mRNA splicing and post-translational processing mechanisms, the two tachykinin genes generate a family of peptides with substantially diverse biological properties.

The sensory nerves of the upper[5] and lower[6] respiratory tract of several species, including humans, contain SP-immunoreactive axons. The terminal varicosities of these unmyelinated C-type fibers are particularly abundant in the airway epithelium and around mucosal arterioles.[7] In addition to SP, C-fibers also contain NKA, NPK and possibly NPγ,[8] all very potent agonists of NK_2 receptors and more potent bronchoconstrictor agents than SP.[9,10] A non-tachykinin peptide also contained in C-fibers is the calcitonin gene-related peptide (CGRP),[11,12] which is a potent vasodilator in the skin[13] and gastrointestinal tract,[14] but does not seem to have a direct effect on microvascular permeability[11] and blood flow[15,16] in the airways. A mixture of these sensory neuropeptides is co-released within the airway mucosa upon afferent stimulation by a variety of physical and chemical stimuli. Other peptide mediators are contained in efferent autonomic nerves, both parasympathetic (vasoactive intestinal polypeptide, VIP; peptide histidine-isoleucine, PHI) and sympathetic (neuropeptide Y, NPY). This complex peptidergic network represents a third nervous pathway serving the airways in parallel to the cholinergic and adrenergic components: the non-cholinergic–non-adrenergic nervous system (NANC).[17,18]

Of the SP produced in the cell bodies of the dorsal root ganglia and of the nodose ganglion, 90% is transported into the peripheral varicosities of afferent C-type fibers,[19] and travels to the lungs within the vagus nerve.[20] Thus, SP acts both as the transmitter of nociceptive information from the lungs to the central nervous system (CNS)[21] and as a potent inflammatory mediator at the peripheral terminal.[22] Upon sensory nerve stimulation, the action potential is conveyed to the spinal cord, but also spreads to the peripheral collaterals, branching in the airway epithelium and around airway vessels and smooth muscle fibers, resulting in a cascade-like amplification of the original stimulus (the 'axon reflex').

Release of neuropeptides from afferent C-fibers can be induced in experimental models by electrical stimulation[23] or by pharmacological stimulation by capsaicin (8-methyl-N-vanillyl-6-nonenamide).[24] This pungent principle of plants of the Capsicum genus exerts a dual action selectively on C-fibers. Its acute effect is the Ca^{2+}-dependent release of neuropeptides from the granules stored inside the nerve varicosities; the chronic effect of exposure to high concentration of capsaicin is the permanent desensitization to capsaicin itself and other stimuli. These effects of capsaicin are mediated by binding to vanilloid-like transient receptor potential channel type 1 ($TRPV_1$), a calcium-permeable channel expressed predominantly by C-type unmyelinated sensory neurons.[25] This receptor responds to a variety of microenvironmental stimuli (chemical irritants, heat, acid pH) by co-releasing multiple neurotransmitters, including SP, neurokinins, CGRP, VIP and somatostatin. Because multiple stimuli can converge on the same TRPV channel, these channels also function as sites of integration of diverse physical and chemical signals towards the same transduction pathway.[26] This property of capsaicin to release and subsequently deplete peptides from sensory nerve endings has been pivotal in understanding the distribution and physiological roles of the tachykinins. Additional information has been obtained from the use of the inorganic dye Ruthenium red[27] as a blocker of the capsaicin-sensitive cation channel, and with the selective vanilloid receptor antagonist capsazepine.[28]

Receptors

Three mammalian neurokinin receptors have been cloned, and their deduced protein sequences with seven putative transmembrane spannin helices are typical of G-protein-coupled receptors.[29] Their activation results in a rise in cytosolic calcium ion (Ca^{2+}) concentration mediated by the phosphatidylinositol pathway.[30] Each of the tachykinin peptides can act as a full agonist on all three receptors, if present at sufficiently high concentrations. However, SP, NKA (also NPK and NPγ) and NKB display preferential affinity for neurokinin NK_1, NK_2 and NK_3 receptors, respectively.[31] The poor selectivity shown by naturally occurring tachykinins is probably due to sequence homology at the carboxy terminus, since synthetic agonists obtained by structural modifications of this domain exhibit high selectivity for individual receptors.

Autoradiographic studies with radiolabeled ligands have visualized SP-binding sites in the respiratory tract of rats, guinea-pigs, rabbits and humans.[32–35] NK_1 receptors have a pivotal role in neurogenic inflammatory responses and are predominantly expressed on epithelial and endothelial cells, submucosal glands and circulating leukocytes. NK_2 receptors affect bronchoconstriction and facilitate pulmonary cholinergic neurotransmission and are expressed at the highest density on airway smooth muscle cells, on neurons in the parasympathetic autonomic ganglia and on post-ganglionic neurons.

Peptidases

The biological effects of tachykinins are modulated by enzymes expressed on the surface of the target cells. This structural arrangement allows these enzymes to degrade peptide agonists in the proximity of their receptors, thus limiting their activity. Most neurogenic inflammatory responses are modulated to a large extent by two membrane-bound peptidases, the neutral endopeptidase (NEP; also called enkephalinase, common acute lymphocytic leukemia antigen, CALLA, EC 3.4.24.11) and the angiotensin converting enzyme (ACE; also called kininase II, dipeptidyl carboxypeptidase I, peptidyl dipeptidase A, EC 3.4.15.1). Inhibition of NEP and/or ACE activity by selective blockers, such as phosphoramidon[36] and captopril,[37] respectively, potentiates neurogenic inflammatory responses.

The lungs contain the highest levels of both NEP and ACE activities in the body.[38,39] Both peptidases are also present in tracheal homogenates, but in markedly reduced concentrations.[40] Immunohistochemical staining and enzyme assays have revealed the presence of NEP in different substructures within the respiratory tract, including the alveolar epithelium,[41] tracheal epithelium,[42,43] tracheal smooth muscle[42,44] and submucosal glands.[45] ACE seems to be concentrated along the luminal surface of the vascular endothelium.[41,46,47] Co-expression of ACE and NEP has been reported in arterial and venous endothelium.[48]

The substrate specificity of NEP and ACE is largely overlapping; however, because both peptidases are membrane-bound, these enzymes can act only in the proximity of the cell surfaces where they are expressed. Thus, their selectivity and efficiency *in vivo* is restricted by the geometrical factors that determine the 'accessibility' of the enzyme to potential substrates. ACE, which is predominantly an endothelial peptidase, modulates the biological activity of blood-borne substrates either injected[49–51] or endogenously released.[52] In contrast, NEP, although expressed in the endothelium, seems to play a more relevant physiological role in the extravascular compartments.

NEUROGENIC INFLAMMATION IN THE AIRWAYS

Plasma extravasation and neutrophil adherence

Electrical stimulation of the cervical vagus nerve or pharmacological stimulation of sensory nerves with capsaicin results in complex changes in the tracheal microvasculature of rodents, leading to increased permeability to plasma macromolecules and an increased number of neutrophils adhering to the endothelium. Both components of this 'neurogenic inflammation' are blocked by selective antagonists of the NK_1 receptor subtype,[53–56] and thus are mediated by the natural NK$_1$ ligand, SP.[31] SP is known to cause complex changes in the endothelium of post-capillary venules, which represent the elective targets of inflammatory mediators.[57,58] SP opens gaps in the endothelial lining,[59,60] presumably by inducing contraction of endothelial cells.[61] SP also promotes endothelium–leukocyte interaction via increased expression of adhesion molecules.[62] Both effects probably involve SP-induced mast cell degranulation with consequent release of tumor necrosis factor α (TNF-α) and cysteinyl leukotrienes.

Selective NK$_1$ receptor antagonists reduce the exudative response to a variety of inhaled irritants that are known to trigger asthma episodes in humans. For example, NK$_1$ antagonism inhibits airway plasma leakage induced by cigarette smoke.[63] Aerosolized hypertonic saline, which reproduces the pathophysiological mechanism of exercise-induced asthma,[64] also causes plasma extravasation in the rat airways that is abolished by pharmacological sensory denervation with capsaicin[65] or by pretreatment with an NK$_1$ receptor antagonist.[56] NK$_1$-mediated plasma extravasation occurs in sensitized guinea-pigs after challenge with aerosolized ovalbumin.[66] The importance of the NK$_1$ receptor in the organization of pulmonary inflammatory reactions has been elucidated further by the observation that gene-targeted deletion of this receptor in mice prevents the acute inflammatory responses associated with immune complex-mediated lung injury, including plasma extravasation and neutrophil influx.[67] Collectively, these studies support the hypothesis that SP and other neuropeptides play an important modulatory role upstream from other inflammatory pathways in the respiratory tract.[68]

NEP and ACE are co-expressed on the postcapillary venular endothelium, the elective site of mediator-induced plasma extravasation and leukocyte adhesion. Inhibition of NEP or ACE potentiates the increase in vascular permeability[69,70] and the adhesion of neutrophils to the vascular endothelium[69,71] produced by sensory nerve stimulation or by exogenous injection of SP. Simultaneous inhibition of both enzymes potentiates these effects more than a maximally effective dose of either inhibitor by itself.[70,71]

Blood flow

Blood flow in the airway microvascular bed is a critical aspect of inflammation. Changes in microvascular blood flow affect the recruitment of inflammatory cells and mediators and the edematous swelling of the respiratory mucosa. On the other hand, the increase in blood flow may also have the protective function of washing away inflammatory mediators and exogenous irritants from inflamed tissues, thus limiting the extent and duration of acute inflammatory and hypersensitivity responses.[72]

The endogenous release of proinflammatory peptides from C-type sensory afferents greatly increases blood flow in the microvascular bed of the rat extrapulmonary airways.[15] Five-fold increase in airway blood flow is produced by a low dose of capsaicin (10^{-7} mol/kg), which does not alter regional blood flow to other organs; thus, the resistance vessels regulating the blood flow to the extrapulmonary airways are more responsive to sensory neuropeptides than similar vessels in other organs. In addition, this dose of capsaicin does not increase airway vascular permeability; thus, the threshold nerve stimulation necessary to induce plasma exudation is much higher than that necessary to increase local blood flow. These observations suggest that the intensity of noxious stimuli qualitatively modulates neurogenic inflammatory responses. Mild stimuli may be eliminated by increased blood flow, whereas stronger, persistent stimuli may require the activation of additional defense mechanisms, such as the recruitment of inflammatory cells and mediators through more permeable vessels. The fact that neuropeptides do not affect intrapulmonary bronchial blood flow,[15] together with previous observations showing that antidromic vagal stimulation evokes plasma extravasation only in the proximal airways,[60] indicates that neurogenic inflammation does not occur in the distal airways of adult lungs, probably due to sparse afferent innervation. In contrast, in young animals the highest density of sensory innervation is found in the distal airways, and this 'inverted' distribution of afferent fibers may explain, at least in part, the different manifestations of airway inflammatory disease in childhood versus adulthood.

The vasodilator effect of capsaicin in the airways is reduced by pretreatment with a cocktail of autonomic inhibitors (atropine, guanethidine and hexamethonium),[15] suggesting that a vasodilator reflex is activated following sensory nerve stimulation, probably mediated by VIP released from parasympathetic efferents. Despite the fact that SP and CGRP immunoreactivities coexist in perivascular C-fibers and are co-released when these nerves are stimulated with capsaicin,[11] only SP increases the blood flow in the airway microvascular bed, whereas CGRP does not produce significant changes.[15] Studies with a selective receptor antagonist have confirmed that neurogenic vasodilatation, like the other vascular effects of sensory nerves in the airways, is due to the effect of SP on NK_1 receptors.[16,73]

In rats pretreated with captopril to inhibit ACE activity, the vasodilator effect of SP on airway microvessels is increased by approximately one order of magnitude.[16] More importantly, ACE inhibition affects the duration of SP-induced vasodilatation. In fact, the vasodilator effect of both SP and capsaicin is very transient, and no change in airway blood flow can be demonstrated 5 minutes after injection of either drug.[15] In contrast, airway blood flow remains elevated 5 minutes after SP is injected in captopril-pretreated animals.[16] Similar potentiation of airway blood flow is obtained using the selective NEP inhibitor phosphoramidon.[74] In contrast, the relaxant effect of SP in isolated pulmonary arteries is potentiated by selective ACE inhibition, but not by inhibition of NEP or other enzymes known to degrade vasoactive peptides,[75]

suggesting regional differences in the endothelial expression and functional importance of peptidases along the respiratory tract. On the basis of the dramatic effect of captopril on the vascular changes produced by SP, it can be speculated that potentiation of neurogenic inflammation may be one cause of the increased bronchial reactivity associated with the chronic therapeutic use of ACE inhibitors in humans.[76]

Bronchomotor tone

Tachykinins released from sensory nerves contract the airway smooth muscle.[77,78] In isolated human bronchi, this effect is mimicked by selective NK_2 agonists[9] and blocked by selective NK_2 antagonists,[79] whereas NK_1 agonists and antagonists are ineffective. Although the NK_2 receptor can be activated by both SP and NKA, the latter is the most potent natural agonist of this receptor.[31]

The contraction induced in isolated segments of ferret tracheal smooth muscle by exogenous tachykinins[42] and by electrical nerve stimulation[44] is potentiated by the NEP inhibitor leucine–thiorphan dose dependently. The effect of electrical stimulation is abolished by atropine and by tachykinin antagonism but is not affected by adrenergic or ganglion blockers; thus this effect is likely to be due to post-ganglionic stimulation of cholinergic nerves by tachykinins. In contrast, electrical nerve stimulation of guinea-pig bronchi evokes early cholinergic contraction followed by long-lasting sensory nerve-dependent contraction that is mediated by NK_1, NK_2[80] and possibly additional NK receptors.[81] NEP inhibitors potentiate the contractile effect of capsaicin and electrical nerve stimulation in guinea-pig bronchi, whereas inhibitors of ACE, aminopeptidases, acetylcholinesterase and serine proteases are without effect.[82]

Mucociliary clearance

Tachykinins stimulate mucus secretion and ciliary beat frequency through activation of NK_1 receptors.[83,84] The first studies on the modulating role of NEP in neurogenic inflammation were *in vitro* studies of airway gland secretion. Inhibitors of NEP potentiate the effect of SP[85] on mucus secretion in the ferret trachea, whereas inhibitors of other proteases (including the ACE inhibitors captopril and teprotide) have no effect. The fact that the N-terminal fragment SP_{1-9} generated by NEP does not induce gland secretion provides additional evidence that NEP cleavage generates inactive SP metabolites in this system. In addition, NEP inhibition potentiates the effect of bradykinin[86] and SP[87] on ciliary motility.

Cough

Although cough is one of the most conspicuous manifestations of lung diseases associated with inflammation (e.g. asthma, bronchitis, cystic fibrosis, viral infections), the mechanisms underlying this protective reflex are poorly understood. In unanesthetized guinea-pigs, inhalation of capsaicin and SP aerosols causes cough,[88] and this effect is potentiated after inhalation of aerosols of NEP inhibitors, presumably by inhibiting the NEP present in the guinea-pig airway epithelium. A similar pathophysiological mechanism can be proposed to explain the dry cough observed in humans as a well-known side-effect of chronic therapy with ACE inhibitors.[89]

VIRUS-INDUCED NEUROGENIC INFLAMMATION

Respiratory infections

Viral respiratory infections frequently cause exacerbations of asthma and chronic obstructive pulmonary disease (COPD), and have been implicated in the pathogenesis of this disease. The following paragraphs review the effects of viral respiratory infections on neurogenically mediated immune, inflammatory and bronchomotor responses in the airways.

The contractile response to SP of ferret tracheal segments increases three-fold following incubation *in vitro* with human influenza virus A1 Taiwan.[90] Pretreatment with an NEP inhibitor increases the response to SP to the same final level in both infected and control tissues, whereas inhibitors of other peptidases (including ACE) are ineffective. Furthermore, NEP activity is decreased in infected tissues. *In vivo*, pathogen-free guinea-pigs selectively infected with murine parainfluenza type I (Sendai) virus[91] develop bronchial hyperreactivity to tachykinins associated with decreased airway NEP activity 4 days after inoculation. These findings suggested that these viral infections may potentiate the contractile response to tachykinins by decreasing the degradative activity of NEP.

The responses induced by tachykinins in the airway microcirculation are similarly affected by respiratory infections. The permeability of tracheal blood vessels to intravascular tracers was initially studied in rats with antibody titers showing natural exposure to three common murine pathogens: Sendai virus, rat coronavirus and *Mycoplasma pulmonis*. Past exposure to these infectious agents is not associated with changes in baseline airway vascular permeability. However, the increase in tracheal vascular permeability evoked by nerve stimulation or by SP is potentiated markedly compared to pathogen-free controls.[92] Similarly, in rats exposed to respiratory infections, nerve stimulation evokes a much larger increase in the number of neutrophils adhering to the venular endothelium, preparing to migrate into the perivascular tissues. Again, NEP inhibition increases the SP-induced change in vascular permeability in pathogen-free rats but does not further amplify the already large increase in rats exposed to infections.[43] NEP activity is decreased in the tracheal epithelium of infected rats compared to pathogen-free rats, but no difference in enzyme activity can be detected in the tracheal submucosa and in the esophagus. Exaggerated neurogenic plasma extravasation and leukocyte adhesion can be reproduced by selectively inoculating pathogen-free rats with

Sendai virus[93] or with *M. pulmonis.*[94] The long-lasting potentiation produced by the latter organism may be due in part to structural changes in the tracheal microvasculature (i.e. increased number of post-capillary venules).[94]

Sendai virus infection potentiates the increase in airway blood flow induced by SP but not histamine.[74] In contrast with the previous observations of the effect of infections on smooth muscle contraction and vascular permeability, after inhibition of the NEP activity alone SP-induced airway vasodilatation in pathogen-free rats is still significantly reduced compared to that in infected rats, whereas inhibition of both NEP and ACE potentiates the effect of SP to the same final level in both infected and control animals. Thus, the effect of Sendai virus infection on airway resistance vessels may be due to a combined down-regulation of the activities of both peptidases.

Collectively, these studies indicated that influenza and parainfluenza viruses potentiate neurogenic inflammatory and hypersensitivity responses, and proposed the associated decrease in peptide-degrading enzyme activity as the cause for the increased responses. The decrease in NEP activity did not appear to be due to the release of a protease inhibitor produced during viral replication because the supernatant from tracheal rings infected with influenza virus did not affect the activity of purified NEP.[90] Since viral infections are commonly associated with extensive damage of the respiratory epithelium, it is possible that the increased responses to endogenous and exogenous tachykinins are due in part to the physical loss of NEP-rich epithelium during viral replication. However, this mechanism alone cannot explain the increased response to intravenous SP,[43,92] the potentiation produced by *M. pulmonis* in the absence of significant epithelial damage[94] or the downregulation of endothelial ACE activity. Therefore, it became progressively evident that other mechanisms have to be involved in the virus-induced airway inflammation and hyperreactivity.

Neuroimmune interactions

Lower respiratory tract infections with respiratory syncytial virus (RSV) cause strong potentiation of neurogenic inflammation, as manifested by the exaggerated increase in microvascular permeability in response to endogenous and exogenous SP observed 5 days after inoculation of the virus.[95] This potentiation of neurogenic inflammation is similar to that outlined above for other respiratory pathogens (influenza and parainfluenza viruses).[93,96] However, RSV does not affect the enzymatic activity of NEP, as seen with the other viruses, and therefore its effect cannot be explained with decreased catabolism of the SP released from nerve fibers. Rather, the potentiation of neurogenic inflammation associated with the presence of RSV in the respiratory tract involves a different post-synaptic mechanism(s), independent of the activity of peptide-degrading enzymes.

SP binds with high affinity to the NK_1 tachykinin receptor subtype.[31] Reverse transcriptase–polymerase chain reaction (RT-PCR) analysis revealed that the expression of the gene encoding this receptor is strongly upregulated in the lung tissues of rats inoculated 5 days previously with RSV.[95] At the same time, the density of binding sites for SP visualized by autoradiography is markedly increased in the bronchial mucosa of RSV-infected lungs (Figure 9.1). Selective antagonism of the NK_1 receptor abolishes the effect of RSV on airway neurogenic inflammation, confirming that this effect requires SP–NK_1 receptor interaction.

In adult rats, the potentiation of capsaicin-induced neurogenic inflammation during RSV infection can be detected in the extrapulmonary, but not in the intrapulmonary airways.[95] This observation implies that the density of capsaicin-sensitive C-type nerves is highest in the proximal airways and progressively decreases in more distal airways, confirming previous observations.[60] However, intrapulmonary airways exposed to RSV respond to exogenous SP with a large increase in vascular permeability, suggesting that

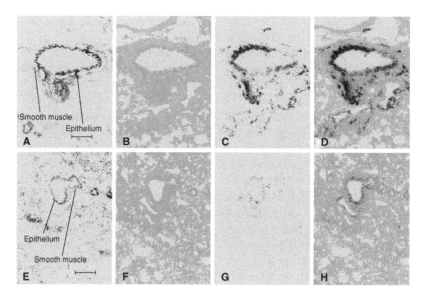

Figure 9.1 Autoradiographic mapping of substance P (SP) binding sites in the lungs of respiratory syncytial virus (RSV)-infected (A-B-C-D) and pathogen-free (E-F-G-H) rats 5 days after inoculation. The illustration shows, from left to right: schematic diagrams (A and E), hematoxylin/eosin (H&E) preparations (B and F), autoradiographic images (C and G) and autoradiography digitally superimposed on H&E (D and H). Specific SP binding was detected over the bronchial mucosa and the wall of adjacent pulmonary vessels and was consistently and markedly increased in infected airways. No significant binding was detected over the airway smooth muscle and the alveolar tissue. Internal scale, 0.5 mm. Reproduced with permission from reference 95. See also Color Plate II

RSV-infected distal airways become hyper-responsive to intravascular SP even in the absence of specific innervation. This is consistent with other studies demonstrating a significant mismatch in the localization of SP-containing nerves and SP receptors in the brain[97] and lungs of adult rats.[98]

Age-dependency

Stimulation of capsaicin-sensitive sensory nerves 5 days after inoculation causes a much larger increase of Evans Blue-labeled albumin extravasation in the intrapulmonary airways of RSV-infected weanling rats compared to age-matched pathogen-free controls.[99] In contrast, analysis of the extrapulmonary airways shows no difference in extravasation between infected and pathogen-free weanling rats (Figure 9.2). Therefore, the response to capsaicin of airway

blood vessels in young rats is qualitatively different from that in adult rats. In separate experiments, we also found that the conversion to the adult-type pattern is completed in rats by 48–50 days of age, which grossly corresponds to adolescence in humans. The differences found between young and adult rats imply age-dependent variability in the distribution of tachykinin-containing sensory nerves along the respiratory tract. Thus, it is possible that the different clinical manifestations of RSV disease in children (lower respiratory tract involvement with bronchiolitis) versus adults (usually upper airway symptoms) may at least in part result from age-related molecular differences in one or more inflammatory pathways, rather than be determined by simple anatomical factors (e.g. airway caliber).

In weanling rats, semiquantitative RT-PCR analysis of the NK_1 receptor mRNA extracted

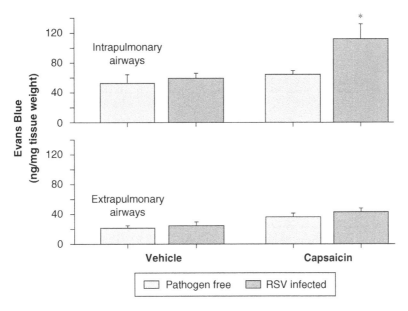

Figure 9.2 Potentiation of airway neurogenic inflammation 5 days after the inoculation of respiratory syncytial virus (RSV) or virus-free medium measured in the intrapulmonary airways (top panel) and extrapulmonary airways (bottom panel) of weanling F-344 rats. In rats injected with vehicle (left columns), RSV did not change vascular permeability compared to pathogen-free controls. However, the increase in vascular permeability elicited in the intrapulmonary airways by capsaicin (right columns) was significantly larger in RSV-infected rats than in pathogen-free controls. In the extrapulmonary airways, vascular permeability did not change significantly. $*p < 0.05$; significantly different from pathogen-free controls. Reproduced with permission from reference 99

from lung tissues consistently revealed a much stronger signal in RSV-infected weanling rats than in pathogen-free controls.[99] Pretreatment with a monoclonal antibody against the F protein of RSV prevented upregulation of the NK_1 receptor (Figure 9.3). In contrast, VIP receptor expression was only slightly elevated in RSV-infected weanling rats compared to the pathogen-free controls. These data indicate that RSV differentially modulates the expression of specific neuropeptide receptors causing an imbalance between the proinflammatory (SP-dependent) and anti-inflammatory (VIP-dependent) components of the NANC nervous system in the respiratory tract and favoring the development and maintenance of airway inflammation. In addition, because SP and VIP modulate several immune functions by exerting opposite influences (stimulatory for SP,

inhibitory for VIP), the peptidergic imbalance caused by RSV might link the neurogenic and immunoinflammatory mechanisms proposed by different authors to explain the pathophysiology of RSV disease and its sequelae.

Bronchomotor tone

The high-affinity NKA receptor (NK_2 subtype) is expressed on smooth muscle cells and mediates NANC bronchoconstriction. RSV does not affect the expression of the NK_2 receptor subtype, as indicated by: the lack of change in the expression of NK_2 receptor mRNA in infected lung tissues;[99] and the sparse binding of radiolabeled ligand to the airway smooth muscle in infected bronchioles.[95]

To confirm these findings, we measured NKA-induced bronchoconstriction in our model

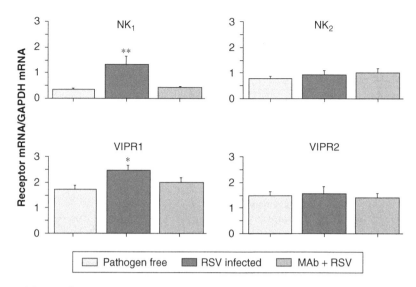

Figure 9.3 Modulation of neuropeptide receptor expression by respiratory syncytial virus (RSV). RT-PCR analysis revealed an approximately four-fold increase in neurokinin NK_1 receptor mRNA from the lungs of RSV-infected rats compared to pathogen-free controls, whereas the vascoactive intestinal peptide (VIP)R_1 receptor mRNA increased by approximately 40%. mRNA levels for the NK_2 VIPR2 receptor subtypes were not affected by the virus. Palivizumab (MAb) prevented upregulation of the NK_1 receptor in RSV-inoculated rats. $*p < 0.05$; $**p < 0.01$; significantly different from pathogen-free controls. Reproduced with permission from reference 95

of RSV bronchiolitis.[100] No significant difference was found in NK_2 receptor mRNA from lung tissues or in NKA-induced bronchospasm between RSV-infected and pathogen-free rats,[100] indicating that RSV does not affect NANC bronchoconstriction. This is consistent with the hypothesis that bronchial obstruction in RSV bronchiolitis is primarily a function of inflammatory edema of the airway mucosa rather than constriction of the airway smooth muscle tone, which would also explain the frequent lack of clinical response to bronchodilators in infants with viral bronchiolitis.

Post-viral inflammation

Despite complete resolution of the infection, the potentiation of neurogenic inflammatory reactions is still present 30 days after inoculation of the virus, as manifested by the exaggerated increase of microvascular permeability in response to sensory nerve stimulation.[101] This potentiation is not only qualitatively but also quantitatively similar to the response measured during the acute phase of the infection. Similar long-term potentiation is observed in adult rats that had developed RSV infection during the weaning period. Surprisingly, the vascular response to exogenous SP is no longer potentiated 30 days after the infection. Although the expression of the NK_1 receptor remains slightly increased after resolution of the acute infection, this effect is no longer statistically significant, and thus it is unlikely to be the primary mechanism responsible for the post-infection changes in neurogenic inflammation. However, enzyme-linked immunoassay reveals a large increase of SP concentration in the lung tissues of rats during and after infection with RSV. Also, capsaicin-induced release of SP remains abnormal after the infection and is approximately twice that measured in pathogen-free controls injected with the same dose of capsaicin at 30 days post-inoculation, suggesting structural and/or functional remodeling of the sensory innervation serving the airways. These findings are consistent with the hypothesis that the mechanism of post-infectious potentiation of neurogenic inflammation operates predominantly at the pre-synaptic level with minor involvement of the post-synaptic component active during the acute phase of the infection. The experimental evidence supporting a pre-synaptic mechanism for the post-viral potentiation of neurogenic inflammation is three-fold: (1) lack of significant vascular response at 30 days post-inoculation of RSV to the same dose of SP that caused large exudation 5 days post-inoculation; (2) lack of persistent elevation of mRNA encoding the NK_1 receptor 30 days post-inoculation; and (3) increased content and increased release of SP from capsaicin-sensitive sensory nerves in lung tissues 30 days post-inoculation.

Neuroimmunomodulation

Immunohistochemical and autoradiographic mapping of NK_1 receptor expression in RSV-infected airways (Figure 9.4) shows clusters of cells staining deeply with an anti-NK_1 antibody and binding radiolabeled SP avidly.[102] Thus, RSV induces overexpression of the NK_1 receptor on selected lymphocyte subpopulations within the bronchus-associated lymphoid tissue (BALT), 'priming' these cells for the immuno-modulatory effects of SP. Release of this peptide from the dense supply of afferent fibers inner-vating the mucosal lymphoid aggregates[103] by airborne irritants inhaled during lower respiratory tract infections initiates a cascade-like sequence by recruiting the immunocytes primed by the virus. Consequently, sensorineural stimulation during RSV infection leads to a markedly increased flux of lymphocytes and monocytes into the airways, with an approximately 20 to 1 monocytes/lymphocytes ratio.[102] This neurogenic recruitment of immunocytes is already measurable 1 day after nerve stimulation, peaks by day 5 and remains significant 10 days after a single stimulus, whereas in the absence of

sensorineural activation immunocyte recruitment by the infection alone is much more limited and transient. Thus, not only is the degree of the cellular response to the virus magnified by concurrent nerve irritation, but this response is also sustained and persists after non-stimulated airways have returned to normal. The simultaneous reduction of both CD4+ and CD8+ cells recovered from infected lung tissues suggests that the lymphocytes flowing into the airways originate from the mucosal immune system.[102]

Neurogenic recruitment of immunocytes into infected airways is abolished by selective phar-macological antagonism of the NK_1 receptor,[102] indicating that SP binding to its high-affinity receptor is primarily responsible for this effect. The influence of SP on immunocyte recruitment during RSV infection appears to be not only quantitative, but also qualitative as shown by the disproportionate number of CD4+ cells versus CD8+ cells found in the BALT. Both lymphocytes and monocytes recruited in the infected airways can amplify and propagate the chemotactic and modulatory functions of sensory nerves in an autocrine and/or paracrine fashion, as they are capable of producing and releasing SP.[104,105] Also, the subsequent activation of these cells with release of cytokines and chemokines is likely to be responsible for the second phase, characterized by the build-up in the airways of a large population of activated lymphocytes and monocytes. The neurogenic recruitment of monocytes is of special interest, as these cells can promote airway inflammation and modulate immune responses via the production of cytokines such as tumor necrosis factor α (TNF-α)[106,107] and interleukins (IL)-1,[108] IL-6,[106] IL-8[106] and IL-10.[109] In addition, RSV-infected monocytes may amplify and spread the infection by delivering a greater load of viral particles to the host tissue than the initial load infecting the monocyte itself.[110]

Mast cells

Histopathological analysis of lung tissues stained with an antibody against tryptase shows

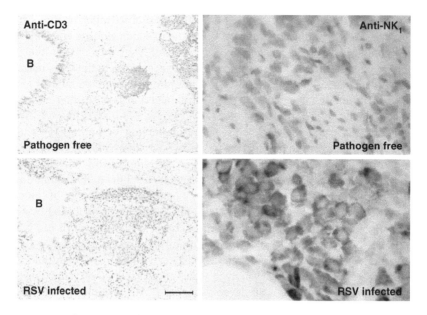

Figure 9.4 Lung sections from rats sacrificed 5 days after the intratracheal inoculation of virus-free medium (upper panels) or respiratory syncytial virus (RSV) (lower panels). Immunoperoxidase staining was performed using antibodies specific for the all-T antigen CD3 (left panels) and the high-affinity substance P receptor NK_1 (right panels). The dark-brown reaction reveals predominance of T cells in the hypertrophic bronchus-associated lymphoid tissue of RSV-infected airways with strong overexpression of the NK_1 receptor on discrete lymphocyte subpopulations. B, bronchiole. Internal scale, 40 µm. Reproduced with permission from reference 102. See also Color Plate III

numerous mast cells in the sections from RSV-infected rats, with an average seven-fold increase compared to the lungs of pathogen-free controls.[111] Most of these mast cells are in close spatial associations with nerve fibers (Figure 9.5), suggesting functional mast cell–nerve interactions similar to those previously reported in other organ systems,[112] particularly the skin, CNS and gastrointestinal tract.[113]

Among mast cell-derived inflammatory mediators, leukotrienes appear to play a particularly important role in virus-infected airways.[111] However, time course analysis of infected lung tissues suggests that the effect of RSV on 5-LO gene expression and leukotriene synthesis is transient, being maximal at 3 days post-inoculation and already resolved at 5 days. Also, a significant increase in transcripts encoding the cys-LT1 receptor can be measured by RT-PCR from RSV-infected lung tissues (Figure 9.6). The

exaggerated neurogenic inflammation in the intrapulmonary airways of young rats infected with RSV involves the concomitant release of cys-LTs and activation of the cys-LT1 receptor, as manifested by the potent inhibitory effect of the receptor antagonist montelukast on capsaicin-induced plasma leakage.[111] Montelukast also has a much smaller, but still significant, inhibitory effect in the intrapulmonary airways of RSV-infected adult rats, whereas no effect can be found in the extrapulmonary airways of either young or adult rats. The increased susceptibility of the intrapulmonary airways of RSV-infected young rats to the inflammatory effects of sensory nerves reflects a higher density of nerve–mast cell synapses compared to older rats. In addition, the anti-inflammatory effect of montelukast in the small airways can be explained by the higher density of mast cells in this section of the respiratory tree.

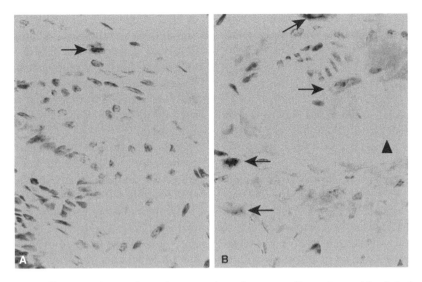

Figure 9.5 Mast cells–nerve interactions. Lung sections from weanling rats sacrificed 5 days after the intranasal inoculation of virus-free medium (A) or respiratory syncytial virus (RSV) suspension (B). Mast cells (arrows) were identified by immunohistochemistry using a monoclonal antibody specific for tryptase. An average seven-fold increase in mast cell density was found in the lung sections from RSV-infected rats compared to pathogen-free controls. These mast cells were always clustered in close proximity to nerve fibers (arrowhead). See also Color Plate IV

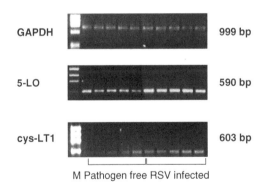

Figure 9.6 Respiratory syncytial virus (RSV)-induced 5-LO and cys-LT1 upregulation. Amplification of 5-LO and cys-LT1 mRNA from the lungs of weanling rats 5 days after intranasal inoculation with RSV ($n=5$) or with virus-free medium ($n=5$). RSV caused a significant increase in 5-LO and cys-LT1 expression compared to pathogen-free weanling rats. Each band was obtained from the lungs of a different animal. M, ladder of molecular weight standards

Collectively, our observations suggest that, following the early phase of the viral infection, leukotriene production/release returns rapidly to baseline levels, but can be reactivated by neurogenic stimulation of the numerous mast cells that had differentiated along the airways during the infection. The consequent release of cys-LTs can in turn amplify the release of inflammatory peptides from sensory nerves[114] forming local neuron–mast cell feedback loops. In addition, since it has been shown that also non-neuronal cells such as monocytes and macrophages express SP and its receptors and release this peptide in response to capsaicin stimulation,[105] it is likely that cells involved in the immune and inflammatory response to the infection contribute to this mechanism of mast cell activation. Finally, RSV may induce qualitative/quantitative changes in mast cell–nerve synapses, such as upregulation of NK_1 receptor expression on mast cell membranes analogous to epithelial cells,[95] vascular endothelial cells[95] and T lymphocytes[115] in infected airways.

Neurotrophins

Recent studies have shown that the expression of nerve growth factor (NGF) and its receptors trkA and p75 in lung tissues decreases progressively with age.[116] Weanling rats have approximately two-fold higher levels of NGF mRNA and protein than adult rats, and the adult expression pattern for these molecules is reached by 8 weeks of age. The expression of the high-affinity receptor trkA parallels that of its ligand, whereas the decline in the expression of the low-affinity p75 receptor is steeper and its mRNA level is more than four-fold lower in adult rats than in weanling rats.[116] These findings are consistent with previous reports of minimal neurotrophin receptor expression in adult lung tissues[117] and show a different profile of developmental maturation in the lungs compared to other non-neuronal tissues, e.g. the thymus, where the expression of neurotrophin receptors peaks at 12 weeks of age in rats.[118]

This genetic blueprint can be modified dramatically by early-life viral infections. In fact, a strong increase of NGF and neurotrophin receptor expression can be found in lungs infected with RSV 5 days after intranasal inoculation of the virus.[116] Furthermore, the characteristic changes in NK_1 receptor expression in rats infected with RSV responsible for the potentiation of neurogenic inflammation are mimicked by the administration of exogenous NGF in the absence of infection, and blockade of NGF activity with a selective antibody inhibits both NK_1 receptor upregulation and the potentiation of neurogenic plasma extravasation in infected lungs, confirming that NGF plays an important role in the mechanism of airway inflammation during RSV infection.[116] These new data explain the report of NGF-induced airway hyperresponsiveness in guinea-pigs, which is completely blocked by selective pharmacological antagonism

of NK_1 receptors.[119] Ultraviolet (UV) inactivation of the viral nucleic acid hinders the effect of RSV on the expression of NGF and its receptors in the lungs, suggesting that the changes observed in the neurotrophin pathways are linked to active viral replication and to expression of the viral genome in the respiratory epithelium.[116]

Although the relative magnitude of the changes caused by RSV in the neurotrophin system is comparable in weanling and adult rats, absolute mRNA levels encoding NGF and its receptors are much higher in RSV-infected weanling rats due to the different baseline. Furthermore, the increase in NGF protein concentration and the inhibitory effect of anti-NGF on neurogenic plasma extravasation is greater in the lungs of weanling rats, suggesting that early-life RSV infections have a more profound influence on neurotrophin systems and lung development. The higher susceptibility of weanling rats appears to derive from a higher degree of plasticity of the peripheral nervous system of young animals.

Because NGF is released from airway epithelial cells,[120,121] increases the production and release of SP and other tachykinins from adult sensory neurons[122] and induces sensory hyperinnervation in the airways of transgenic mice,[123] it represents the ideal link between virus-infected respiratory epithelium and the dense subepithelial network of unmyelinated sensory fibers. Overexpression of NGF and its low- and high-affinity receptors during RSV infection can generate long-term consequences via: (1) upregulation of the preprotachykinin A (PPT-A) gene encoding the precursors of SP and NKA; and (2) upregulation of the genes encoding vanilloid-type TRPV channels, which increases the responsiveness of sensory fibers and the release of proinflammatory peptides upon stimulation by airborne irritants.

Measurements of microvascular permeability in the intrapulmonary airways have confirmed that neurogenic inflammation is more prominent in the lungs of RSV-infected weanling rats and it is abolished by NGF blockade, whereas in the lungs of RSV-infected adult rats the magnitude of the neurogenic plasma extravasation and the inhibitory effect of NGF blockade are relatively small. These findings are consistent with the hypothesis that NGF plays an important role in the mechanism of neurogenic inflammation during RSV infection and that the magnitude of its effect is age-dependent, thus justifying the different distribution of sensory afferents across the respiratory tract at different ages.

The RSV–asthma link

RSV is the most important respiratory pathogen in infancy and can cause serious lower respiratory tract infections, particularly in prematurely born infants and children with underlying cardiorespiratory conditions.[124] Epidemiological studies have indicated that RSV infection in infancy is associated with recurrent wheezing later in life, giving rise to the theory that there is a link between RSV and asthma.[125] However, the pathogenetic mechanisms of RSV-induced airway inflammation and hyperreactivity remain largely unknown and no effective therapeutic option is currently available to manage the acute and chronic clinical manifestations of this infection. It has been suggested that RSV may enhance the development of allergic inflammatory responses following early-life episodes of bronchiolitis. This hypothesis is supported by several studies showing an imbalance between Th1 and Th2 lymphocytes following the infection, suggesting that RSV may create a persistent atopic state by skewing immunity towards Th2-type responses. An alternative hypothesis is that abnormal neural control and/or complex neuroimmune interactions may result from the infection, generating a persistent state of airway hyperreactivity.

We have shown that RSV markedly increases the expression of the NK_1 tachykinin receptor in the respiratory epithelium and vascular endothelium, whereas the expression of the NK_2 tachykinin receptor and of VIP receptors

is affected minimally. The physiological manifestation of this receptor imbalance is represented by exaggerated neurogenic inflammation in the airways during the acute viral infection. After resolution of the infection, NK_1 receptor expression progressively returns to baseline, but airway neurogenic inflammation remains abnormal, owing to remodeling of the sensory innervation, which involves amplification of peptide synthesis and release. RSV infections occurring in the early postnatal period have a profound impact on the development of neuropeptide-mediated responses, which remain potentiated into adulthood. Also, neurogenic inflammation in infected young rats is prominent in the intrapulmonary airways, whereas it is observed almost exclusively in the extrapulmonary airways during adulthood, reflecting age-dependent differences in the pattern of sensorineural innervation across the respiratory tract.

Extending these studies, we have identified additional important modes of interaction between sensory nerves and cellular effectors playing critical roles in inflammatory and allergic disorders, particularly lymphocytes, monocytes and mast cells, and we have shown that all these neuroimmune interactions are amplified by RSV infection. Finally, we have found evidence that NGF is essential for the integration of the different neuroimmune interactions and represents the ideal link between virus-infected respiratory epithelium and the dense subepithelial network of unmyelinated sensory fibers. Figure 9.7 illustrates the general model of neuroimmune interactions in RSV-infected airways emerging from our studies.

This model implies that, in the airways as in other organ systems (e.g. gastrointestinal tract, skin), there is close anatomical juxtaposition and functional interaction of sensory nerves with mucosal lymphoid tissue and mast cells. NGF has a profound impact on the distribution and function of sensory nerves, as well as on the regulation of multiple immunoinflammatory pathways, and infections such as RSV can alter both sensorineural and immunoinflammatory

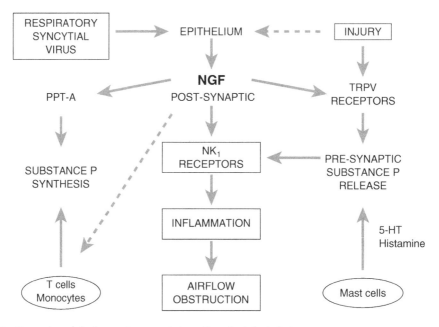

Figure 9.7 General model of neuroimmune interactions in infected airways

pathways in the respiratory tract, with a final effect exquisitely dependent on chronological age and developmental window.

THERAPEUTIC STRATEGIES

Corticosteroids

Several investigators have demonstrated that corticosteroids induce ACE activity in cultured alveolar macrophages,[126] in endothelial cells and in the rat lung *ex vivo*.[127] In human monocytes, dexamethasone has been shown to induce the activity of ACE, but not that of other ectoenzymes,[128] suggesting that the glucocorticoid effect may be rather selective. Similarly, the corticosteroid budesonide induces a gradual increase of NEP gene expression in transformed human airway epithelial cells.[129] The increase in ACE and NEP activities has a long latency and peaks after 5–6 days of incubation. The effects of corticosteroids on other components of the neurogenic inflammatory pathway

have different time courses; corticosteroid inhibition of NK_1 receptor mRNA transcription peaks within a few hours,[130] whereas the increase in the SP content of dorsal root ganglia following adrenalectomy can be detected at 10 days, but not at 5 days.[131]

In vivo, dexamethasone inhibits in a dose- and time-dependent fashion the increase of vascular permeability produced in the rat trachea by endogenous and exogenous tachykinins.[96] Marked inhibition can be obtained with doses of dexamethasone within the clinical therapeutic range. The inhibitory effect of dexamethasone has a latency of several hours and reaches its maximum after a 5-day course of dexamethasone injections, thus resembling the time dependency of corticosteroid-induced upregulation of ACE and NEP activities *in vitro*. This time dependency suggests that the effect of corticosteroids on peptidase activity is predominant over the effects on NK_1 receptors and neuropeptide content. The administration of dexamethasone can prevent the potentiation of neurogenic plasma extravasation induced in the trachea by Sendai virus infection.[96] Furthermore, the inflammatory infiltrates and the epithelial damage associated with this acute viral infection are virtually absent after treatment with dexamethasone.

The simultaneous inhibition of NEP and ACE completely reverses the protective effect of dexamethasone against neurogenic inflammation. The dose of dexamethasone that inhibits by more than 50% the SP-induced extravasation (0.5 mg/kg per day for 2 days) has no effect on the plasma extravasation induced by an intravenous injection of a non-peptide mediator, the platelet-activating factor (PAF). Furthermore, PAF-induced extravasation is not affected by the combined inhibition of NEP and ACE. These observations suggest that low-dose dexamethasone protects tracheal post-capillary venules by increasing tachykinin degradation without affecting the responsiveness of the venular endothelium to non-peptide inflammatory mediators. However, the inhibitory effect of corticosteroids against sensory nerve-mediated extravasation may also affect a variety of other inflammatory mediators indirectly. For example, it is known that histamine and bradykinin cause antidromic stimulation of sensory nerves in the lung, thus releasing SP and other neuropeptides,[132] and that the elimination of these nerves reduces histamine's effect on airway vascular permeability.[133,134] Thus, corticosteroids may inhibit plasma extravasation produced by non-peptide inflammatory mediators by inhibiting the effect of secondarily released tachykinins.

Leukotriene modifiers

Recent studies outlined above have shown that acute RSV infection is associated with a marked increase in the number of mast cells in the airway mucosa and transiently increased expression of the 5-LO gene with production of cysteinyl leukotrienes, probably derived from the expanded mast cell population. Interestingly, the mast cells in the infected mucosa appeared to form clusters around nerve fibers, suggesting functional interactions through the formation of local neuron–mast cell feedback loops. In fact, the leukotriene receptor antagonist montelukast potently inhibited neurogenic inflammation in the intrapulmonary airways of infected weaning rats, and to a much lesser degree of adult rats.[21]

Consistent with our findings in animal models, therapy with a leukotriene receptor antagonist was effective in reducing respiratory symptoms in RSV-infected children up to 3 years of age.[135] An important similarity between Bisgaard's data and ours is that a post-hoc analysis revealed a stronger effect of anti-leukotriene therapy in younger children (≤ 9 months of age).[136] An ongoing randomized controlled trial will probably clarify whether there is a group of patients who could particularly benefit by an early treatment with leukotriene receptor antagonist.

The great clinical relevance of these studies derives from the fact that at present there is no evidence-based therapy against acute viral bronchiolitis or chronic post-viral wheeze. The usefulness of bronchodilators is controversial,[23] and steroids are ineffective on the acute and long-term clinical outcome, whether administered systemically[24–26] or topically.[27–29] Therefore, confirmation of the therapeutic efficacy of leukotriene and identification of patients over-producing leukotrienes may provide a new, targeted therapeutic approach to this common disease. Also, since RSV infection influences the risk of subsequent asthma,[18–20] the follow-up of these patients will elucidate whether increased leukotriene synthesis during the acute infection is predictive of the development of post-bronchiolitis complications, particularly childhood asthma.

β₂-Adrenergic agonists

For decades, short-acting β_2-adrenergic agonists have been the first-line therapy in the management of acute bronchospasm. The most used drug in this class is albuterol, a racemic mixture containing a 50 : 50 ratio of two isomers, designated as S (*sinister*) for the left-handed orientation and R (*rectus*) for the right-handed orientation. These stereoisomers are identical in chemical and physical properties but have distinct pharmacological characteristics because the β_2-adrenoceptor binds only the (R)-isomer with high affinity (IC_{50} 1 µmol/l), whereas the receptor binding affinity of (S)-albuterol is approximately 150-fold lower. Thus, essentially all of the β_2-receptor binding and therapeutic effect of racemic albuterol derives from the (R)-isomer. Unfortunately, most studies exploring the efficacy of albuterol or other β_2-adrenergic agonists in viral bronchiolitis have failed to demonstrate clinical benefit.

Many clinical benefits of β_2-agonists may depend not on the bronchodilatory property of these drugs, but rather on their anti-inflammatory effects. Studies in our animal models suggest that (R)-albuterol has a marked inhibitory effect on neurogenic inflammation during acute lower respiratory tract infections. Interestingly, the potentiation of capsaicin-induced neurogenic inflammation in the extrapulmonary airways was totally abolished by the administration of 1.25 mg (R)-albuterol, whereas an equivalent dose of racemic albuterol was able to reduce the effect of capsaicin only by half. No inhibitory effect on vascular permeability was seen with low-dose (S)-albuterol (0.31 mg), whereas we found significant inhibition at high doses, suggesting that (S)-albuterol might act as a partial receptor agonist.

(S)-albuterol is considered to be devoid of clinical benefits, but it opposes the bronchodilator activity of (R)-albuterol,[137] may be proinflammatory[138] and exacerbates airway reactivity to spasmogens. The presence of (S)-albuterol may explain why racemic albuterol is not as potent as (R)-albuterol. The mechanism of the anti-inflammatory effect of (R)-albuterol is probably due to a direct effect on the specialized endothelium of the post-capillary venules, decreasing the formation of the endothelial gaps necessary for the leakage of plasma macromolecules.[139]

This anti-inflammatory effect is generally not present when β_2-agonists are used parenterally, whereby a high concentration in the airways is avoided[140] and may not be evident clinically with the currently recommended dosages. In addition, this effect is not likely to wane with frequent or repeated use, as there is no evidence of tolerance to the anti-leakage effect in rats treated with β_2-agonists.[141]

Tachykinin antagonists

Several studies have shown that atopic individuals have increased levels of immunoreactive SP in bronchoalveolar and nasal lavage fluids compared with non-allergic controls, both at baseline and following allergen provocation.[142] In addition, there is evidence that NK_1 receptor gene expression may be amplified.[143] Another study found an increased supply of SP-immunoreactive fibers in the airway mucosa of asthmatics compared to non-asthmatics,[144] although this observation was not confirmed by subsequent studies.[145,146] Inhaled NKA causes bronchoconstriction in asthmatics[147] and tachykinins enhance mucus secretion from isolated human bronchi.[148] Collectively, these observations support the hypothesis that tachykinins released from sensory C-fibers by inhaled irritants may contribute to the pathophysiology of airway inflammation in diseases such as asthma and chronic bronchitis.

Of course, this hypothesis needs to be confirmed by clinical studies exploring the effect of selective antagonists of tachykinin receptors. In the first clinical trial involving an NK receptor antagonist, a dual NK_1/NK_2 antagonist was shown to block the decrease in specific airway conductance induced by inhaled aerosolized bradykinin in asthmatic patients.[149] The findings of this clinical trial suggested that neurogenic mechanisms play a relevant role in human airway inflammation and encouraged further clinical evaluation of tachykinin antagonists. On the other hand, preliminary studies with the selective NK_1 receptor antagonist CP-99,994 failed to show significant protection against hypertonic saline-induced bronchoconstriction and cough in asthmatic subjects.[150]

A possible explanation for these discordant findings is that selective blockade of a single NK receptor subtype may be bypassed by over-activation of the other subtypes, which may also assume the roles of the blocked receptor. This biological redundancy is well established in other inflammatory systems (e.g. cytokines), and it is likely that clinically effective tachykinin antagonists will have to resemble in part the lack of specificity typical of glucocorticoids. Another important issue is that the pharmacokinetics of the molecules tested may have been inadequate to provide significant results; as an example, the half-life of CP-99,994 is quite short, and therefore unlikely to exert a sustained anti-inflammatory effect during a bronchoprovocation experiment. However, perhaps the most important flaw of the clinical studies performed to date resides in the choice of the test population, e.g. adult patients with atopic asthma. From our most recent studies, the message emerges consistently that the structure and function of the sensory innervation of the respiratory tract is exquisitely age-dependent and that neurogenic inflammatory mechanisms in the airways are much more active and important earlier rather than later in life, when the predominant asthma phenotype is non-atopic transient wheezing triggered by viral infections. Thus, future clinical trials should focus on pediatric patients and infectious wheezing to understand whether the information obtained in experimental cellular and animal models can be transferred to the clinical arena.

CONCLUSIONS

Peptide neurotransmitters released primarily from vagal sensory afferents cause powerful inflammatory effects in the airways of several species, including humans. These effects are mediated by specific G-protein-coupled receptors and are modulated by membrane-bound peptidases. These peptides have extensive localization in the respiratory tract, where they have been shown to evoke a constellation of biological responses termed 'neurogenic inflammation'.

In virus-infected airways, exaggerated inflammation and hyperreactivity results from both pre-synaptic (changes in the peptide content and activation threshold of sensory nerve fibers) and post-synaptic (over-expression of NK receptors on target tissues) amplification of otherwise physiological defense mechanisms. New studies in animal models and in humans indicate that these changes in airway innervation are caused by altered expression of critical neurotrophic factors and receptors, which are initiated during viral respiratory infections and can persist long after the infection is cleared. As neurogenic inflammatory mechanisms are operational in human airways and other organ systems, selective pharmacological interventions modulating this pathway may provide useful therapy in numerous human diseases where neuropeptides play a pathogenetic role.

REFERENCES

1. Cascieri MA, Huang RR, Fong, TM, et al. Determination of the amino acid residues in substance P conferring selectivity and specificity for the neurokinin receptors. Mol Pharmacol 1992; 41: 1096–9
2. Nakanishi S. Substance P precursor and kininogen: their structures, gene organizations, and regulation. Phys Rev 1987; 67: 1117–42
3. MacDonald MR, Takeda J, Rice CM, Krause JE. Multiple tachykinins are produced and secreted upon post-translational processing of three substance P precursor proteins, α-, β-, and γ-preprotachykinin. J Biol Chem 1989; 264: 15578–92
4. Kage R, McGregor GP, Thim L, Conlon JM. Neuropeptide γ: a peptide isolated from rabbit intestine that is derived from γ-preprotachykinin. J Neurochem 1988; 50: 1412–17
5. Baraniuk JN, Lundgren JD, Mullol J, et al. Substance P and neurokinin A in human nasal mucosa. Am J Respir Cell Mol Biol 1991; 4: 228–36
6. Lundberg JM, Hokfelt T, Martling C-R, et al. Substance P-immunoreactive sensory nerves in the lower respiratory tract of various mammals including man. Cell Tissue Res 1984; 235: 251–61
7. Baluk P, Nadel JA, McDonald DM. Substance P-immunoreactive sensory axons in the rat respiratory

tract: a quantitative study of their distribution and role in neurogenic inflammation. J Compar Neurol 1992; 319: 586–98

8. Martling CR, Theodorsson-Norheim E, Lundberg JM. Occurrence and effects of multiple tachykinins: substance P, neurokinin A, and neuropeptide K in human lower airways. Life Sci 1987; 40: 1633–43

9. Advenier C, Naline E, Drapeau G, Regoli D. Relative potencies of neurokinins in guinea-pig and human bronchus. Am Rev Respir Dis 1987; 139: 133–7

10. Palmer JBD, Barnes PJ. Neuropeptides and airway smooth muscle function. Am Rev Respir Dis 1987; 136 (Suppl): 50–4

11. Lundberg JM, Franco-Cereceda A, Hua X, et al. Co-existence of substance P and calcitonin gene-related peptide-like immunoreactivities in sensory nerves in relation to cardiovascular and bronchoconstrictor effects of capsaicin. Eur J Pharmacol 1985; 108: 315–19

12. Baraniuk JN, Merida M, Linnoila I, et al. Calcitonin gene related peptide (CGRP) in human nasal mucosa. J Allergy Clin Immunol 1989; 83: 304

13. Brain SD, Williams TJ, Tippins JR, et al. Calcitonin gene-related peptide is a potent vasodilator. Nature 1985; 313: 54–6

14. Bauerfeind P, Hof R, Hof A, et al. Effects of hCGRP I and II on gastric blood flow and acid secretion in anesthetized rabbits. Am J Physiol 1989; 256: G145–G149

15. Piedimonte G, Hoffman JIE, Husseini WK, et al. Effect of neuropeptides released from sensory nerves on blood flow in the rat airway microcirculation. J Appl Physiol 1992; 72: 1563–70

16. Piedimonte G, Hoffman JIE, Husseini WK, et al. NK_1 receptors mediate neurogenic inflammatory increase in blood flow in rat airways. J Appl Physiol 1993; 74: 2462–8

17. Barnes PJ, Baraniuk JN, Belvisi MG. Neuropeptides in the respiratory tract (part I). Am Rev Respir Dis 1991; 144: 1187–98

18. Barnes PJ, Baraniuk JN, Belvisi MG. Neuropeptides in the respiratory tract (part II). Am Rev Respir Dis 1991; 144: 1391–9

19. Brimijoin S, Lundberg JM, Brodin E, et al. Axonal transport of substance P in the vagus and sciatic nerves of the guinea-pig. Brain Res 1980; 191: 443–57

20. Lundberg JM, Brodin E, Saria A. Effects and distribution of vagal capsaicin-sensitive substance P neurons with special reference to the trachea and lungs. Acta Physiol Scand 1983; 119: 243–52

21. Otsuka M, Konishi S, Takahasi T. Hypothalamic substance P as a candidate for transmitter of primary afferent neurons. Fed Proc 1975; 34: 1922–8

22. Lembeck F, Holzer P. Substance P as neurogenic mediator of antidromic vasodilation and neurogenic

plasma extravasation. Naunyn Schmiedebergs Arch Pharmacol 1979; 310: 175–83

23. Olgart L, Gazelius B, Brodin E, Nilsson G. Release of substance P-like immunoreactivity from the dental pulp. Acta Physiol Scand 1977; 101: 510–12

24. Holzer P. Capsaicin: cellular targets, mechanisms of action, and selectivity for thin sensory neurons. Pharmacol Rev 1991; 43: 143–201

25. Caterina MJ, Julius D. The vanilloid receptor: a molecular gateway to the pain pathway. Annu Rev Neurosci 2001; 24: 487–517

26. O'Neil RG, Brown RC. The vanilloid receptor family of calcium-permeable channels: molecular integrators of microenvironmental stimuli. News Physiol Sci 2003; 18: 226–31

27. Amann R, Maggi CA. Ruthenium red as a capsaicin antagonist. Life Sci 1991; 49: 849–56

28. Urban L, Dray A. Capsazepine, a novel capsaicin antagonist, selectively antagonizes the effects of capsaicin in the mouse spinal cord in vitro. Eur J Pharmacol 1991; 134: 9–11

29. Nakanishi S. Mammalian tachykinin receptors. Ann Rev Neurosci 1991; 14: 123–36

30. Guard S, Watson SP. Tachykinin receptor types: classification and membrane signalling mechanisms. Neurochem Int 1991; 18: 149–65

31. Regoli D, Drapeau G, Dion S, Couture R. New selective agonists for neurokinin receptors: pharmacological tools for receptor characterization. Trends Pharmacol Sci 1988; 9: 290–5

32. Carstairs JR, Barnes PJ. Autoradiographic mapping of substance P receptors in lung. Eur J Pharmacol 1986; 127: 295–6

33. Hoover DB, Hancock JC. Autoradiographic localization of substance P binding sites in guinea-pig airways. J Auton Nerv Syst 1987; 19: 171–4

34. Black JL, Diment LM, Aloan LA, et al. Tachykinin receptors in rabbit airways: characterization by functional, autoradiographic and binding studies. Br J Pharmacol 1992; 107: 429–36

35. Sertl K, Wiedermann CJ, Kowalski ML, et al. Substance P: the relationship between receptor distribution in rat lung and the capacity of substance P to stimulate vascular permeability. Am Rev Respir Dis 1988; 138: 151–9

36. Hudgin RL, Charleson SE, Zimmerman M, et al. Enkephalinase: selective peptide inhibitors. Life Sci 1981; 29: 2593–601

37. Ondetti MA, Rubin B, Cushman DW. Design of specific inhibitors of angiotensin-converting enzyme: new class of orally active antihypertensive agents. Science 1977; 196: 441–4

38. Llorens C, Schwartz J-C. Enkephalinase activity in rat peripheral organs. Eur J Pharmacol 1981; 69: 113–16

39. Patchett AA, Cordes EH. The design properties of N-carboxyalkyldipeptide inhibitors of angiotensin converting enzyme. Adv Enzym 1985; 57: 1–84

40. Dusser D, Nadel J, Sekizawa K, et al. Neutral endopeptidase angiotensin converting enzyme inhibitors potentiate kinin-induced contraction of ferret trachea. J Pharmacol Exp Ther 1988; 244: 531–6

41. Johnson AR, Ashton J, Schulz WW, et al. Neutral metalloendopeptidase in human lung tissue and cultured cells. Am Rev Respir Dis 1985; 132: 564–8

42. Sekizawa K, Tamaoki J, Graf P, et al. Enkephalinase inhibitor potentiates mammalian tachykinin-induced contraction in ferret trachea. J Pharmacol Exp Ther 1987; 243: 1211–17

43. Borson D, Brokaw J, Sekizawa K, et al. Neutral endopeptidase and neurogenic inflammation in rats with respiratory infections. J Appl Physiol 1989; 66: 2653–8

44. Sekizawa K, Tamaoki J, Nadel J, Borson D. Enkephalinase inhibitor potentiates substance P-electrically induced contraction in ferret trachea. J Appl Physiol 1987; 63: 1401–5

45. Nadel JA. Regulation of neurogenic inflammation by neutral endopeptidase. Am Rev Respir Dis 1992; 145: S48–S52

46. Caldwell PRB, Seegal BC, Hsu KC, et al. Angiotensin-converting enzyme: vascular endothelial localization. Science 1976; 191: 1050–1

47. Ryan US, Ryan JW, Whitaker C, Chiu A. Localization of angiotensin converting enzyme (kininase II). II. Immunocytochemistry immunofluorescence. Tissue Cell 1976; 8: 125–45

48. Llorens-Cortes C, Huang H, Vicart P, et al. Identification characterization of neutral endopeptidase in endothelial cells from venous arterial origins. J Biol Chem 1992; 267: 14012–18

49. Shore SA, Stimler-Gerard NP, Coats SR, Drazen JM. Substance P-induced bronchoconstriction in the guinea-pig: enhancement by inhibitors of neutral metalloendopeptidase angiotensin-converting enzyme. Am Rev Respir Dis 1988; 137: 331–6

50. Ichinose M, Barnes PJ. The effect of peptidase inhibitors on bradykinin-induced bronchoconstriction in guinea-pigs in vivo. Br J Pharmacol 1990; 101: 77–80

51. Bertrand C, Geppetti P, Baker J, et al. Role of peptidases and NK_1 receptors in vascular extravasation induced by bradykinin in the rat nasal mucosa. J Appl Physiol 1993; 74: 2456–61

52. Lötvall JO, Tokuyama K, Lofdahl CG, et al. Peptidase modulation of noncholinergic vagal bronchoconstriction and airway microvascular leakage. J Appl Physiol 1991; 70: 2730–5

53. Eglezos A, Giuliani S, Viti G, Maggi CA. Direct evidence that capsaicin-induced plasma protein extravasation is mediated through tachykinin NK1 receptors. Eur J Pharmacol 1991; 209: 277–9

54. Lei YH, Barnes PJ, Rogers DF. Inhibition of neurogenic plasma exudation in guinea-pig airways by CP-96,345, a new non-peptide NK1 receptor antagonist. Br J Pharmacol 1992; 105: 261–2

55. Lembeck F, Donnerer J, Tsuchiya M, Nagahisa A. The non-peptide tachykinin antagonist, CP-96,345, is a potent inhibitor of neurogenic inflammation. Br J Pharmacol 1992; 105: 527–30

56. Piedimonte G, Bertrand C, Geppetti P, et al. A new NK1 receptor antagonist (CP-99,994) prevents the increase in tracheal vascular permeability produced by hypertonic saline. J Pharmacol Exp Ther 1993; 266: 270–3

57. Majno G, Palade GE, Schoefl GI. Studies on inflammation, II. The site of action of histamine serotonin along the vascular tree: a topographic study. J Biophys Biochem Cytol 1961; 11: 607–25

58. Messadi DV, Pober JS, Fiers W, et al. Induction of an activation antigen on postcapillary venular endothelium in human skin organ culture. J Immunol 1987; 139: 1557–62

59. Majno G, Palade GE. Studies on inflammation, I. The effect of histamine serotonin on vascular permeability: an electron microscopy study. J Biophys Biochem Cytol 1961; 11: 571–604

60. McDonald DM. Neurogenic inflammation in the rat trachea. I. Changes in venules, leucocytes, and epithelial cells. J Neurocytol 1988; 17: 583–603

61. Majno G, Shea SM, Leventhal M. Endothelial contraction induced by histamine-type mediators. J Cell Biol 1969; 42: 647–72

62. Matis WL, Lavker RM, Murphy GF. Substance P induces the expression of an endothelial-leukocyte adhesion molecule by microvascular endothelium. J Invest Dermatol 1990; 94: 492–5

63. Delay GP, Lundberg JM. Cigarette smoke-induced airway oedema is blocked by the NK1 antagonist, CP-96,345. Eur J Pharmacol 1991; 203: 157–8

64. Smith CM, Anderson SD. Hyperosmolarity as the stimulus to asthma induced by hyperventilation? J Allergy Clin Immunology 1986; 77: 729–36

65. Umeno E, McDonald DM, Nadel JA. Hypertonic saline increases vascular permeability in the rat trachea by producing neurogenic inflammation. J Clin Invest 1990; 85: 1905–8

66. Bertrand C, Geppetti P, Baker J, et al. Role of neurogenic inflammation in antigen-induced vascular extravasation in guinea pig trachea. J Immunol 1993; 150: 1479–85

67. Bozic CR, Lu B, Hopken UE, et al. Neurogenic amplification of immune complex inflammation. Science 1996; 273: 1722–5

68. Colten HR, Krause JE. Pulmonary inflammation: a balancing act. N Engl J Med 1997; 336: 1094–6

69. Umeno E, Nadel J, Huang H-T, McDonald D. Inhibition of neutral endopeptidase potentiates neurogenic inflammation in the rat trachea. J Appl Physiol 1989; 66: 2647–52

70. Piedimonte G, McDonald DM, Nadel JA. Neutral endopeptidase and kininase II mediate glucocorticoid inhibition of neurogenic inflammation in the rat trachea. J Clin Invest 1991; 88: 40–4

71. Katayama M, Nadel JA, Piedimonte G, McDonald DM. Peptidase inhibitors reverse steroid-induced suppression of neutrophil adhesion in rat tracheal blood vessels. Am J Physiol 1993; 264: L316–L322

72. Wagner EM, Mitzner WA. Bronchial circulatory reversal of methacholine-induced airway constriction. J Appl Physiol 1990; 69: 1220–4

73. Piedimonte G, Hoffman JIE, Husseini WK, et al. Neurogenic vasodilation in the rat nasal mucosa involves neurokinin$_1$ tachykinin receptors. J Pharmacol Exp Ther 1993; 265: 36–40

74. Yamawaki I, Geppetti P, Bertrand C, et al. Sendai virus infection potentiates the increase in airway blood flow induced by substance P. J Appl Physiol 1995; 79: 398–404

75. Rouissi N, Nantel F, Drapeau G, et al. Inhibitors of peptidases: how they influence the biological activities of substance P, neurokinins, kinins and angiotensin in isolated vessels. Pharmacology 1990; 40: 185–95

76. Lindgren BR, Andersson RG. Angiotensin-converting enzyme inhibitors and their influence on inflammation, bronchial reactivity and cough. A research review. Med Toxicol Adverse Drug Exp 1989; 4: 369–80

77. Lundberg JM, Saria A. Bronchial smooth muscle contraction induced by stimulation of capsaicin-sensitive sensory neurons. Acta Physiol Scand 1982; 116: 473–6

78. Lundberg JM, Saria A, Brodin E, et al. A substance P antagonist inhibits vagally induced increase in vascular permeability bronchial smooth muscle contraction in the guinea-pig. Proc Natl Acad Sci USA 1983; 80: 1120–4

79. Advenier C, Naline E, Toty L, et al. Effects on the isolated human bronchus of SR 48968, a potent selective nonpeptide antagonist of the neurokinin A (NK$_2$) receptors. Am Rev Respir Dis 1992; 146: 1177–81

80. Maggi CA, Patacchini R, Rovero P, Santicioli P. Tachykinin receptors and noncholinergic bronchoconstriction in the guinea-pig isolated bronchi. Am Rev Respir Dis 1991; 144: 363–7

81. McKnight AT, Maguire JJ, Varney MA, Williams BJ. Characterization of receptors for tachykinins using selectivity of agonists and antagonists: evidence for a NK-4 receptor in guinea pig isolated trachea. J Physiol 1989; 409: 30P

82. Djokic T, Nadel J, Dusser D, et al. Inhibitors of neutral endopeptidase potentiate electrically capsaicin-induced noncholinergic contraction in guinea-pig bronchi. J Pharmacol Exp Ther 1989; 248: 7–11

83. Meini S, Mak JCW, Rohde JAL, Rogers DF. Tachykinin control of ferret airways – mucus secretion, bronchoconstriction and receptor mapping. Neuropeptides 1993; 24: 81–9

84. Lindberg S, Dolata J. NK1 receptors mediate the increase in mucociliary activity produced by tachykinins. Eur J Pharmacol 1993; 231: 375–80

85. Borson D, Gold M, Varsano S, et al. Enkephalinase inhibitors potentiate tachykinin-induced release $^{35}SO_4$-labeled macromolecules from ferret trachea. Fed Proc 1986; 45: 626

86. Tamaoki J, Kobayashi K, Sakai N, et al. Effect of bradykinin on airway ciliary motility and its modulation by neutral endopeptidase. Am Rev Respir Dis 1989; 140: 430–5

87. Kondo M, Tamaoki J, Takizawa T. Neutral endopeptidase inhibitor potentiates the tachykinin-induced increase in ciliary beat frequency in rabbit trachea. Am Rev Respir Dis 1990; 142: 403–6

88. Kohrogi H, Graf P, Sekizawa K, et al. Neutral endopeptidase inhibitors potentiate substance P and capsaicin-induced cough in awake guinea pigs. J Clin Invest 1988; 82: 2063–8

89. McEwan JR, Fuller RW. Angiotensin converting enzyme inhibitors and cough. J Cardiovasc Pharmacol 1989; 13 (Suppl 3): S67–S69

90. Jacoby DB, Tamaoki J, Borson DB, Nadel JA. Influenza infection causes airway hyperresponsiveness by decreasing enkephalinase. J Appl Physiol 1988; 64: 2653–8

91. Dusser D, Jacoby D, Djokic T, et al. Virus induces airway hyperresponsiveness to tachykinins: role of neutral endopeptidase. J Appl Physiol 1989; 67: 1504–11

92. McDonald D. Respiratory tract infections increase susceptibility to neurogenic inflammation in the rat trachea. Am Rev Respir Dis 1988; 137: 1432–40

93. Piedimonte G, Nadel JA, Umeno E, McDonald DM. Sendai virus infection potentiates neurogenic inflammation in the rat trachea. J Appl Physiol 1990; 68: 754–60

94. McDonald DM, Schoeb TR, Lindsey JR. Mycoplasma pulmonis infections cause long-lasting potentiation of neurogenic inflammation in the respiratory tract of the rat. J Clin Invest 1991; 87: 787–99

95. Piedimonte G, Rodriguez MM, King KA, et al. Respiratory syncytial virus upregulates expression of the substance P receptor in rat lungs. Am J Physiol 1999; 277: L831–L840

96. Piedimonte G, McDonald DM, Nadel JA. Glucocorticoids inhibit neurogenic plasma extravasation and prevent virus-potentiated extravasation in the rat trachea. J Clin Invest 1990; 86: 1409–15

97. Liu H, Brown JL, Jasmin L, et al. Synaptic relationship between substance P and substance P receptor: light and electron microscopic characterization of the mismatch between neuropeptides and their receptors. Proc Natl Acad Sci USA 1994; 91: 1009–13

98. Ichikawa S, Sreedharan SP, Owen RL, Goetzl EI. Immunochemical localization of type I VIP receptor and NK-1-type substance P receptor in rat lung. Am J Physiol 1995; 268: L584–L588

99. King KA, Hu C, Rodriguez MM, et al. Exaggerated neurogenic inflammation and substance P receptor upregulation in RSV-infected weanling rats. Am J Respir Cell Mol Biol 2001; 24: 101–7

100. Piedimonte G. Neuro-immune interactions in respiratory syncytial virus-infected airways. Pediatr Infect Dis J 2002; 21: 462–7

101. Piedimonte G, Hegele RG, Auais A. Persistent airway inflammation after resolution of respiratory syncytial virus infection in rats. Pediatr Res 2004; 55: 657–65

102. Auais A, Adkins B, Napchan G, Piedimonte G. Immuno-modulatory effects of sensory nerves during respiratory syncytial virus infection in rats. Am J Physiol 2003; 285: L105–L113

103. Maggi CA. The effects of tachykinins on inflammatory immune cells. Regul Pept 1997; 70: 75–90

104. Lai JP, Douglas SD, Ho WZ. Human lymphocytes express substance P and its receptor. J Neuroimmunol 1998; 86: 80–6

105. Ho WZ, Lai JP, Zhu XH, et al. Human monocytes and macrophages express substance P and neurokinin-1 receptor. J Immunol 1997; 159: 5654–60

106. Becker S, Quay J, Soukup J. Cytokine (tumor necrosis factor, IL-6, IL-8) production by respiratory syncytial virus-infected human alveolar macrophages. J Immunol 1991; 147: 4307–12

107. Panuska JR, Midulla F, Cirino N, et al. Virus induced alteration in macrophage production of tumor necrosis factor prostaglandin E2. Am J Physiol 1990; 259: L396–L402

108. Salkind AR, Nichols JE, Roberts NJ Jr. Suppressed expression of ICAM-1 and LFA-1 abrogation of leukocyte collaboration after exposure of human mononuclear leukocytes to respiratory syncytial virus in vitro. Comparison with exposure to influenza virus. J Clin Invest 1991; 88: 505–11

109. Panuska JR, Merolla R, Rebert NA, et al. Respiratory syncytial virus induces interleukin-10 by human alveolar macrophages. Suppression of early cytokine production and implications for incomplete immunity. J Clin Invest 1995; 96: 2445–53

110. Panuska JR, Cirino NM, Midulla F, et al. Productive infection of isolated human alveolar macrophages by respiratory syncytial virus. J Clin Invest 1990; 86: 113–19

111. Wedde-Beer K, Hu C, Rodriguez MM, Piedimonte G. Leukotrienes mediate neurogenic inflammation in lungs of young rats infected with respiratory syncytial virus. Am J Physiol 2002; 282: L1143–L1150

112. Theoharides TC. The mast cell: a neuroimmunoendocrine master player. Int J Tissue React 1996; 18: 1–21

113. Bauer O, Razin E. Mast cell–nerve interactions. News Physiol Sci 2000; 15: 213–18

114. McAlexander MA, Myers AC, Undem BJ. Inhibition of 5-lipoxygenase diminishes neurally evoked tachykinergic contraction of guinea pig isolated airway. J Pharmacol Exp Ther 1998; 285: 602–7

115. Romaguera RL, Rodriguez MM, Jiang X, et al. T-lymphocyte subpopulations in bronchial lymphoid tissue of RSV-infected rats overexpress substance P receptors. Am J Respir Crit Care Med 2000; 159: A656

116. Hu C, Wedde-Beer K, Auais A, et al. Nerve growth factor and nerve growth factor receptors in respiratory syncytial virus-infected lungs. Am J Physiol 2002; 283: L494–L502

117. Lomen-Hoerth C, Shooter EM. Widespread neurotrophin receptor expression in the immune system and other nonneuronal rat tissues. J Neurochem 1995; 64: 1780–89

118. Garcia-Suarez O, Germana A, Hannestad J, et al. Changes in the expression of the nerve growth factor receptors trkA and p75^{LNGR} in the rat thymus with ageing and increased nerve growth factor plasma levels. Cell Tissue Res 2000; 301: 225–34

119. deVries A, Dessing MC, Engels F, et al. Nerve growth factor induces a neurokinin-1 receptor-mediated airway hyperresponsiveness in guinea pigs. Am J Respir Crit Care Med 1999; 159: 1541–4

120. Fox AJ, Barnes PJ, Belvisi MG. Release of nerve growth factor from human airway epithelial cells. Am J Respir Crit Care Med 1998; 155: A157

121. Hunter DD, Stellato C, Undem BJ. Constitutive expression of nerve growth factor by human airway epithelial cells. Am J Respir Crit Care Med 2001; 163: A825

122. Lindsay RM, Harmar AJ. Nerve growth factor regulates expression of neuropeptide genes in adult sensory neurons. Nature 1989; 337: 362–4

123. Hoyle G, Graham R, Finkelstein J, et al. Hyperinnervation of the airways in transgenic mice overexpressing nerve growth factor. Am J Respir Cell Mol Biol 1998; 18: 149–57

124. Hall CB. Respiratory syncytial virus. In Feigin RD, Cherry JD, eds. Textbook of Pediatric Infectious Diseases, 4th edn. Philadelphia: WB Saunders, 1998: 2084–111

125. Piedimonte G, Simoes EA. Respiratory syncytial virus and subsequent asthma: one step closer to unravelling the Gordian knot? Eur Respir J 2002; 20: 515–17

126. Friedland J, Setton C, Silverstein E. Angiotensin converting enzyme: induction by steroids in rabbit alveolar macrophages in culture. Science 1977; 197: 64–5

127. Mendelsohn FAO, Lloyd CJ, Kachel C, Funder JW. Induction by glucocorticoids of angiotensin converting enzyme production from bovine endothelial cells in culture and rat lung in vivo. J Clin Invest 1982; 70: 684–92

128. Vuk-Pavlovic Z, Kreofsky TJ, Rohrbach MS. Characteristics of monocyte angiotensin-converting enzyme (ACE) induction by dexamethasone. J Leuk Biol 1989; 45: 503–9

129. Borson DB, Gruenert DC. Glucocorticoids induce neutral endopeptidase in transformed human tracheal epithelial cells. Am J Physiol 1991; 260: L83–L89

130. Ihara H, Nakanishi S. Selective inhibition of expression of the substance P receptor mRNA in pancreatic acinar AR42J cells by glucocorticoids. J Biol Chem 1990; 265: 22441–5

131. Smith GD, Seckl JR, Sheward WJ, et al. Effect of adrenalectomy and dexamethasone on neuropeptide content of dorsal root ganglia in the rat. Brain Res 1991; 564: 27–30

132. Saria A, Martling C-R, Yan Z, et al. Release of multiple tachykinins from capsaicin-sensitive sensory nerves in the lung by bradykinin, histamine, dimethylphenyl piperazinium, and vagal nerve stimulation. Am Rev Respir Dis 1988; 137: 1330–5

133. Saria A, Lundberg JM, Skofitsch G, Lembeck F. Vascular protein leakage in various tissues induced by substance P, capsaicin, bradykinin, serotonin, histamine, and by antigen challenge. Naunyn Schmiedebergs Arch Pharmacol 1983; 324: 212–18

134. Lundberg JM, Saria A. Capsaicin-induced desensitization of airway mucosa to cigarette smoke, mechanical and chemical irritants. Nature 1983; 302: 251–3

135. Bisgaard H. A randomized trial of montelukast in respiratory syncytial virus postbronchiolitis. Am J Respir Crit Care Med 2004; 167: 379–83

136. Bisgaard H. Montelukast in RSV bronchiolitis. Am J Respir Crit Care Med 2004; 169: 542–3

137. Mitra S, Ugur M, Ugur O, et al. (S)-Albuterol increases intracellular free calcium by muscarinic receptor activation and a phospholipase C-dependent mechanism in airway smooth muscle. Mol Pharmacol 1998; 53: 347–54

138. Leff AR, Herrnreiter A, Naclerio RM, et al. Effect of enantiomeric forms of albuterol on stimulated secretion of granular protein from human eosinophils. Pulm Pharmacol Ther 1997; 10: 97–104

139. Sulakvelidze I, McDonald DM. Anti-edema action of formoterol in rat trachea does not depend on capsaicin-sensitive sensory nerves. Am J Respir Crit Care Med 1994; 149: 232–8

140. Boschetto P, Roberts NM, Rogers DF, Barnes PJ. Effect of antiasthma drugs on microvascular leakage in guinea pig airways. Am Rev Respir Dis 1989; 139: 416–21

141. Bowden JJ, Anderson GP, Lefevre PM, et al. Characterization of tolerance to the anti-leakage effect of formoterol in rat airways. Eur J Pharmacol 1997; 338: 83–7

142. Nieber K, Baumgarten CR, Rathsack R, et al. Substance P and β-endorphin-like immunoreactivity in lavage fluids of subjects with and without allergic asthma. J Allergy Clin Immunol 1992; 90: 646–52

143. Peters MJ, Adcock IM, Gelder CM, et al. NK1 receptor gene expression is increased in asthmatic lung reduced by corticosteroids. Am Rev Res Dis 1992; 145: A835

144. Ollerenshaw SL, Jarvis D, Sullivan CE, Woolcock AJ. Substance P immunoreactive nerves in airways from asthmatics and non-asthmatics. Eur Respir J 1991; 4: 673–82

145. Howarth PH, Djukanovic R, Wilson JW, et al. Mucosal nerves in endobronchial biopsies in asthma and non-asthma. Int Arch Allergy Appl Immunol 1991; 94: 330–3

146. Lilly CM, Bai TR, Shore SA, et al. Neuropeptide content of lungs from asthmatic and nonasthmatic patients. Am J Respir Crit Care Med 1995; 151: 548–53

147. Joos G, Pauwels R, Van Der Straeten M. Effect of inhaled substance P and neurokinin A on the airways of normal asthmatic subjects. Thorax 1987; 42: 779–83

148. Rogers DF, Aursudkij B, Barnes PJ. Effects of tachykinins on mucus secretion in human bronchi in vitro. Eur J Pharmacol 1989; 174: 283–6

149. Ichinose M, Nakajima N, Takahashi T, et al. Protection against bradykinin-induced bronchoconstriction in asthmatic patients by neurokinin receptor antagonist. Lancet 1992; 340: 1248–51

150. Fahy JV, Wong HH, Geppetti P, et al. Effect of an NK1 receptor antagonist (CP-99,994) on hypertonic saline-induced bronchoconstriction and cough in male asthmatic subjects. Am J Respir Crit Care Med 1995; 152: 879–84

Susceptibility to asthma exacerbations: antiviral immunity and protection against asthma exacerbations

Marco Contoli, Luminita A Stanciu, Simon Message, Alberto Papi and Sebastian L Johnston

Epidemiological studies show that respiratory virus infections are associated with the great majority of asthma exacerbations in both adults and children,[1-6] and that rhinoviruses are the most frequent viruses detected.[1]

Rhinoviruses infect the lower airways[7] and, in experimental studies, rhinovirus infection leads to long-lasting airway narrowing,[8] reductions in lung function in asthmatic volunteers[9] and increased bronchial hyperreactivity in allergic subjects.[10] A recent study indicates that asthmatic subjects are more susceptible to rhinovirus infection than normal subjects, in that they develop more severe and more prolonged lower respiratory tract symptoms and falls in lung function following naturally occurring rhinovirus infection than do normal individuals.[2] The reasons for this increased susceptibility in asthmatics are still largely unknown. An emerging hypothesis to explain the increased clinical susceptibility of asthmatic patients to viral infection is that asthmatic subjects have an impaired antiviral immunity in terms of innate immune and acquired immune responses. Therefore, we review antiviral mechanisms in normal subjects, emphasizing data on antiviral defence against respiratory viruses (mainly rhinovirus and respiratory syncytial virus; RSV) and we then review the relatively few available data specifically investigating immune responses of asthmatic patients to respiratory viral infections. Identification of differences between normal and asthmatic subjects in terms of antiviral responses to respiratory virus infections may identify novel pharmacological approaches for prevention and/or treatment of virus-induced asthma exacerbations.

ANTIVIRAL DEFENSE IN HUMANS

The immune system can be broadly divided into non-specific and specific components, with non-specific elements being called into play against all viruses, while the specific components demonstrate a limited reactivity to a single virus and its close relatives. Non-specific immune elements include cells such as phagocytes (neutrophils and macrophages), natural killer (NK) cells, mast cells, basophils and epithelial cells and components of body fluids such as complement, innate interferons (IFNs), defensins and surfactant proteins as well as apoptosis of virus-infected cells.[11-14] A critical aspect of non-specific immunity (also known as innate immune response) is its lack of memory. However, it is present immediately for early protection and its specificity is very broad. The specific component of the immune system consists of B and T cells that express antigen-specific receptors (immunoglobulin (Ig) and and the T-cell receptor (TCR)) on their surface, reacting in a highly specific manner with a limited set of antigens. Specific immunity is built up by experience and, for primary infections, it is weak or absent; however, once developed (acquired/memory responses) it has the advantage of being rapid and highly specific.[11,12]

In primary infection, virus replicates in the respiratory tract, and replication is considered to occur principally in bronchial epithelial cells. Type 1 IFN responses are detected early and are antiviral directly as well as via activating NK cells. In addition to destruction of virally infected cells, NK cells release cytokines, including IFN-γ, which activate additional inflammatory cells including macrophages in the airway. Such non-specific immune mechanisms are essential in early defense against virus in the first few days.[14] In addition, innate immune responses influence the nature of the acquired immune response: stronger innate responses towards a type 1 or weaker towards a type 2 response. Meanwhile, viral antigens are processed locally and in regional lymph nodes by dendritic cells and are presented to T cells. T-cell responses take days to develop, but memory CD4+ and CD8+ responses may persist for life. Tissue T-cell recruitment is dependent on the production of chemokines and on alterations in the expression of adhesion molecules on the endothelium of inflamed tissues. Time is also required to generate B-cell responses: mucosal IgA and serum IgM may be detected after a few days, while IgG takes around a week to be detectable, increasing in amount and avidity over the following 2–3 weeks, and may remain detectable for life. Specific immune mechanisms such as CD8+ T cells and immunoglobulin are responsible for the eradication of infectious

virus in the later stages of infection. Secondary infection with the same virus results in rapid mobilization of B and T cell-specific immunity with an earlier T-cell response, coinciding with the NK cell response. If re-infection is with the same serotype, a rapid increase in levels of pre-existing, neutralizing antibodies may limit viral replication to such an extent that infection is clinically silent.[14]

We more particularly review the data available in the literature on cellular and soluble components of innate and specific immune responses to viral infections. Little is known on the immunological responses to naturally occurring respiratory virus infections in asthmatic patients. However, we focus on data investigating whether an impaired antiviral response underlies the increased susceptibility of asthmatic subjects to respiratory viral infection.

INNATE IMMUNE RESPONSE

Macrophages

Alveolar macrophages, present in large numbers in the lower airway (up to 90% of the cells seen in bronchoalveolar lavage (BAL) from normal volunteers),[15] are ideally placed for early phagocytosis of virus particles and of virus-infected cells. They are also likely to play an important role in the immune response through antigen-presentation to T cells and through the production of cytokines, chemokines and other mediators with innate antiviral properties such as innate IFNs, interleukin (IL)-12, leukotriene B$_4$ (LTB$_4$), toxic oxygen species (O$_2^-$, H$_2$O$_2$), tumor necrosis factor (TNF)-α, IL-1, IL-8, membrane co-factor protein (MCP)-1, IL-15.[16–20]

Natural killer cells

NK cells respond to virus infection in an antigen-independent manner, eliminating virus-infected cells and modulating adaptive immunity towards viruses.[21–23]

Several cytokines produced by virus-infected cells including IL-12, IL-15, IL-18, IL-21 and IFN-α/β can activate NK cell proliferation, cytotoxicity or IFN-γ production.[23]

The function of NK cells is regulated by a balance between signals transmitted by activating and inhibitory receptors.[22] Cell-surface major histocompatibility complex (MHC) class I molecules provide an inhibitory signal that protects healthy host cells from NK cell-mediated lysis. Virus-infected cells and malignant cells often express MHC class I molecules at reduced levels and thus are less able to generate inhibitory NK cell signals, rendering them more susceptible to attack by NK cells.[23–25] NK cell inhibitory receptors appear to contain intracytoplasmic tyrosine-based inhibition motifs and to antagonize NK cell activation pathways through protein tyrosine phosphatases.[23,26] NK cells kill infected cells through the release of perforin and granzymes from granular storage compartments and through binding of the death receptors Fas and TRAIL-R on target cells through their respective NK cell ligands.[23,27] Perforin inserts into the membrane of target cells where it assembles into a pore that allows granzyme access to the cytosol, where it triggers apoptosis.[28] Binding of the death receptors also activates cell apoptosis.[23]

NK cells engage in several kinds of interaction with other cells of the immune system, including dendritic cells and other antigen-presenting cells (APCs). Dendritic cells can influence the proliferation and activation of NK cells both through release of cytokines, including IL-12, and through cell-surface interactions, including CD40/CD40 ligand, leukocyte functional antigen (LFA)-1/intercellular adhesion molecule 1 (ICAM-1) and CD27/CD70.[29] In return, NK cells can provide signals that result in either dendritic cell maturation or apoptosis.[23,24]

NK cells should be considered as a potential component of antiviral defence to respiratory viruses. Indeed, NK-like cytotoxicity is increased by incubation of human rhinovirus with peripheral blood monuclear leukocytes from healthy donors.[30] In primary RSV infection NK cells have been shown to infiltrate the lung early in infection, with peak cytolytic activity detected at day 3 post-infection,[31] and depletion of NK cells resulted in prolonged shedding of RSV from infected mice.[32] In another study, NK cells were the predominant population at day 4 post-RSV infection and the recruitment of IFN-γ-secreting NK cells preceded the activation and recruitment of CD8+ T cells.[33] NK T cells also contribute to the efficient induction of CD8+ T-cell immune responses against RSV,[34] although little else is known regarding the role of NK T cells in antiviral responses to respiratory viruses and asthma.

It has also been shown that NK cells can be divided into type 1 (NK1 secreting IFN-γ) and type 2 (NK2 secreting IL-4) cells,[35] although, similarly to NK T cells, little is known regarding their role in respiratory viral infections and asthma.

Interferons

Human IFNs are grouped into type I IFNs (IFN-α, IFN-β, IFN-ε, IFN-κ and IFN-ω) and type II IFN (IFN-γ).[36–40] Most types of virus-infected cells are capable of synthesizing IFN-α/β in cell culture. By contrast, IFN-γ is synthesized principally by type 1 NK and T cells.[40] IL-12, IL-15 and IL-18 are important cytokines able to induce the production of IFN-γ and to promote type 1 responses.[41–44]

Human type I IFN genes include 13 IFN-α genes and single genes for IFN-β, IFN-ε IFN-κ and IFN-ω, respectively.[45–48] All IFN genes lack introns and are clustered on the short arm of chromosome 9. The human IFN-γ gene possesses three introns and maps to the long arm of chromosome 12. When the IFN-β gene is deleted by targeted disruption, the resultant mice are highly susceptible to viral infection. The IFN-α subspecies do not compensate for the loss of IFN-β, suggesting a unique role for IFN-β that is essential for a fully effective antiviral response.[49]

IFNs exert their actions through cognate cell-surface receptors that are largely species specific. Type I IFNs have a common receptor consisting of two subunits, IFNAR-1 and IFNAR-2. The IFN-γ receptor is characterized by a ligand-binding IFNGR-1 subunit and the accessory IFNGR-2. IFN signaling involves an IFN-mediated heterodimerization of the cell-surface receptor subunits, IFNAR-1 and IFNAR-2 with IFN-α/β and IFNGR-1, and IFNGR-2 with IFN-γ.[50,51] IFN binding to its cognate receptor subunits leads to activation of overlapping pairs of Jak and STAT transcription factors by tyrosine phosphorylation. The Jak-1 and Tyk-2 kinases are activated by IFN-α/β, which leads to the phosphorylation and dimerization of the STAT1 (p91) and STAT2 (p113) proteins and subsequent translocation, along with IRF-9 (p48), to the nucleus. The complex of these three proteins, known as IFN-stimulated gene factor 3 (ISGF-3), activates the transcription of IFN-α/β-inducible genes through the IFN-stimulated response element (ISRE). The Jak-1 and Jak-2 kinases are activated by IFN-γ, which leads to the phosphorylation and homodimerization of the STAT1 protein and subsequent translocation to the nucleus. The STAT1 dimer complex, known as GAF (for gamma activation factor), activates the transcription of IFN-γ-inducible genes through the IFN-γ activation site (GAS) enhancer element[40] (Figure 10.1).

IFN-γ affects diverse aspects of innate immunity, such as the activation of macrophages, and has strong effects on acquired immune responses, promoting the development of type 1 while suppressing type 2 T cell functions.[52–55]

Also, type I IFNs induce the transcription of several antiviral genes such as protein kinase R (PKR), which inhibits translation initiation through the phosphorylation of protein synthesis initiation factor eIF-2α;[56–58] the oligoadenylate synthetase family (OAS) and RNase L nuclease, which mediate RNA degradation; the family of Mx protein GTPases, which appear to target viral nucleocapsids and inhibit RNA synthesis; and adenosine deaminase (ADAR), which edits dsRNA by deamination of adenosine to yield

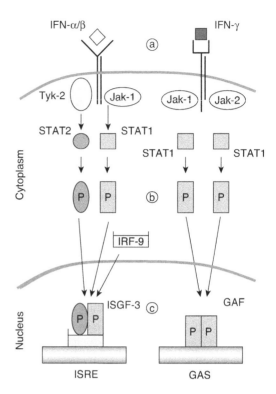

Figure 10.1 Schematic diagram of interferon (IFN) signaling. The signaling process is initiated by binding of IFN to its receptor (a). IFN binding leads to the activation of STAT transcription factors by tyrosine phosphorylation (b). IFN-stimulated gene factor 3 complex (ISGF-3) consists of STAT1, STAT2 and IRF-9, while gamma activation factor (GAF) is a STAT1 dimer complex. These complexes bind to the IFN-stimulated response element (ISRE) and IFN-γ activation site (GAS) elements of the DNA, respectively (c) inducing the activation and transcription of several genes involved in antiviral defense including: protein kinase R (PKR); oligoadenylate synthetase family (OAS); RNase L nuclease; Mx protein GTPases; adenosine deaminase (ADAR) and nitric oxide synthase (iNOS). See text for details

inosine.[59] Moreover, IFNs contribute to the antiviral responses by the induction of MHC class I and class II antigens and, especially IFN-γ, through the induction of inducible nitric oxide synthase (iNOS) that leads to increased production of nitric oxide (NO).[60]

In addition to these direct effects, virus-induced IFN-α/β are also known to contribute indirectly to the antiviral response by affecting cells of the immune system. IFN-α/β are crucial in the activation of NK cells and macrophages and, recently, attention has been focused on the role of IFN-α/β as the key cytokines that link the innate and adaptive immune systems.[61,62] IFN-α/β directly affect the fate of the CD8+ T-cell proliferation and they may be the key cytokines that induce effective B-cell responses.[63] In this context, it is interesting to note that IFN-α/β are also induced by non-viral, pathogen-associated molecules, such as lipopolysaccharide (LPS).[64]

Another pathway of IFN-α/β antiviral function is to induce apoptosis, or programmed cell death, in virus-infected cells.[65–69] Early apoptosis of infected cells may greatly reduce virus yields. Recent work has demonstrated a link between IFN-α/β signaling, the transcriptional activation through ISGF-3 of p53 (a 53 kDa multifunctional nuclear phosphoprotein with a role in the maintenance of genomic stability) and the induction of its proapoptotic target genes in virus-infected cells.[69–71] If apoptosis occurs within a few hours of virus infection of a cell, that cell is not available for successful virus replication, which therefore aborts. In addition, the infected cell is phagocytosed as a result of undergoing apoptosis, rather than dying by cell necrosis as a result of virus replication. Phagocytosis will therefore remove infected cells without stimulating inflammatory pathways, while death by necrosis, in addition to releasing new viruses to infect other cells, will also result in release of many mediators of inflammation – leading to a robust inflammatory response to infection (Figure 10.2).

A new family of interferons, called type III IFN-λs, and characterized by three elements: λ1, λ2 and λ3, also termed IL-29, IL-28A and IL-28B, has been recently described.[72,73] The three highly homologous IFN-λ proteins demonstrate limited (about 20%) homology to cytokines from both type I IFNs and IL-10 families.[74] Human IFN-λs bind to a unique heterodimeric receptor (IFN-λR), composed of CRF2-12 (also designated IFN-λR1) and CRF2-4 (also designated IL-10R2) shared with other class II cytokine-receptor ligands including IL-10, IL-22 and IL-26.[73]

Viral infection induces upregulation of IFN-λ mRNA in epithelial cells, peripheral blood mononuclear cells (PBMCs) and dendritic cells.[72,73,75–78] IFN-λs exhibit some similar biological properties to type I IFNs: they induce IFN-stimulated genes, signal via Jak/STAT pathways that lead to the upregulation of several antiviral proteins and enzymes including 2',5'-OAS and MxA, have antiviral activity *in vitro*[72,73,76] and have also exhibited antiviral activity in an *in vivo* model of vaccinia virus-infected mice.[79] Based on current knowledge, it thus appears that both IFN-α/β and IFN-λ ligand-receptor systems can independently induce an antiviral state by engaging similar participants of the antiviral response, though the signaling pathways involved in IFN-λ production are currently largely unknown. Recent data suggest that IFN-λ may be involved in antiviral immune responses against rhinovirus. *In vitro* rhinovirus infection of a bronchial epithelial cell line (BEAS-2B) led to IFN-λ production and this cytokine demonstrated a dose-dependent antiviral effect against rhinovirus (M. Contoli *et al.*, Nat Med 2006; in press). Moreover, IFN-λ production occurred after *in vitro* rhinovirus infection of primary bronchial epithelial cells, macrophages and BAL cells from healthy volunteers.

Defensins

Defensins are small, cationic, antimicrobial peptides, which have the capacity to kill bacteria, fungi and enveloped viruses by disruption of the microbial membrane.[80] Defensins are structurally characterized by the presence of six cysteine residues that form three intramolecular disulfide bonds. Based on the pairing of cysteines in these disulfide bridges, defensins are divided into the α- and β-defensin subfamilies. Although the human genome project implies that there are over 20 potentially expressed genes, six members of the α-defensin family and four β-defensins

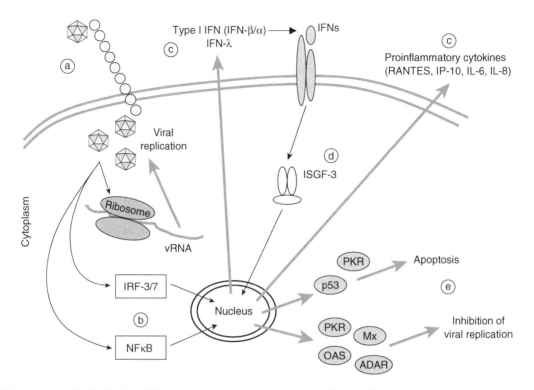

Figure 10.2 Viral infection (a) induces activation of transcription factors (b) (NFκB, IRF-3, IRF-7) that leads to proinflammatory cytokine and interferon (IFN) production (c). Interferons (d), through autocrine and paracrine activities, build up an antiviral state by the production of several proteins and enzymes able to inhibit viral replication (e) and to induce cellular apoptosis (e). See text for details

have been characterized to date.[80] Human α-defensins 1–4 are major components of the human neutrophil azurophilic granules,[81] whereas human α-defensins 5 and 6 are found in the secretory granules of intestinal Paneth cells.[82] Human β-defensins (HBD)1–4 are commonly found in epithelial cells including respiratory epithelium,[83,84] and evidence suggests that these molecules may be involved in lung host defense against both bacteria and viruses.[85]

While there is compelling evidence that defensins permeabilize bacterial cell membranes the mechanism is not known. Defensins may act by forming oligomeric membrane-spanning pores, by disrupting lipid membranes or through a combination of such effects.[86–88] Also, HBD-2 has been shown to be chemotactic for immature

dendritic cells and memory T cells via interactions with the chemokine receptor CCR6.[89] Moreover, HBD-2 has been reported to be able to induce Toll-like receptor 4 (TLR4)-dependent activation of immature dendritic cells.[90]

HBD-2 expression was induced by rhinovirus infection *in vitro* in primary bronchial epithelial cells and *in vivo* in nasal lavage,[91,92] suggesting a role for defensins in host defense against rhinovirus infection.

TOLL-LIKE RECEPTORS AND ANTIVIRAL DEFENSES

Toll-like receptors (TLRs) are a family of receptors that recognize and respond to a variety of pathogen-associated molecular patterns (PAMPs).[93,94] Currently, 13 TLRs have been identified from mammalian genes: TLRs 1–9 are common to mouse and human, while TLR10 is functional only in humans, and TLRs 11–13 are unique to the mouse.[95] TLRs are present on the cell surface and/or intracellularly.

Engagement of TLRs by PAMPs on cells such as macrophages and neutrophils drives innate immune effector function, such as inflammation and induction of microbicidal activity, while activation of TLRs expressed on APCs (most notably dendritic cells) leads to the initiation of adaptive immunity through induction of IL-12 and the co-stimulatory molecules involved in T-cell activation.[94] These events occur through PAMPs triggering TLR signaling cascades, leading to activation of transcription factors and mitogen-activated protein (MAP) kinases, and subsequent altered gene expression.[96] TLRs 'recognize' viral PAMPs and trigger antiviral signaling pathways leading to the induction of the type I IFN response. All TLRs tested so far lead to NFκB activation, while IRF-3 activation is restricted to certain family members. TLR-mediated signaling pathways to both NFκB and IRF-3, leading to type I IFN production, have been identified as a crucial link in understanding how viral infection leads to the IFN response. In response to viral infection, TLR3,[97–100] -7[101,102], -8[101,102] and -9[101–103] have been implicated in induction of type I IFNs. Much less is known about IFN-λ; however, it has recently been demonstrated that TLRs 3, 4, 7, 8 and 9 mediate virus induction of IFN-λs, as well as α/β IFN.[102]

While it has been documented how LPS interacts with the TLR4 receptor complex,[104] very little is known about how viral PAMPs engage with TLRs. The first indication of a viral PAMP being recognized by a TLR was the case of RSV fusion (F) protein and TLR4.[105] F protein stimulated secretion of IL-6 from wild-type monocytes, but not from cells isolated from mice with a mutation in the TLR4 domain or from TLR4 knockout mice. RSV infection in TLR4-deficient mice leads to impaired NK cell trafficking, deficient NK cell function, impaired IL-12 expression and impaired virus clearance, with longer RSV persistence in the lung of TLR4-deficient compared to normal mice.[106] However, a recent study found no significant role for TLR4 in primary murine RSV infection.[107] In other studies, the production by epithelial cells of IL-8 and RANTES elicited by RSV replication correlated with RSV-induced disease severity[108,109] and was NFκB-[110,111] and TLR3-dependent.[112] Double-stranded (ds)RNA is a molecular pattern produced by many viruses, including RSV, and TLR3-mediated responses to poly(I:C) (a synthetic analog of viral dsRNA) including activation of NFκB, IRF3 and the production of type I IFNs[98] (Figure 10.3).

Several studies have documented that TLRs are expressed in vivo in bronchial epithelial cells suggesting a relevant role in host defense against pulmonary infections.[113] TLR2 is the predominant TLR expressed on the apical surface of the bronchial airway epithelial cell, while TLR3 and TLR4 also reside intracellularly and TLR5 is located at the basolateral surface. TLR4 can be mobilized to the apical membrane following stimulation with RSV. TLR1 and TLR9 have been detected on the apical surface.[114] Recently it has been shown that TLR3 plays an important role in antiviral defense against rhinovirus in epithelial cells: in vitro rhinovirus infection of epithelial cells leads to the upregulation of TLR3 and blocking TLR3 causes increased viral replication.[97]

SPECIFIC IMMUNITY: ROLE OF T LYMPHOCYTES

T cells are believed to be key cells in the pathogenesis of asthma. αβ TCR T cells recognize allergens via MHC class II (helper CD4+ T cells), and newly synthesized viral proteins via MHC class I molecules (CD8+ T cells) on antigen-presenting cells. Helper T cells provide help to CD8+ T cells and B cells. CD8+ T cells are classically considered to fight viruses via

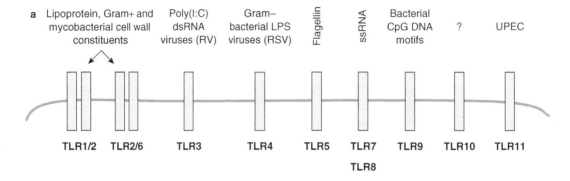

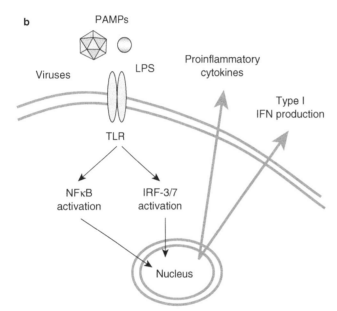

Figure 10.3 (a) Schematic representation of the principal microbial Toll-like receptor (TLR) ligands. dsRNA, double-stranded RNA; RV, rhinovirus; LPS, lipopolysaccharide; RSV, respiratory syncytial virus; ssRNA, single-stranded RNA; CpG DNA, unmethylated CpG dinucleotide motifs; UPEC, uropathogenic *Escherichia coli*. (b) TLR induces proinflammatory cytokines and type I interferon (IFN) production through the activation of NFκB and IRF transcription factors. PAMPs, pathogen-associated molecular patterns

direct lysis of virus-infected cells and via IFN-γ production. Both helper CD4+ and cytotoxic CD8+ T cells have been subdivided into type 1 (Th1 and Tc1, producing IFN-γ and IL-2) and type 2 (Th2 and Tc2, producing IL-4, IL-5 and IL-13) subpopulations. Type 1 cells are driven to differentiation by the presence of the cytokines IL-12, IL-15 and IL-18, and type 2 cells are primarily driven to differentiation by the presence of IL-4. The type 1 cytokine IFN-γ, along with type I IFNs, plays a crucial role in establishing an antiviral state in neighboring

cells.[40] Type 2 cytokines promote B lymphocyte responses (in particular switching antibody production to IgG1a and IgE) and also lead to recruitment and activation of basophils and eosinophils.

The normal T-cell response to virus infection is characterized by type 1 CD4+ and CD8+ T cell responses[11] but different RSV viral proteins may induce either type 1 or type 2 responses.[115] Production of IFN-γ was increased in rhinovirus-stimulated PBMCs and nasal secretions during rhinovirus infections[116–119] and in human

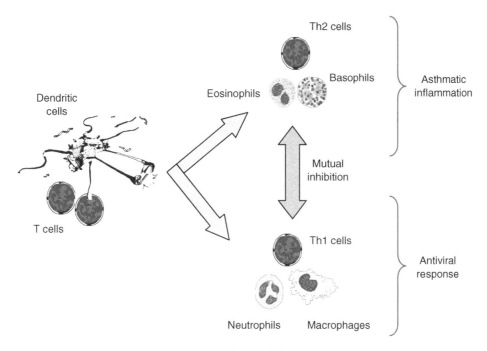

Figure 10.4   Th1 and Th2 immune responses in asthma and during antiviral responses

and animal models of influenza, parainfluenza and RSV infection.[120]

Asthma is characterized by a type 2 cell infiltration and many studies have demonstrated mutual inhibition of Th1 and Th2 cells. Therefore, it is possible that, within a pre-existing type 2 cytokine allergic asthmatic microenvironment, there may be inhibition of the normal effective type 1 antiviral immune responses, or that responses may be skewed towards inappropriate and potentially harmful type 2 responses (Figure 10. 4).

T cell recruitment into the airway is at least partly under the influence of chemokines, including those whose production by epithelial cells is upregulated by viruses. The type of chemokines produced by airway epithelial cells may influence the nature and the effectiveness of the specific immune response. Following experimental rhinovirus infection an increase in CD3+, CD4+ and CD8+ within the epithelium and submucosa of both normal and asthmatic subjects

was reported.[121] By contrast, rhinovirus infection is usually accompanied by peripheral-blood lymphopenia, and the degree of lymphopenia correlates with the severity of cold symptoms[122] and changes in airway responsiveness.[121] These data suggest increased recruitment of T cells to the airway, although alternative mechanisms such as reduced apoptosis could also contribute to an increase in the number of activated T cells in the airway.

T cells expressing the γδ T cell receptor are particularly associated with defense at epithelial surfaces and have a different mode of recognizing foreign antigens, but they are also involved in lung immunity. The role of γδ T cells in protection from respiratory pathogens is less well characterized than that of αβ T cells.[123–127] Mitogen-stimulated γδ T cells from the peripheral blood of infants with acute RSV infection produced significantly less IFN-γ and more IL-4 than γδ T cells from infants with acute reovirus infection.[128] During convalescence, the percentage of γδ T cells increased in children who recovered fully but failed to do so in children who developed post-bronchiolitic wheezing.[128] These results suggest an important role for γδ T cells not only in the pathogenesis of acute RSV disease in human infants, but also in the development of recurrent wheezing after bronchiolitis.

ANTIVIRAL IMMUNITY IN ASTHMATIC PATIENTS

Recent studies indicate that individuals with asthma are more susceptible to naturally occurring rhinovirus infection than normal individuals, in that lower respiratory tract symptoms and changes in peak expiratory flow were both more severe and of longer duration in the asthmatic subjects than in the normal subjects.[2] However, the reasons for this increased susceptibility in individuals with asthma have to date been largely unknown, but an emerging hypothesis supported by *in vitro* and *in vivo* experimental viral models is that asthmatic patients have a deficient innate and acquired antiviral defense against respiratory virus infections.

DECREASED INTERFERON-β PRODUCTION AND APOPTOSIS IN EPITHELIAL CELLS IN ASTHMA

We have recently described a novel mechanism for increased susceptibility to rhinovirus infection in asthmatic subjects. Asthmatic bronchial epithelial cells were found to have a defect in innate immune responses to rhinovirus infection, with profoundly impaired production of IFN-β and apoptosis in response to rhinovirus infection, resulting in greatly increased virus replication.[129] In contrast, normal bronchial epithelial cells rapidly produced IFN-β and underwent apoptosis, rendering them almost completely resistant to rhinovirus replication. Impaired responses in asthmatic cells were specifically restricted to innate immunity as

measured as IFN-β production and apoptosis, while the production of inflammatory mediators (IL-6 and RANTES) was not affected.[129] Impaired innate immune responses were observed in primary bronchial epithelial cells from both steroid-naive and steroid-treated asthmatic patients,[129] and in the presence of dexamethasone, indicating that the defects in antiviral immunity were not a result of steroid treatment, and that steroids have no effects on apoptotic responses and on IFN-β production in bronchial epithelial cells after rhinovirus infection, in accordance with the clinical observation of relative ineffectiveness of steroids in virus-induced asthma exacerbations.[130] Finally, exposure of bronchial epithelial cells from asthmatics to exogenous IFN-β restored innate immune responses and limited virus replication to levels observed in normal individuals.[129] Thus, signaling pathways downstream of the type I interferon receptor that lead to activation of programmed cell death and interferon production are intact. This has important implications for therapy, indicating that pharmacological replacement/augmentation of IFN-β to promote innate immune responses could be proposed as a novel approach to prevent and treat virus-induced asthma exacerbations (Figure 10.5).

DECREASED INTERFERON-λ PRODUCTION IN EPITHELIAL CELLS AND MACROPHAGES IN ASTHMA

The reasons why IFN-β production from bronchial epithelial cells is deficient in asthma are currently unknown. However, two possibilities among many others include polymorphisms in the IFN-β gene or promoter in asthma, leading to impaired production, as well as a defect specific to asthmatic bronchial epithelial cells. Since the IFN-λ genes are on chromosome 19, they are unlikely to be closely linked genetically with the type I IFN genes on chromosome 9. We therefore extended our studies to provide further insight into mechanisms

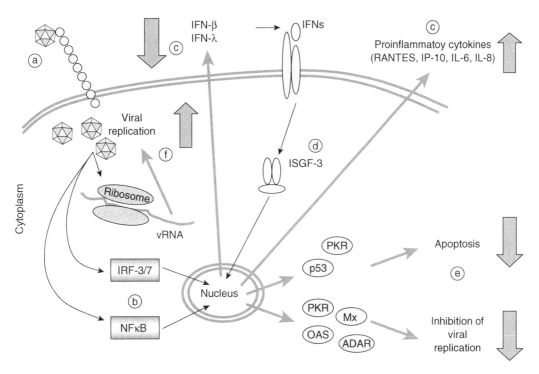

Figure 10.5 A defective innate immune response occurs in asthmatic bronchial epithelial cells both in terms of interferon production (c) (IFN-β and IFN-λ) and in terms of apoptosis (e). The impaired antiviral response leads to increased viral replication (f) and increased proinflammatory cytokine production (c)

of deficient innate immunity in asthma, to investigate IFN-λ production in response to rhinovirus infection of both primary bronchial epithelial cells and BAL cells from asthmatic and normal subjects. *In vitro* rhinovirus infection of both primary bronchial epithelial cells and BAL cells (90% macrophages) revealed deficient production of IFN-λ1 and -λ2/3 in asthmatic subjects as compared to normal subjects (M. Contoli *et al.*, unpublished observations), confirming that impaired innate immune responses in asthma are not restricted to IFN-β production and apoptotic responses in epithelial cells, but also extend to this distantly related novel antiviral cytokine family, and to other lung host defense cells including macrophages. Further, we found that induction of IFN-λs by rhinovirus infection of bronchial epithelial cells was strongly inversely related

to rhinovirus replication *in vitro*. Finally, to determine whether IFN-γ production was important in determining responses to rhinovirus infection *in vivo*, the same volunteers were then experimentally infected with rhinovirus-16, the severity of symptoms and reductions in lung function were monitored and the virus load was determined in BAL. *In vitro* production of IFN-λs by rhinovirus infection of BAL cells was strongly inversely correlated with both common cold symptoms and *in vivo* virus load, and strongly positively correlated with severity of falls in lung function, in asthmatic and normal volunteers, experimentally infected with rhinovirus-16. Asthmatic patients, in whom *in vitro* IFN-λ production in BAL cells was significantly lower than in normal subjects, exhibited increased common cold symptoms, and reductions in lung function and virus load after *in vivo* rhinovirus-16 infection. In marked contrast, normal subjects had robust IFN-λ responses, less severe cold symptoms, lower virus load and no significant changes in lung function (M. Contoli *et al.*, unpublished observations). These results document the importance of IFN-λ in the host defense against rhinovirus infection *in vitro* and *in vivo*, and indicate that deficient IFN-λ production in addition to deficient IFN-β is likely to be important in the pathogenesis of virus-induced asthma exacerbations (Figure 10.5).

DECREASED ANTIBACTERIAL IMMUNE RESPONSES IN ASTHMA

On the innate immune side, not only may the antiviral but also the antibacterial response be impaired in asthmatic patients. A recent study documented that asthma is a risk factor for invasive pneumococcal disease, indicating increased risk of bacterial infection in asthma,[131] while other studies have indicated increased detection of *Chlamydophila* and *Mycoplasma pneumoniae* in asthma.[132,133] The mechanisms of increased susceptibility to bacterial infections in asthma are unknown. However, it is likely that innate IFN production is also important in host defense against both Gram-negative (including *Streptococcus pneumoniae*) and Gram-positive bacterial infections,[134–141] although their role in this regard is much less well understood than in the context of viral infections.[142] We therefore investigated IFN-λ production in response to bacterial LPS stimulation of BAL cells from asthmatic subjects as compared to normal subjects. As we had observed with rhinovirus infection, IFN-λ production in response to LPS was also profoundly reduced in BAL cells from asthmatic subjects as compared to normal subjects and was inversely related to fall in forced expiratory volume (FEV_1) after *in vivo* rhinovirus infection (M. Contoli *et al.*, unpublished observations).

Taken together, these studies, including references 129 and 131, indicate that the deficiencies in components of innate immune responses in asthmatic subjects are surprisingly broad and involve defective responses against both viruses and LPS in two IFN families (IFN-β and IFN-λ) (Figure 10.5). Deficiency in any of the signaling intermediates or of transcription factors involved in the induction of the IFN genes (involving NFκB, IRF-3 and ATF/c-Jun transcription factors)[143–145] could potentially explain deficient production of IFNs in asthma. Moreover, as TLRs are common key elements of the innate immune response against both viruses and LPS, further investigations are clearly required to evaluate whether TLR expression or function is impaired in asthmatic patients (Figure 10.3b).

DECREASED TYPE 1 AND INCREASED TYPE 2 NATURAL KILLER CELL RESPONSES IN ASTHMA

An interesting field of investigation in the innate immune responses to viral infection is represented by the antiviral actions exerted by NK cells. There are some data in the literature suggesting a role of NK2 cells in the pathogenesis of asthma. Indeed, it has been shown that in blood the percentage of IFN-γ-producing NK1 cells is much lower and the percentage of IL-4-producing NK2 cells is much higher in asthmatic patients as compared to healthy individuals.[146] Therefore, it may be proposed that, in an airway environment rich in type 2 cytokines, NK1 cell functions and effective antiviral innate immunity might be impaired. If this is the case, then a key component of the early immune response would be deficient, and viral clearance would be impaired. In addition, if NK2 function is favored by the asthmatic microenvironment, production of type 2 cytokines by NK cells in response to virus infection might be one mechanism for amplification of type 2 and impairment of type 1 T-cell responses. However, there are no studies of NK cell function in the airway in asthma or in virus-induced asthma.

DECREASED TYPE 1 T-CELL ANTIVIRAL RESPONSES IN ASTHMA

In addition to innate immune responses, acquired immune responses are also important in contributing to antiviral immunity. Efficient T-cell responses to virus infection are thought to be predominantly of type 1. It has been suggested that, in the lower airways of allergic asthmatics with a pre-existing Th2-type allergic inflammation microenvironment, the T-cell responses to viral infection may be skewed towards inappropriate and potentially harmful type 2 responses. Indeed, in a murine model of asthma in transgenic mice expressing virus (lymphocytic choriomeningitis virus; LCMV)-specific CD8+ T cells, the induction of a Th2 immune response to ovalbumin (OVA) was able to switch the virus-specific CD8+ T cell response to IL-5 production, leading to accumulation of eosinophils in the lung.[147] By contrast, the virus peptide-specific CD8+ T cell-induced responses in non- or sham-immunized transgenic mice resulted in an accumulation of neutrophils, without any detectable eosinophil recruitment. Moreover, virus peptide-specific lung CD8+ T cells from OVA-immunized mice produced IL-5 and reduced levels of IFN-γ, whereas CD8+ T cells from sham-immunized mice secreted large amounts of IFN-γ and no detectable IL-5.[147] These data indicate that a Th2 environment in the lung can switch virus-specific CD8+ T cell responses to IL-5 production, leading to impaired secretion of IFN-γ and delayed clearance of the virus from the lung. *In vitro* human data indicate that exposure of PBMCs to rhinovirus results in an upregulation of IFN-γ and IL-12 (type 1 cytokines produced by T cells and monocytes, respectively) production in both normal and atopic asthmatic subjects. However, PBMCs from asthmatic subjects produced significantly lower levels of IFN-γ and IL-12, demonstrating a deficient type 1 cytokine production.[118] IL-4 (type 2 cytokine produced by T cells) production in PBMCs was induced by rhinovirus only in the atopic asthmatic group.[118]

There is also evidence *in vivo* that imbalances in type 1/type 2 immune responses influence the outcome of rhinovirus infection. Gern *et al.* showed an inverse relationship between the ratio of IFN-γ/IL-5 mRNA in sputum and cold symptoms and time to virus clearance from sputum in asthmatics and atopics experimentally infected with rhinovirus, indicating that a stronger type 1 immune response is associated with less severe symptoms and faster viral clearance.[119] Moreover, it has been shown that the higher the *in vitro* Th1 response to rhinovirus infection in PBMCs, measured as IFN-γ production or IFN-γ/IL-5 ratio, the lower the bronchial hyperresponsiveness and the higher the per cent predicted FEV_1 in stable asthmatic patients.[148] These data suggest that an impaired Th1 antiviral immune response not only is a characteristic of asthmatic patients but it might indirectly reflect the severity of the disease. Taken together, these studies suggest that an increased level of type 2 cytokines in asthmatic subjects is likely to be associated with deficient type 1 responses and that this may also play a role in the increased susceptibility of asthmatic patients to viral infections. Studies on airway T-cell responses to rhinovirus infections in asthmatic and normal subjects will be required to confirm whether this is indeed the case.

A defective Th1 immune response has been implicated in the pathogenesis and severity of RSV bronchiolitis both in animal models and in humans. Mice with type 2 cytokine responses after RSV infection develop enhanced disease with pulmonary hemorrhage and eosinophilia, whereas those with type 1 responses have reduced immunopathology and enhanced viral clearance.[149] Children with a deficient Th1 and a relatively increased Th2 immune response, in both airway secretions and peripheral blood after RSV upper respiratory tract infection, manifest acute bronchiolitis as compared to children with stronger type 1 responses, who develop mild clinical illness without bronchiolitis and clear virus more effectively.[150] Several studies have documented that a relatively increased Th2 cytokine profile during RSV bronchiolitis is associated not only with increased severity of the disease itself, but also with increased risk of wheezing during follow-up (most of which is likely to be caused by rhinovirus infections).[151,152]

Taken together these data suggest that, in asthmatic patients, characterized by a predominant Th2 inflammation in the airways, a deficient type 1 antiviral response occurs. A defective type 1 immune response to rhinoviruses may be implicated in the pathogenesis of virus-induced exacerbations of asthma.

CONCLUSIONS

Acute exacerbations are the major cause of morbidity in asthma and, despite optimized currently available therapy for asthma, exacerbations still occur.[153–155] The majority are precipitated by rhinovirus infections.[1] Asthmatics have increased susceptibility to rhinovirus infections and increased risk of invasive bacterial infection.[2,131] Results coming from *in vitro* and *in vivo* studies indicate that a deficient immune response to viral infection, both in the innate immune response and in the adaptive immune response, occurs in asthmatic patients (M. Contoli *et al.*, unpublished observations, and references 118, 119 and 129). The mechanisms of this impaired antiviral immune response are unknown. In particular, it is unknown whether this is a genetically induced impairment and/or whether it is due to the pre-existing asthmatic airway Th2 immune response, able to inhibit the naturally occurring Th1 immune response that follows viral infection. Interestingly, a recent *in vitro* study indicates that the asthmatic defective immune response to rhinovirus in bronchial epithelial cells can be restored by provision of exogenous IFN-β, restoring innate immune responses and limiting virus replication to levels observed in normal individuals.[129] Further studies are needed to evaluate the complex immunological events that follow viral infection

in asthmatic patients, in order to identify possible mechanisms responsible for the increased susceptibility of asthmatic patients to viral infection. The identification of these mechanisms could provide novel pharmacological targets able to prevent or to treat viral-induced asthma exacerbations.

REFERENCES

1. Johnston SL, Pattemore PK, Sanderson G, et al. Community study of role of viral infections in exacerbations of asthma in 9–11 year old children. BMJ 1995; 310: 1225–9

2. Corne JM, Marshall C, Smith S, et al. Frequency, severity, and duration of rhinovirus infections in asthmatic and non-asthmatic individuals: a longitudinal cohort study. Lancet 2002; 359: 831–4

3. Johnston SL, Pattemore PK, Sanderson G, et al. The relationship between upper respiratory infections and hospital admissions for asthma: a time-trend analysis. Am J Respir Crit Care Med 1996; 154: 654–60

4. Johnston SL, Xie P, Johnson W. Comparison of standard virology and PCR in diagnosis of rhinovirus and respiratory syncytial virus infections in nasal aspirates from children hospitalized with wheezing illness and bronchiolitis. Am J Respir Crit Care Med 1996; 153: A503

5. Tan WC, Xiang X, Qiu D, et al. Epidemiology of respiratory viruses in patients hospitalized with near-fatal asthma, acute exacerbations of asthma, or chronic obstructive pulmonary disease. Am J Med 2003; 115: 272–7

6. Contoli M, Caramori G, Mallia P, et al. Mechanisms of respiratory virus-induced asthma exacerbations. Clin Exp Allergy 2005; 35: 137–45

7. Papadopoulos NG, Bates PJ, Bardin PG, et al. Rhinoviruses infect the lower airways. J Infect Dis 2000; 181: 1875–84

8. Cheung D, Dick EC, Timmers MC, et al. Rhinovirus inhalation causes long-lasting excessive airway narrowing in response to methacholine in asthmatic subjects in vivo. Am J Respir Crit Care Med 1995; 152: 1490–6

9. Bardin PG, Fraenkel DJ, Sanderson G, et al. Peak expiratory flow changes during experimental rhinovirus infection. Eur Respir J 2000; 16: 980–5

10. Gern JE, Calhoun W, Swenson C, et al. Rhinovirus infection preferentially increases lower airway responsiveness in allergic subjects. Am J Respir Crit Care Med 1997; 155: 1872–6

11. Yewdell JW, Bennink JR. Immune responses to viruses. In Richman DR, Whiteley RJ, Hayden FG, eds. Clinical

Virology, 2nd edn. Washington, DC: ASM Press, 1997: 271–306

12. Whitton JL, Oldstone MBA. Immune responses to viruses. In Fields BN, Knipe DN, Howley PM, eds. Field's Virology, 3rd edn. Philadelphia: Lippincott-Raven, 1996: 345–74

13. Tosi MF. Innate immune responses to infection. J Allergy Clin Immunol 2005; 116: 241–9; quiz 50

14. Message SD, Johnston SL. The immunology of virus infection in asthma. Eur Respir J 2001; 18: 1013–25

15. Reynolds HY. Bronchoalveolar lavage. Am Rev Respir Dis 1987; 135: 250–63

16. Gern JE, Dick EC, Lee WM, et al. Rhinovirus enters but does not replicate inside monocytes and airway macrophages. J Immunol 1996; 156: 621–7

17. Johnston SL, Papi A, Monick MM, Hunninghake GW. Rhinoviruses induce interleukin-8 mRNA and protein production in human monocytes. J Infect Dis 1997; 175: 323–9

18. Hall DJ, Bates ME, Guar L, et al. The role of p38 MAPK in rhinovirus-induced monocyte chemoattractant protein-1 production by monocytic-lineage cells. J Immunol 2005; 174: 8056–63

19. Laza-Stanca V, Stanciu LA, Message S, et al. Rhinovirus infection of human macrophages induces IL-15 production. Proc Am Thorac Soc 2005; 2: A584

20. Gordon SB, Read RC. Macrophage defences against respiratory tract infections. Br Med Bull 2002; 61: 45–61

21. Biron CA, Nguyen KB, Pien GC, et al. Natural killer cells in antiviral defense: function and regulation by innate cytokines. Annu Rev Immunol 1999; 17: 189–220

22. Moretta L, Biassoni R, Bottino C, et al. Human NK-cell receptors. Immunol Today 2000; 21: 420–2

23. Smyth MJ, Cretney E, Kelly JM, et al. Activation of NK cell cytotoxicity. Mol Immunol 2005; 42: 501–10

24. Cerwenka A, Lanier LL. Natural killer cells, viruses and cancer. Nat Rev Immunol 2001; 1: 41–9

25. Lodoen MB, Lanier LL. Viral modulation of NK cell immunity. Nat Rev Microbiol 2005; 3: 59–69

26. Regunathan J, Chen Y, Wang D, Malarkannan S. NKG2D receptor-mediated NK cell function is regulated by inhibitory Ly49 receptors. Blood 2005; 105: 233–40

27. Sato K, Hida S, Takayanagi H, et al. Antiviral response by natural killer cells through TRAIL gene induction by IFN-alpha/beta. Eur J Immunol 2001; 31: 3138–46

28. Trapani JA, Smyth MJ. Functional significance of the perforin/granzyme cell death pathway. Nat Rev Immunol 2002; 2: 735–47

29. Degli-Esposti MA, Smyth MJ. Close encounters of different kinds: dendritic cells and NK cells take centre stage. Nat Rev Immunol 2005; 5: 112–24

30. Levandowski RA, Horohov DW. Rhinovirus induces natural killer-like cytotoxic cells and interferon alpha in mononuclear leukocytes. J Med Virol 1991; 35: 116–20

31. Anderson JJ, Norden J, Saunders D, et al. Analysis of the local and systemic immune responses induced in BALB/c mice by experimental respiratory syncytial virus infection. J Gen Virol 1990; 71: 1561–70

32. Harrop JA, Anderson JJ, Hayes P, et al. Characteristics of the pulmonary natural killer (NK) cell response to respiratory syncytial virus infection in BALB/c mice. Immunol Infect Dis 1994; 4: 179–84

33. Hussell T, Openshaw PJ. Intracellular IFN-gamma expression in natural killer cells precedes lung CD8+ T cell recruitment during respiratory syncytial virus infection. J Gen Virol 1998; 79: 2593–601

34. Johnson TR, Hong S, Van Kaer L, et al. NK T cells contribute to expansion of CD8(+) T cells and amplification of antiviral immune responses to respiratory syncytial virus. J Virol 2002; 76: 4294–303

35. Peritt D, Robertson S, Gri G, et al. Differentiation of human NK cells into NK1 and NK2 subsets. J Immunol 1998; 161: 5821–4

36. Clemens MJ. Interferons and apoptosis. J Interferon Cytokine Res 2003; 23: 277–92

37. Basler CF, Garcia-Sastre A. Viruses and the type I interferon antiviral system: induction and evasion. Int Rev Immunol 2002; 21: 305–37

38. Katze MG, He Y, Gale M Jr. Viruses and interferon: a fight for supremacy. Nat Rev Immunol 2002; 2: 675–87

39. Biron CA. Role of early cytokines, including alpha and beta interferons (IFN-alpha/beta), in innate and adaptive immune responses to viral infections. Semin Immunol 1998; 10: 383–90

40. Samuel CE. Antiviral actions of interferons. Clin Microbiol Rev 2001; 14: 778–809

41. Hsieh CS, Macatonia SE, Tripp CS, et al. Development of TH1 CD4+ T cells through IL-12 produced by Listeria-induced macrophages. Science 1993; 260: 547–9

42. Macatonia SE, Hosken NA, Litton M, et al. Dendritic cells produce IL-12 and direct the development of Th1 cells from naive CD4+ T cells. J Immunol 1995; 154: 5071–9

43. Munder M, Mallo M, Eichmann K, Modolell M. Murine macrophages secrete interferon gamma upon combined stimulation with interleukin (IL)-12 and IL-18: a novel pathway of autocrine macrophage activation. J Exp Med 1998; 187: 2103–8

44. Akira S. The role of IL-18 in innate immunity. Curr Opin Immunol 2000; 12: 59–63

45. Perry AK, Chen G, Zheng D, et al. The host type I interferon response to viral and bacterial infections. Cell Res 2005; 15: 407–22

46. Pestka S, Krause CD, Walter MR. Interferons, interferon-like cytokines, and their receptors. Immunol Rev 2004; 202: 8–32

47. Chen J, Baig E, Fish EN. Diversity and relatedness among the type I interferons. J Interferon Cytokine Res 2004; 24: 687–98

48. Roberts RM, Liu L, Guo Q, et al. The evolution of the type I interferons. J Interferon Cytokine Res 1998; 18: 805–16

49. Deonarain R, Alcami A, Alexiou M, et al. Impaired antiviral response and alpha/beta interferon induction in mice lacking beta interferon. J Virol 2000; 74: 3404–9

50. Bach EA, Aguet M, Schreiber RD. The IFN gamma receptor: a paradigm for cytokine receptor signaling. Annu Rev Immunol 1997; 15: 563–91

51. Mogensen KE, Lewerenz M, Reboul J, et al. The type I interferon receptor: structure, function, and evolution of a family business. J Interferon Cytokine Res 1999; 19: 1069–98

52. Muller U, Steinhoff U, Reis LF, et al. Functional role of type I and type II interferons in antiviral defense. Science 1994; 264: 1918–21

53. Shtrichman R, Samuel CE. The role of gamma interferon in antimicrobial immunity. Curr Opin Microbiol 2001; 4: 251–9

54. Huang S, Hendriks W, Althage A, et al. Immune response in mice that lack the interferon-gamma receptor. Science 1993; 259: 1742–5

55. Parronchi P, De Carli M, Manetti R, et al. IL-4 and IFN (alpha and gamma) exert opposite regulatory effects on the development of cytolytic potential by Th1 or Th2 human T cell clones. J Immunol 1992; 149: 2977–83

56. Schneider RJ, Shenk T. Impact of virus infection on host cell protein synthesis. Annu Rev Biochem 1987; 56: 317–32

57. Samuel CE. The eIF-2 alpha protein kinases, regulators of translation in eukaryotes from yeasts to humans. J Biol Chem 1993; 268: 7603–6

58. Clemens MJ, Elia A. The double-stranded RNA-dependent protein kinase PKR: structure and function. J Interferon Cytokine Res 1997; 17: 503–24

59. Samuel CE. Antiviral actions of interferon. Interferon-regulated cellular proteins and their surprisingly selective antiviral activities. Virology 1991; 183: 1–11

60. Gao J, Morrison DC, Parmely TJ, et al. An interferon-gamma-activated site (GAS) is necessary for full expression of the mouse iNOS gene in response to interferon-gamma and lipopolysaccharide. J Biol Chem 1997; 272: 1226–30

61. Chan CW, Crafton E, Fan HN, et al. Interferon-producing killer dendritic cells provide a link between innate and adaptive immunity. Nat Med 2006; 12: 207–13

62. Biron CA. Interferons alpha and beta as immune regulators – a new look. Immunity 2001; 14: 661–4

63. Le Bon A, Schiavoni G, D'Agostino G, et al. Type i interferons potently enhance humoral immunity and can promote isotype switching by stimulating dendritic cells in vivo. Immunity 2001; 14: 461–70

64. Kirchner H, Weyland A, Storch E. Local interferon induction by bacterial lipopolysaccharide in mice after pretreatment with Corynebacterium parvum. J Interferon Res 1986; 6: 483–7

65. Everett H, McFadden G. Apoptosis: an innate immune response to virus infection. Trends Microbiol 1999; 7: 160–5

66. Shen Y, Shenk TE. Viruses and apoptosis. Curr Opin Genet Dev 1995; 5: 105–11

67. Teodoro JG, Branton PE. Regulation of apoptosis by viral gene products. J Virol 1997; 71: 1739–46

68. Hilleman MR. Strategies and mechanisms for host and pathogen survival in acute and persistent viral infections. Proc Natl Acad Sci USA 2004; 101 (Suppl 2): 14560–6

69. Takaoka A, Hayakawa S, Yanai H, et al. Integration of interferon-alpha/beta signalling to p53 responses in tumour suppression and antiviral defence. Nature 2003; 424: 516–23

70. Vousden KH, Lu X. Live or let die: the cell's response to p53. Nat Rev Cancer 2002; 2: 594–604

71. Shao RG, Cao CX, Nieves-Neira W, et al. Activation of the Fas pathway independently of Fas ligand during apoptosis induced by camptothecin in p53 mutant human colon carcinoma cells. Oncogene 2001; 20: 1852–9

72. Sheppard P, Kindsvogel W, Xu W, et al. IL-28, IL-29 and their class II cytokine receptor IL-28R. Nat Immunol 2003; 4: 63–8

73. Kotenko SV, Gallagher G, Baurin VV, et al. IFN-lambdas mediate antiviral protection through a distinct class II cytokine receptor complex. Nat Immunol 2003; 4: 69–77

74. Kotenko SV. The family of IL-10-related cytokines and their receptors: related, but to what extent? Cytokine Growth Factor Rev 2002; 13: 223–40

75. Robek MD, Boyd BS, Chisari FV. Lambda interferon inhibits hepatitis B and C virus replication. J Virol 2005; 79: 3851–4

76. Osterlund P, Veckman V, Siren J, et al. Gene expression and antiviral activity of alpha/beta interferons and interleukin-29 in virus-infected human myeloid dendritic cells. J Virol 2005; 79: 9608–17

77. Coccia EM, Severa M, Giacomini E, et al. Viral infection and Toll-like receptor agonists induce a differential expression of type I and lambda interferons in human plasmacytoid and monocyte-derived dendritic cells. Eur J Immunol 2004; 34: 796–805

78. Spann KM, Tran KC, Chi B, et al. Suppression of the induction of alpha, beta, and lambda interferons by the NS1 and NS2 proteins of human respiratory syncytial virus in human epithelial cells and macrophages [corrected]. J Virol 2004; 78: 4363–9

79. Bartlett NW, Buttigieg K, Kotenko SV, Smith GL. Murine interferon lambdas (type III interferons) exhibit potent antiviral activity in vivo in a poxvirus infection model. J Gen Virol 2005; 86: 1589–96

80. Selsted ME, Ouellette AJ. Mammalian defensins in the antimicrobial immune response. Nat Immunol 2005; 6: 551–7

81. Welling MM, Hiemstra PS, van den Barselaar MT, et al. Antibacterial activity of human neutrophil defensins in experimental infections in mice is accompanied by increased leukocyte accumulation. J Clin Invest 1998; 102: 1583–90

82. Ouellette AJ IV. Paneth cell antimicrobial peptides and the biology of the mucosal barrier. Am J Physiol 1999; 277: G257–61

83. Bals R, Wang X, Wu Z, et al. Human beta-defensin 2 is a salt-sensitive peptide antibiotic expressed in human lung. J Clin Invest 1998; 102: 874–80

84. McCray PB Jr, Bentley L. Human airway epithelia express a beta-defensin. Am J Respir Cell Mol Biol 1997; 16: 343–9

85. Schutte BC, McCray PB Jr. Beta-defensins in lung host defense. Annu Rev Physiol 2002; 64: 709–48

86. Lehrer RI, Barton A, Daher KA, et al. Interaction of human defensins with Escherichia coli. Mechanism of bactericidal activity. J Clin Invest 1989; 84: 553–61

87. Sawai MV, Jia HP, Liu L, et al. The NMR structure of human beta-defensin-2 reveals a novel alpha-helical segment. Biochemistry 2001; 40: 3810–16

88. Ganz T, Lehrer RI. Antibiotic peptides from higher eukaryotes: biology and applications. Mol Med Today 1999; 5: 292–7

89. Yang D, Chertov O, Bykovskaia SN, et al. Beta-defensins: linking innate and adaptive immunity through dendritic and T cell CCR6. Science 1999; 286: 525–8

90. Biragyn A, Ruffini PA, Leifer CA, et al. Toll-like receptor 4-dependent activation of dendritic cells by beta-defensin 2. Science 2002; 298: 1025–9

91. Duits LA, Nibbering PH, van Strijen E, et al. Rhinovirus increases human beta-defensin-2 and -3 mRNA expression in cultured bronchial epithelial cells. FEMS Immunol Med Microbiol 2003; 38: 59–64

92. Proud D, Sanders SP, Wiehler S. Human rhinovirus infection induces airway epithelial cell production of human beta-defensin 2 both in vitro and in vivo. J Immunol 2004; 172: 4637–45

93. Cook DN, Pisetski DS, Schwartz DA. Toll-like receptors in the pathogenesis of human disease. Nat Immunol 2004; 5: 975–9

94. Bowie AG, Haga IR. The role of toll-like receptors in the host response to viruses. Mol Immunol 2005; 42: 859–67

95. Takeda K, Kaisho T, Akira S. Toll-like receptors. Ann Rev Immunol 2003; 21: 335–76

96. Aderem A, Ulevitch RJ. Toll-like receptors in the induction of the innate immune response. Nature 2000; 406: 782–7

97. Hewson CA, Jardine A, Edwards MR, et al. Toll-like receptor 3 is induced by and mediates antiviral activity against rhinovirus infection of human bronchial epithelial cells. J Virol 2005; 79: 12273–9

98. Alexopoulou L, Holt AC, Medzhitov R, Flavell RA. Recognition of double-stranded RNA and activation of NF-kappaB by Toll-like receptor 3. Nature 2001; 413: 732–8

99. Tabeta K, Georgel P, Janssen E, et al. Toll-like receptors 9 and 3 as essential components of innate immune defense against mouse cytomegalovirus infection. Proc Natl Acad Sci USA 2004; 101: 3516–21

100. Schulz O, Diebold SS, Chen M, et al. Toll-like receptor 3 promotes cross-priming to virus-infected cells. Nature 2005; 433: 887–92

101. Heil F, Hemmi H, Hochrein H, et al. Species-specific recognition of single-stranded RNA via toll-like receptor 7 and 8. Science 2004; 303: 1526–9

102. Yang K, Puel A, Zhang S, et al. Human TLR-7-, -8-, and -9-mediated induction of IFN-alpha/beta and -lambda is IRAK-4 dependent and redundant for protective immunity to viruses. Immunity 2005; 23: 465–78

103. Hochrein H, Schlatter B, O'Keeffe M, et al. Herpes simplex virus type-1 induces IFN-alpha production via Toll-like receptor 9-dependent and -independent pathways. Proc Natl Acad Sci USA 2004; 101: 11416–21

104. Miyake K. Innate recognition of lipopolysaccharide by Toll-like receptor 4-MD-2. Trends Microbiol 2004; 12: 186–92

105. Kurt-Jones EA, Popova L, Kwinn L, et al. Pattern recognition receptors TLR4 and CD14 mediate response to respiratory syncytial virus. Nat Immunol 2000; 1: 398–401

106. Haynes LM, Moore DD, Kurt-Jones EA, et al. Involvement of Toll-like receptor 4 in innate immunity to respiratory syncytial virus. J Virol 2001; 75: 10730–7

107. Ehl S, Bischoff R, Ostler T, et al. The role of Toll-like receptor 4 versus interleukin-12 in immunity to respiratory syncytial virus. Eur J Immunol 2004; 34: 1146–53

108. Miller AL, Strieter RM, Gruber AD, et al. CXCR2 regulates respiratory syncytial virus-induced airway hyperreactivity and mucus overproduction. J Immunol 2003; 170: 3348–56

109. Tekkanat KK, Maassab H, Miller A, et al. RANTES (CCL5) production during primary respiratory syncytial virus infection exacerbates airway disease. Eur J Immunol 2002; 32: 3276–84

110. Casola A, Garofalo RP, Haeberle H, et al. Multiple cis regulatory elements control RANTES promoter activity in alveolar epithelial cells infected with respiratory syncytial virus. J Virol 2001; 75: 6428–39

111. Fiedler MA, Wernke-Dollries K, Stark JM. Inhibition of viral replication reverses respiratory syncytial

virus-induced NF-kappaB activation and interleukin-8 gene expression in A549 cells. J Virol 1996; 70: 9079–82

112. Rudd BD, Burstein E, Duckett CS, et al. Differential role of TLR3 in respiratory syncytial virus-induced chemokine expression. J Virol 2005; 79: 3350–7

113. Basu S, Fenton MJ. Toll-like receptors: function and roles in lung disease. Am J Physiol 2004; 286: L887–L92

114. Greene CM, McElvaney NG. Toll-like receptor expression and function in airway epithelial cells. Arch Immunol Ther Exp 2005; 53: 418–27

115. Openshaw PJ. Antiviral immune response and lung inflammation after respiratory syncytial virus infection. Proc Am Thorac Soc 2005; 2: 121–5

116. Lau L, Corne J, Scott S. Nasal cytokines in the common cold. Am J Respir Crit Care Med 1996; 153: A866

117. Hsia J, Goldstein AL, Simon GL, et al. Peripheral blood mononuclear cell interleukin-2 and interferon-gamma production, cytotoxicity, and antigen-stimulated blastogenesis during experimental rhinovirus infection. J Infect Dis 1990; 162: 591–7

118. Papadopoulos NG, Stanciu LA, Papi A, et al. A defective type 1 response to rhinovirus in atopic asthma. Thorax 2002; 57: 328–32

119. Gern JE, Vrtis R, Grindle KA, et al. Relationship of upper and lower airway cytokines to outcome of experimental rhinovirus infection. Am J Respir Crit Care Med 2000; 162: 2226–31

120. Folkerts G, Nijkamp FP. Virus-induced airway hyperresponsiveness. Role of inflammatory cells and mediators. Am J Respir Crit Care Med 1995; 151: 1666–73; discussion 1673–4

121. Fraenkel DJ, Bardin PG, Sanderson G, et al. Lower airways inflammation during rhinovirus colds in normal and in asthmatic subjects. Am J Respir Crit Care Med 1995; 151: 879–86

122. Levandowski RA, Ou DW, Jackson GG. Acute-phase decrease of T lymphocyte subsets in rhinovirus infection. J Infect Dis 1986; 153: 743–8

123. Chen ZW. Immune regulation of gammadelta T cell responses in mycobacterial infections. Clin Immunol 2005; 116: 202–7

124. Tam S, King DP, Beaman BL. Increase of gammadelta T lymphocytes in murine lungs occurs during recovery from pulmonary infection by Nocardia asteroides. Infect Immun 2001; 69: 6165–71

125. Moore TA, Moore BB, Newstead MW, Standiford TJ. Gamma delta-T cells are critical for survival and early proinflammatory cytokine gene expression during murine Klebsiella pneumonia. J Immunol 2000; 165: 2643–50

126. Moreau JF, Taupin JL, Dupon M, et al. Increases in CD3+CD4–CD8– T lymphocytes in AIDS patients with disseminated Mycobacterium avium-intracellulare complex infection. J Infect Dis 1996; 174: 969–76

127. Carding SR, Allan W, Kyes S, et al. Late dominance of the inflammatory process in murine influenza by gamma/delta T cells. J Exp Med 1990; 172: 1225–31

128. Aoyagi M, Shimojo N, Sekine K, et al. Respiratory syncytial virus infection suppresses IFN-gamma production of gammadelta T cells. Clin Exp Immunol 2003; 131: 312–17

129. Wark P, Johnston SL, Bucchieri F, et al. Asthmatic bronchial epithelial cells have a deficient innate immune response to infection with rhinovirus. J Exp Med 2005; 201: 937–47

130. Grunberg K, Sharon RF, Sont JK, et al. Rhinovirus-induced airway inflammation in asthma: effect of treatment with inhaled corticosteroids before and during experimental infection. Am J Respir Crit Care Med 2001; 164: 1816–22

131. Talbot TR, Hartert TV, Mitchel E, et al. Asthma as a risk factor for invasive pneumococcal disease. N Engl J Med 2005; 352: 2082–90

132. Biscione GL, Corne J, Chauhan AJ, Johnston SL. Increased frequency of detection of Chlamydophila pneumoniae in asthma. Eur Respir J 2004; 24: 745–9

133. Martin RJ, Kraft M, Chu HW, et al. A link between chronic asthma and chronic infection. J Allergy Clin Immunol 2001; 107: 595–601

134. Rothfuchs AG, Trumstedt C, Wigzell H, Rottenberg ME. Intracellular bacterial infection-induced IFN-gamma is critically but not solely dependent on Toll-like receptor 4-myeloid differentiation factor 88-IFN-alpha beta-STAT1 signaling. J Immunol 2004; 172: 6345–53

135. Weigent DA, Huff TL, Peterson JW, et al. Role of interferon in streptococcal infection in the mouse. Microb Pathog 1986; 1: 399–407

136. Schiavoni G, Mauri C, Carlei D, et al. Type I IFN protects permissive macrophages from Legionella pneumophila infection through an IFN-gamma-independent pathway. J Immunol 2004; 173: 1266–75

137. Freudenberg MA, Merlin T, Kalis C, et al. Cutting edge: a murine, IL-12-independent pathway of IFN-gamma induction by gram-negative bacteria based on STAT4 activation by Type I IFN and IL-18 signaling. J Immunol 2002; 169: 1665–8

138. Gold JA, Hoshino Y, Hoshino S, et al. Exogenous gamma and alpha/beta interferon rescues human macrophages from cell death induced by Bacillus anthracis. Infect Immun 2004; 72: 1291–7

139. Niesel DW, Hess CB, Cho YJ, et al. Natural and recombinant interferons inhibit epithelial cell invasion by Shigella spp. Infect Immun 1986; 52: 828–33

140. Carlin JM, Weller JB. Potentiation of interferon-mediated inhibition of Chlamydia infection by interleukin-1 in human macrophage cultures. Infect Immun 1995; 63: 1870–5

141. Devitt A, Lund PA, Morris AG, Pearce JH. Induction of alpha/beta interferon and dependent nitric oxide

synthesis during Chlamydia trachomatis infection of McCoy cells in the absence of exogenous cytokine. Infect Immun 1996; 64: 3951–6

142. Decker T, Muller M, Stockinger S. The yin and yang of type I interferon activity in bacterial infection. Nat Rev Immunol 2005; 5: 675–87

143. Du W, Maniatis T. An ATF/CREB binding site is required for virus induction of the human interferon beta gene [corrected]. Proc Natl Acad Sci USA 1992; 89: 2150–4

144. Falvo JV, Parekh BS, Lin CH, et al. Assembly of a functional beta interferon enhanceosome is dependent on ATF-2-c-jun heterodimer orientation. Mol Cell Biol 2000; 20: 4814–25

145. Thanos D, Maniatis T. The high mobility group protein HMG I(Y) is required for NF-kappa B-dependent virus induction of the human IFN-beta gene. Cell 1992; 71: 777–89

146. Wei H, Zhang J, Xiao W, et al. Involvement of human natural killer cells in asthma pathogenesis: natural killer 2 cells in type 2 cytokine predominance. J Allergy Clin Immunol 2005; 115: 841–7

147. Coyle AJ, Erard F, Bertrand C, et al. Virus-specific CD8+ cells can switch to interleukin 5 production and induce airway eosinophilia. J Exp Med 1995; 181: 1229–33

148. Brooks GD, Buchta KA, Swenson CA, et al. Rhinovirus-induced interferon-gamma and airway responsiveness in asthma. Am J Respir Crit Care Med 2003; 168: 1091–4

149. Alwan WH, Kozlowska WJ, Openshaw PJ. Distinct types of lung disease caused by functional subsets of antiviral T cells. J Exp Med 1994; 179: 81–9

150. Legg JP, Hussian IR, Warner JA, et al. Type 1 and type 2 cytokine imbalance in acute respiratory syncytial virus bronchiolitis. Am J Respir Crit Care Med 2003; 168: 633–9

151. Roman M, Calhoun WJ, Himton KL, et al. Respiratory syncytial virus infection in infants is associated with predominant Th-2-like response. Am J Respir Crit Care Med 1997; 156: 190–5

152. Renzi PM, Turgeon JP, Yang JP, et al. Cellular immunity is activated and a Th2-response is associated with early wheezing in infants after bronchiolitis. J Pediatr 1997; 130: 584–93

153. Pauwels RA, Lofdahl CG, Postma DS, et al. Effect of inhaled formoterol and budesonide on exacerbations of asthma. Formoterol and Corticosteroids Establishing Therapy (FACET) International Study Group. N Engl J Med 1997; 337: 1405–11

154. Rabe KF, Adachi M, Lai CK, et al. Worldwide severity and control of asthma in children and adults: the global asthma insights and reality surveys. J Allergy Clin Immunol 2004; 114: 40–7

155. Harrison TW, Oborne J, Newton S, Tattersfield AE. Doubling the dose of inhaled corticosteroid to prevent asthma exacerbations: randomised controlled trial. Lancet 2004; 363: 271–5

Pathophysiology. Lessons from human respiratory syncytial virus bronchiolitis and acute wheezing episodes in infants

Malcolm G Semple and Rosalind L Smyth

WHEEZING IS COMMON

Illness where wheeze is the major symptom is the commonest reason for children to present to doctors in primary and secondary care. In the UK approximately 30% of all children will have attended their primary care general practitioner with wheeze before their fifth birthday. In 2002 general practitioner-diagnosed asthma accounted for 5% of primary care consultations in children, and 14% of all hospital admissions for childhood illnesses in the UK.[1] Children under the age of 5 years suffer disproportionately more from wheeze than older children aged 5–16 years with 68 versus 49 general practitioner weekly consultations per 100 000 children.[2]

WHEEZING IN INFANCY IS MOST OFTEN CAUSED BY VIRUS INFECTION

Most acute wheeze in childhood is associated with viral lower respiratory tract infection. In a 21-month prospective study of children who were hospitalized in Finland for acute expiratory wheeze, a potential causative viral agent was detected in 88% of cases ($n=293$, median age 1.6 years, range 3 months to 16 years).[3] Although 11 different viruses were described, the most

frequent viruses described in the whole group were human respiratory syncytial virus (hRSV) (27%), enteroviruses (25%), rhinovirus (24%) and non-typable rhino/enterovirus (16%). In infants (children under 12 months), hRSV was found in 54%, respiratory picornaviruses (rhinovirus and enteroviruses) in 42% and human metapneumovirus (hMPV) in 11% of cases. In older children, the respiratory picornaviruses were the most frequently detected viruses (65% age 1–2 years, 82% over 2 years) and, in sharp contrast, hMPV was detected in less than 4% of infants over 1 year old. Comparisons of viruses detected between age groups showed that hRSV and hMPV infection was observed more frequently in wheezing infants than in wheezing children of any other age group.

INFANTS WHO WHEEZE EXHIBIT DISTINCT PHENOTYPES IN CHILDHOOD

Large prospective longitudinal studies have demonstrated that infants who wheeze in infancy fall into distinct phenotypes in later childhood.[4–6] Stein and colleagues have described the phenotypes of these 'childhood wheezers' by sketching the prevalence of wheezing in childhood at different ages (Figure 11.1).[4] In infants, there is

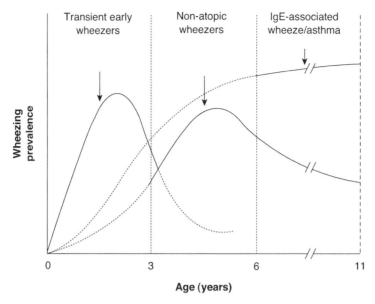

Figure 11.1 Hypothetical schematic of yearly prevalence of wheezing in childhood by phenotype. Reproduced from reference 4 with permission from the BMJ Publishing Group

no relationship between circulating IgE and the prevalence of lower respiratory illness with wheeze, indicating that most wheeze in infants is not an early manifestation of atopy nor an allergic predisposition.[7] This is quite different in older children and adults, where recurrent episodic wheeze (asthma) is strongly associated with elevated serum IgE and skin-prick allergen sensitivity.

BRONCHIOLITIS IS COMMON AND HAS A SIGNIFICANT MORTALITY AND MORBIDITY

Acute respiratory infections remain the most important cause of pediatric mortality, accounting for about 3 million deaths each year, and rank first among the causes of disability-adjusted life-years lost in developing countries (90 million, 6.1% of total). hRSV is the single most important cause of severe lower respiratory tract infections in infants and young children causing significant morbidity and mortality (64 million cases pa,

160 000 deaths pa).[8] The hRSV disease spectrum includes a wide array of respiratory symptoms from rhinitis and otitis media to pneumonia and bronchiolitis; the latter two diseases are associated with substantial morbidity and some mortality. hRSV is a global health problem affecting infants and the elderly. The World Health Organization (WHO) has designated hRSV as a major target of research and therapy throughout the globe.[9]

EPIDEMICS OF hRSV ARE SEASONAL AND PREDICTABLE, PERMITTING HOSPITAL CAPACITY PLANNING AND PRAGMATIC CLINICAL RESEARCH

Winter epidemics of pneumonia in infants were recognized as viral infections in 1939 and histology consistent with a syncytium-forming virus was described in 1941.[10,11] In 1957 Chanock *et al.* isolated a novel virus from infants with respiratory illness which appeared to be similar to chimpanzee coryza agent: a virus known to cause coryza in captive chimpanzees.[12] It was later discovered that the two viruses were the same and that the chimpanzees had probably caught the virus from their keepers.[13] The chimpanzee coryza agent would later be named human respiratory syncytial virus (hRSV). In 1961 hRSV was identified as being the main causal pathogen in winter bronchiolitis epidemics.[14,15] Community surveillance of hRSV and influenza virus was described by Hall and Douglas in 1976. Since then it has been possible for hospitals to be proactive in managing seasonal variation in admissions due to respiratory virus epidemics by increasing capacity.[16] More recently passive immunization for hRSV and vaccination for influenza virus has been given to patients at risk of severe disease based upon prior knowledge of the seasonal nature of hRSV and influenza virus epidemics.[17]

hRSV BRONCHIOLITIS AND WHEEZE: THE ASSOCIATION

Most pediatricians have listened to parents making an association between a significant lower respiratory tract infection during infancy and subsequent wheezing in early years of childhood.

In 2000 Bont *et al.* undertook a systematic review of the long-term consequences of bronchiolitis.[18] Thirteen prospective follow-up studies were selected which included 1161 infants followed for 1–14 years after an episode of bronchiolitis in the first 2 years of life. A clinical diagnosis of bronchiolitis was used in all studies but hRSV infection was confirmed by assay in only eight of the 13. Controls were included in seven of the studies. In the majority of the studies (11 of 13) a total of 777 infants were recruited following admission to hospital for bronchiolitis. The conclusions of these studies are most relevant to infants who suffered a moderate or severe bronchiolitis, rather than the larger number of infants in the community who experienced an uncomplicated upper respiratory tract infection or mild bronchiolitis. Two

studies recruited from the community and followed a total of 384 infants for 8 and 13 years. Both of these studies included controls.[19,20]

Table 11.1 describes the 13 studies reviewed by Bont and five studies published since. Despite the heterogeneous nature of these studies over a period of 40 years, they consistently find a strong and significant relationship between bronchiolitis in infancy and subsequent airway obstruction, whether defined by physician-diagnosed wheeze, parentally recorded wheeze, recurrent wheeze, airway hyperresponsiveness or reduced lung function. In the 11 studies where a relationship between bronchiolitis and atopy was investigated in childhood only one has found a relationship between hRSV infection in infancy and increased risk of developing atopy in later childhood.[21]

Two studies in infants support the hypothesis that RSV infection in infancy is associated with elevated specific IgE in early childhood, but the association with atopy is not clear. In one of these, a large prospective community-based study ($n=609$), hRSV-specific serology was used as a surrogate marker for prior hRSV infection.[22] On follow-up at 1 year, raised aeroallergen-specific IgE to house dust mite ($n=3$), birch ($n=5$) and grass pollen ($n=9$) was always associated with a previous hRSV-seropositive IgG or IgM but the number of affected cases were few, the effect was not seen on follow-up at 2 years and there were no differences in the clinical manifestations of allergy between RSV-seropositive and -seronegative infants. In the other, a much smaller prospective study of infants hospitalized with severe hRSV infection ($n=42$) using age- and sex-matched controls ($n=84$), an association was described between sensitization against food allergens and recurrent wheeze in the second year of life.[23] It would appear that severe respiratory syncytial virus bronchiolitis during the first year of life is an important risk factor associated with development of recurrent wheezing and sensitization to common allergens during the subsequent year of life, but that the association with the development of atopy in

Table 11.1 Summary characteristics and findings of 18 prospective follow-up studies of children who, as infants, experienced bronchiolitis

Study year and reference	hRSV proven	Hospital admission	Controls	Age at enrollment (months)	Follow-up (years)	Outcome	Relationship of parental history of atopy to wheeze if studied
1963[76]	No	Yes	No	< 24	14	Bronchiolitis related to recurrent wheeze in 49% of patients	None found
1978[77,78]	Yes	Yes	Yes	< 12	8	Wheeze in 56% of patients. Reduced PFT	None found
1971–1974[79]	Yes	Yes	Yes	< 12	7	hRSV bronchiolitis related to recurrent wheeze, cough and days off school and reduced PFT	None found
1981[80]	Yes	Yes	'Infants from non-atopic families'	< 24	20	No difference in prevalence of asthma. Reduction in PFT	Not studied
1981[81]	No	Yes	No	< 24	8	Wheeze in 52% of patients. Reduced PFT	Not studied
1982[26]	Yes	Yes	Yes	< 12	10	Wheeze in 42% of patients. Reduced PFT	None found
1984[19]	No	No	Yes	< 24	8	Wheeze in 44% of patients	None found
1984[82]	Yes	Yes	Yes	< 24	8	Wheeze in 45% of patients, and reduced PFT	None found
1986[83,84]	Yes	Yes	No	< 6	2	Nasal hRSV-specific IgE predicts wheeze. 53% of cases wheeze	Not studied
1989[85]	Yes	Yes	No	< 12	5	Wheeze in 71% of patients	None found

(Continued)

(*Continued*)

Study year and reference	hRSV proven	Hospital admission	Controls	Age at enrollment (months)	Follow-up (years)	Outcome	Relationship of parental history of atopy to wheeze if studied
1992[86,87]	Yes	Yes	No	< 12	5 and 10	Wheeze in 43% then 34% of patients, reduced PFT	None found
1993[88]	Yes	Yes	Yes	< 12	2	Wheeze in 44% of cases compared with only 12.9% of controls ($p=0.001$)	None found
1995[21,27,29]	Yes	Yes	Yes	< 12	3, 7 and 13	Wheeze in 60%, 30% then 43% of patients. hRSV risk factor for allergy	Yes
1997[89]	No	Yes	No	< 12	3 months	Wheeze in 65% of patients. Th2 cytokine profile predicts wheeze	Not studied
1999[24]	Yes	Yes	No	< 13	3	Reduced PFT during acute bronchiolitis predictive of recurrent wheeze during follow-up	None found
1999[20]	Yes	No	Yes	< 36	13	Wheeze in hRSV patients up to 11 but not at 13 years	None found
2000[90,91]	Yes	Yes	Yes	< 12	1 and 3	Monocyte IL-10 related to recurrent wheeze at 1 year. Reduced health-related quality of life at 3 years	None found
1999–2001[23]	Yes	Yes	Yes	Mean 4 Range 2–9 months	Age 1 year	hRSV bronchiolitis a risk for recurrent wheeze and atopic sensitization	None found to wheeze

PFT, pulmonary function testing included in study

later childhood has not been convincingly described.

Bont *et al.* described a large prospective community-based 3-year follow-up study of daily respiratory symptoms in 140 infants who had been admitted to hospital with hRSV bronchiolitis in infancy and which has generated a unique record of respiratory morbidity and seasonal variation in wheeze.[24] Bont *et al.* demonstrated that airway morbidity following severe hRSV bronchiolitis has a seasonal pattern, peaking in winter, which suggests that viral infections are the predominant trigger for wheezing.[24] Serum IgE was measured in infants at conclusion of the study. No association was found between total IgE or allergen-specific IgE and the occurrence of wheeze during follow-up. Eczema in the infant and parental history of atopy (asthma, eczema and hayfever) were not associated with wheezing during the 3 years of follow-up. Eczema in the infant was associated with parental history of atopy but not with total or specific IgE. The authors concluded that parental atopy appears to be a risk factor for atopy in infants, but atopy in infants and their parents is not related to airway morbidity following significant hRSV infection. Kneyber *et al.*, in a quantitative review of the long-term affects of hRSV bronchiolitis, concluded that hRSV infection in infancy caused recurrent wheeze but did not cause atopy or atopic asthma in later childhood.[25]

These findings are consistent with those of two large community-based studies. Pullan *et al.* reported a 10-year follow-up study of 164 children in the North East of England, UK affected by severe bronchiolitis in infancy compared with 111 controls.[26] Pullan described an increase in bronchial hyperreactivity but no increase in atopy. Stein *et al.* followed a large birth cohort of 517 infants from birth to 13 years old in Tucson, AZ, USA.[20] They concluded that hRSV infection in children under 4 years old, regardless of disease severity, was not associated with subsequent allergic sensitization. Sigurs *et al.* have serially reported one smaller cohort study of 47 children raised in Sweden. This is the only long-term cohort study that has found an association between hRSV bronchiolitis in infancy and development of atopy in later life.[21,27–29]

hRSV INFECTION CAUSES DISEASE AND WHEEZE THROUGHOUT LIFE

The clinical picture of bronchiolitis is rarely seen after the second year of life, and with such interest in hRSV bronchiolitis it would be easy to infer that hRSV infection is only a problem in infancy. The unique age distribution of bronchiolitis may be a function of airway caliber as much as acquisition of immunity. hRSV is unusual in that it can cause severe disease in infants born to mothers with moderate levels of circulating anti-hRSV immunoglobulin. Primary hRSV infection usually protects against recurrence of severe disease but the naturally acquired immunity is poor and hRSV reinfection is recognized throughout childhood and adult life.[3] hRSV is unlike many other viruses in this respect. hRSV reinfection is often associated with wheeze and exacerbations of asthma throughout life (though rhinovirus infection is the most frequent provocation of exacerbations of asthma).[24,30] hRSV infection continues to be a major cause of morbidity and mortality, on a par with influenza virus, in all who are immunocompromised, those who have chronic lung or heart disease and both the frail and healthy elderly population.[31]

DOES hRSV INFECTION CAUSE ASTHMA?

The answer to this question depends upon the definition of asthma. This is not a pedantic point. If it can be shown that hRSV infection alone or severe hRSV disease is a direct cause of recurrent wheeze in childhood then significant investment in the prevention or treatment of hRSV disease in the general population would be justified.

The problem with the question is the rather vague but popular definition of asthma as '*a chronic inflammatory pulmonary disorder that is characterized by reversible obstruction of the airways*'. This simple definition suggests that asthma is a well-defined clinical disorder, which it is not. A collaboration between the National Heart, Lung, and Blood Institute, National Institutes of Health, USA and the World Health Organization resulted in The Global Initiative For Asthma (GINA). GINA's definition of asthma is based on the functional consequences of airway inflammation:

Asthma is a chronic inflammatory disorder of the airways in which many cells and cellular elements play a role. The chronic inflammation causes an associated increase in airway hyperresponsiveness that leads to recurrent episodes of wheezing, breathlessness, chest tightness, and coughing, particularly at night or in the early morning. These episodes are usually associated with widespread but variable airflow obstruction that is often reversible either spontaneously or with treatment. (GINA 2004)

This definition acknowledges the key role of complex inflammatory processes underlying a clinical condition which appears in many guises. The most consistent symptom described by patients with asthma is wheeze, and then nocturnal cough.

There are at least 16 recent studies supporting a strong association between severe bronchiolitis in early infancy and subsequent recurrent wheeze in childhood, although this association appears to be lost in the early teenage years. It is easy to jump to the conclusion that bronchiolitis in infancy causes asthma, especially if wheeze is what we call asthma. This conclusion oversimplifies a number of complex issues.

One problem is that hRSV infection is very common in infancy. Recent seroprevalence studies in Japan and Thailand have shown that approximately half of all infants have been infected with hRSV in the first year of life

and all have been infected before their fifth birthday.[32,33] There are no hRSV-uninfected cohorts of children in the general population to compare their prevalence of asthma (or wheeze for that matter) with infants who are seropositive or have had severe bronchiolitis.

The strong association between severe hRSV disease in infancy (bronchiolitis) and subsequent wheeze need not be a direct consequential effect but due to a shared genetic predisposition.[34] There is mounting evidence that the infants who experience severe hRSV bronchiolitis have an impaired Th1 response to the virus, characterized by reduced IFN-γ production by blood monocytes and reduced IFN-γ concentrations in respiratory secretions.[35–38] Infants with a subtle impairment in their Th1 response may remain predisposed to inefficient clearance of respiratory virus infections or experience a relatively unopposed Th2 inflammatory response to these infections. Such mechanisms would explain why these infants appear to be more prone to symptomatic respiratory virus infections, experiencing wheeze during childhood, until they acquire immunity to these ubiquitous viruses. The majority of relevant studies indicate that these infants are not disproportionately atopic and do not go on to develop classical asthma.

There are many genetic epidemiological studies which describe associations between common polymorphisms in the genes for cytokines,[39–41] cytokine receptors,[42] Toll-like receptors[43] and surfactant proteins[44,45] and severe hRSV disease in infants and adults.[46] The 'genetic predisposition' to severe hRSV disease does not require a unique impairment in the innate immunity. Instead the interplay of polygenic polymorphisms in diverse parts of the immune system (mucosal, innate and adaptive) may contribute to susceptibility to severe disease. Any combination of these polymorphisms could contribute to a common causal link between bronchiolitis in infancy and wheeze in later childhood.

There is also the possibility that wheeze in childhood is a direct consequence of hRSV infection. Fascinating studies of hRSV infection in mice reported by Culley et al. have shown that the age of mice when they experience primary hRSV infection determines the polarity of T cell-mediated disease during reinfection in later life. Infection in the neonatal mouse results in a Th2 dominant response to subsequent reinfection which lasts into adulthood.[47] This raises the possibility that deferring the age at which infants experience hRSV infection until later childhood could reduce their risk of subsequent wheeze.

O'Donnell has described how mice infected with hRSV and influenza virus are acutely susceptible to sensitization to aeroallergen (ovalbumin). CD8+ splenocytes from these sensitized mice exhibited a Th2 skewed cytokine response and allergen-specific IgG1 production.[48] In a similar mouse study Barends et al. described how RSV infection enhanced an allergic response to ovalbumin, but only when the immune system had already been primed by the allergen.[49] This RSV-enhanced allergic response was not attenuated by prior infection with RSV. If such a mechanism of synergy between aeroallergen sensitization and virus infection exists in human infants then priming by hRSV in infancy in the presence of a common aeroallergen could lead to bronchial hyperreactivity to aeroallergen and virus in later life. Two studies of human infants have shown an increase in sensitization to aeroallergens in infants who were hospitalized by hRSV bronchiolitis but the effect was only evident for the first 2 years of life.[22,23]

It is generally accepted that hRSV, like many other respiratory pathogens, causes wheeze during acute infection. It is much harder to demonstrate that a direct consequence of an endemic infection in infancy is associated with a disease state in a proportion of the population many years later. One solution to this problem would be to undertake prospective placebo-controlled studies in normal infants involving anti-hRSV interventions to acute hRSV disease followed by long-term follow-up of respiratory symptoms. In such studies, observation of a reduction in wheeze in childhood in the treatment group would be evidence of a causal role for hRSV infection. Potential agents would include prophylactic interventions: immunization (whether passive by immunoglobulin or active by vaccination), and therapies such as inhibitors of hRSV replication and immunomodulators.

Again, hRSV presents several stumbling blocks in this avenue of research. It is unlikely that large randomized controlled trials (RCTs) involving prophylactic agents will be run in normal infants. As severe bronchiolitis affects only 1–2% of the normal infant population, studies would require massive recruitment to achieve statistical power.

A pragmatic approach has been to recruit high-risk infants to prospective prophylactic studies, but this method limits applicability of the results to the general infant population. Studies involving a therapeutic intervention involving severely affected previously well infants will have more relevance, and the ideal scenario will be a RCT of a vaccine with long-term follow-up.

Investigators must be satisfied with the effectiveness of the chosen intervention for these studies to have any chance of success. Unfortunately, hRSV has proven to be a fickle foe. Despite many years of research the therapeutic value and role of the few available interventions have not been clearly described.

IMMUNIZATION: ACTIVE VACCINATION

There is no licensed hRSV vaccine. In the 1960s a formalin-inactivated whole-virus vaccine was trialed in infants and children. Tragically, the vaccine did not protect against infection, and when some of the vaccinated children became naturally infected they experienced severe and sometimes fatal RSV disease.[50,51] This immunopathological phenomenon has been reproduced in cattle vaccinated against bovine RSV, a virus closely related to hRSV.[52] Development of a suitable vaccine has been hampered by an incomplete understanding of which immune responses to viral epitopes stimulate protection against serious hRSV disease and which epitopes promote an excessive inflammatory response. Both live attenuated vaccines and subunit vaccines are being cautiously evaluated in humans.

IMMUNIZATION: PASSIVE IMMUNIZATION

The suggestion that passive immunization may provide some protection against severe bronchiolitis came from a study of breast-feeding practice in a case-controlled cohort of infants admitted to hospital.[53] A number of socioeconomic factors may have confounded the study but the investigators found high levels of hRSV-neutralizing IgA, detectable IgG-neutralizing antibody and the absence of specific IgM in the colostrum of the nursing mothers. The data suggested that previous maternal hRSV infection provided protection by passive transfer of IgA via the colostrum. The socioeconomic confounders associated with breast-feeding prevent the use of breast-feeding as a pre-exposure intervention to hRSV infection in a long-term study of wheeze in childhood.

Two immune globulin products (RSV-IGIV (Respigam™) and palivizumab (Synagis™)) have been licensed for prophylactic use in infants at high risk of severe hRSV disease.[54,55] Administration of immunoglobulin does not prevent infection or disease but does provide protection against severe hRSV disease in some patients in high-risk groups. High-risk infants are typically prematurely born and have chronic lung disease of prematurity (CLD; bronchopulmonary dysplasia) but other infants such as those with significant congenital cardiac lesions also benefit.

In a small retrospective study, 13 children who received RSV-IGIV in infancy were compared with 26 age- and gestational age-matched controls at approximately 9 years of age.[56] Pulmonary function was better in the treatment group, there were fewer episodes of wheeze, less atopy was reported and fewer days of school were missed. This study gave the first indication that prophylaxis of hRSV infection in infancy might reduce the risk of recurrent wheeze in childhood, but the quality of evidence from small retrospective studies is considered poor. Better evidence is needed from double-blind RCTs.

RSV-IGIV prophylaxis involved slow intravenous infusion over several hours repeated monthly during the endemic hRSV season. In the PREVENT study 13% of infants with chronic lung disease required extra diuretics for fluid overload due to the immunoglobulin infusion.[57] RSV-IGIV has largely been superseded by palivizumab (a humanized monoclonal) which is 50–100 times more potent per weight.[55] Palivizumab is given as a monthly intramuscular injection and avoids fluid overload.

There are two large prospective studies of the long-term effects of palivizumab prophylaxis on recurrent wheeze. One case-controlled study involves several centers in America and Europe (Protocol W00-353; Abbott Laboratories).[58] The other study in Canada compared two cities with similar social and demographic features.[59] One city used palivizumab prophylaxis in high-risk infants for four seasons while the other did not. Preliminary data reported orally and in abstracts from these two studies suggest that palivizumab given in infancy and prior to natural hRSV infection modulates the severity of disease and reduces the risk of recurrent wheeze in childhood. Both studies suggested that hRSV prophylaxis reduced the risk of subsequent wheeze and supported the existence of a causal mechanism between hRSV infection in infancy and wheeze in childhood.

Two animal models of hRSV disease support these preliminary findings. Mejias *et al.* described a mouse model where hRSV inoculation induced a significant inflammatory response in the lungs which progressed into a chronic disease characterized by airway hyperresponsiveness.[60] The airway inflammation persisted for 22 weeks despite absence of detectable virus after 6 weeks. Using this model palivizumab or a control antibody was administered once at 24 hours before inoculation,

1 hour after inoculation or 48 hours after inoculation. Regardless of the timing of administration, all mice treated with palivizumab showed significantly decreased RSV loads in bronchoalveolar lavage (BAL) and lung specimens compared with those of infected–untreated controls. Pulmonary histopathology scores, airway obstruction measured by plethysmography and airway hyperresponsiveness after methacholine challenge were significantly reduced in mice treated with palivizumab antibody 24 hours before inoculation compared with those for untreated controls. Concentrations of interferon-γ, interleukin-10, macrophage inflammatory protein 1α, regulated on activation normal T-cell expressed and secreted (RANTES) and eotaxin in BAL fluids were also significantly reduced in mice treated with palivizumab 24 hours before inoculation. This study demonstrates that the reduced RSV replication associated with palivizumab was associated with significant modulation of inflammatory and clinical markers of acute disease severity and subsequent pulmonary function abnormalities.[60]

Piedimonte et al. have described a model of hRSV infection in the Fischer F-344 strain rat which explores the non-adrenergic non-cholinergic (NANC) nervous system and its role in the modulation of local inflammatory and immune responses in the distal airways.[61] Historically the parasympathetic nervous system has been viewed as providing excitory innervation to pulmonary smooth muscle, with inhibitory stimulation of adrenergic receptors on smooth muscle being mediated by circulating adrenergic agonists. The NANC innervation is now recognized as providing the majority of innervation to the distal airways in animal models.[62] NANC innervation includes excitatory (eNANC) and inhibitory (iNANC) fibers. The excitatory fibers produce peptide neurotransmitters including substance P (SP), also known as neurokinin-1, which interacts with a specific receptor to stimulate smooth muscle contraction. SP also has potent proinflammatory cytokine-like effects upon lymphocytes, mast cells and neutrophils. This mechanism whereby eNANC

innervation produces inflammation is called 'neurogenic inflammation'.

Piedimonte et al. described upregulation of SP receptor gene expression in the distal airways of rats following hRSV infection suggesting that hRSV infection increases the susceptibility of distal airways to the excitatory and proinflammatory effects of SP.[63] The group later reported that palivizumab administration to weanling rats before and up to 72 hours after hRSV inoculation prevented the upregulation of the SP receptor and abolished acute neurogenic inflammatory changes in the distal airways. This effect persisted for at least 30 days after inoculation.[64] Using the same rat model the group has described reduction in the severity of capsaicin-induced apnea by selective blockade of the SP receptor and GABA type A receptor, suggesting that apnea, a common problem in neonates suffering hRSV bronchiolitis, is influenced by the eNANC pathway.[64,65]

These animal models describe how hRSV infection results in chronic airway hyperresponsiveness through two distinct inflammatory mechanisms and supports the direct consequential hypothesis that hRSV infection potentiates chronic airway reactivity. Studies in these models offer hope that long-term immunomodulation is possible through effective early intervention or prophylaxis.

DISEASE MODIFICATION: ANTIVIRAL THERAPY

Ribavirin is a synthetic guanosine analog and broad-spectrum antiviral agent. Ribavirin is the only approved (licensed) drug for treatment of hRSV infection. Its use is controversial because of questions regarding efficacy, concerns about occupational exposure, difficulties in administration and high cost.[66] The efficacy of this therapy for the treatment of acute disease has been the subject of systematic review by the Cochrane collaboration. This review published in 2004 included 12 RCTs in the meta-analyis.[67] All trials enrolled infants below the age of 6 months. In

Table 11.2 Summary characteristics and findings of antiviral intervention studies upon post-bronchiolitis wheeze

Year, type, reference	Treatment	Controls	Age at enrollment	Follow-up	Primary outcome
1986–87, Retrospective[92]	Ribavirin ($n=33$)	No Rx, age and risk matched ($n=67$)		5 years	No differences in RAD or PFT
1997, DB PC RCT[93]	Ribavirin ($n=28$)	Placebo ($n=26$)		9 years	No differences in number of URTIs, RAD or PFT
1983–85, DB PC RCT[68]	Ribavirin ($n=24$) 13 had PFTs	Placebo ($n=11$) 6 had PFTs	1–33 months	6 years	No difference in methacholine reactivity. Excess abnormal PFTs in placebo group
1994–95, Retrospective, no blinding[94]	Ribavirin ($n=22$)	Conservative ($n=19$)	<6 months	1 year	Reduced wheeze and asthma medications in Ribavirin group
1997–99, Blinded, randomized, uncontrolled[95]	Ribavirin ($n=24$)	Conservative ($n=21$)	<6 months	1 year	Reduced respiratory symptoms and hospitalizations in Ribavirin group

PFT, pulmonary function test; DB, double-blind; PC, placebo-controlled; RCT, randomized controlled trial; URTI, upper respiratory tract infection; RAD, reactive airways disease; Rx, treatment

four trials with 158 patients, mortality with ribavirin was 5.8% compared with 9.7% with placebo (odds ratio (OR) 0.58; 95% confidence interval (CI) 0.18–1.85). In three trials with 116 patients the probability of respiratory deterioration with ribavirin was 7.1% compared with 18.3% with placebo (OR 0.37; 95% CI 0.12–1.18). In three studies with 104 ventilated patients, the weighted mean difference in days of hospitalization was 1.9 fewer days with ribavirin (95% CI −4.6 to +0.9) and the weighted mean difference in days of ventilation was 1.8 fewer days with ribavirin (95% CI −3.4 to −0.2). While the power of the studies was poor, the cumulative results of these small trials showed that ribavirin has benefits on some short-term clinical outcomes. This needs to be set against its high cost, difficulties in administration and safety concerns.

In this Cochrane review one placebo-controlled RCT reported by Rodriguez et al. examined the effect of ribavirin upon the long-term respiratory sequelae of severe hRSV bronchiolitis.[68] Rodriguez et al. found that significantly fewer children in the ribavirin group ($n = 24$) had moderate or severely abnormal pulmonary function and fewer episodes of wheeze than the placebo group ($n = 11$) over the 6-year period of follow-up. The beneficial effects in this study were statistically significant but the differences between groups were small. The study by Rodriguez et al. and four other follow-up studies have specifically examined the effect of ribavirin upon the long-term respiratory sequelae of severe hRSV bronchiolitis (Table 11.2). Two studies following 154 children for between 5 and 7 years found no difference in lung function or wheeze. Two studies following 86 infants for 1 year found reduced wheeze, reduced asthma medication and reduced hospitalizations in the ribavirin-treated groups. Unfortunately, there are conflicting conclusions from a handful of small studies addressing the value of ribavirin treatment upon the long-term respiratory sequelae of hRSV bronchiolitis.

Table 11.3 Summary characteristics and findings of anti-inflammatory intervention studies upon post-bronchiolitis respiratory symptoms

Year, type, reference	Treatment, group size and duration	Controls	Age at enrollment	Follow-up	Primary outcome
1996, RCT no blinding, no placebo[71]	Cromolyn neb (n=34) or budesonide neb (n=34), 4 months	No therapy (n=34)	1–23 months	16 weeks on therapy	Less wheeze and fewer hospitalizations
1998, RCT no blinding, no placebo[72]	Cromolyn (n=29), budesonide neb (n=31), 4 months	No therapy (n=28)	1–23 months	1 year	No differences in wheeze or asthma symptoms
1998, PC DB RCT[74]	Budesonide neb (n=21), 6 weeks	Saline neb (n=19), 6 weeks	0–12 months	6 months	No differences in wheeze. Significantly more infants in treatment group admitted with respiratory problems
1999, PC DB RCT[96]	Budesonide mdi (n=26), 8 weeks	Placebo mdi (n=28), 8 weeks	0–12 months	12 months	No differences in symptoms nor hospitalization
2000, PC DB RCT[97]	Prednisolone oral (n=24), 7 days	Placebo (n=23), 7 days	0–24 months	3–7 years	No difference in wheeze
2000, RCT no blinding, no placebo[73]	Budesonide neb (n=40), 7 days Budesonide neb (n=36), 8 weeks	No therapy (n=41)	0–9 months	2 years	Fewer children in treatment groups receiving asthma medication than controls
2000, PC DB RCT[98]	Budesonide neb (n=83), 2 weeks	Placebo neb (n=82), 2 weeks	0–12 months	12 months	No differences in symptoms or readmission rates

neb, nebulizer; mdi, metered dose inhaler

DISEASE MODIFICATION: ANTI-INFLAMMATORY THERAPY

Oral cysteinyl-leukotriene antagonists and inhaled corticosteroids are two groups of drugs recognized as being effective in the treatment of asthma. Studies have been performed using both groups of drugs in the acute and convalescent phases of bronchiolitis.

Bisgaard described outcomes over 28 days of treatment with montelukast initiated within 7 days of the onset of bronchiolitis symptoms.[69] A total of 130 infants admitted with hRSV bronchiolitis were randomized to receive montelukast or placebo. Infants with a suspected history of asthma were excluded; 116 infants (median age 9 months) provided diary card data for the treatment period. Infants in the treatment group were free of any symptoms on 22% of the days and nights compared with 4% of the infants in the placebo group ($p = 0.015$). A total of 87 infants completed 2 months of follow-up, at which time there were no significant differences in respiratory symptoms between the treatment and control groups.

In 2001, Simoes reviewed the treatment and prevention of hRSV bronchiolitis with a particular view to long-term effects on respiratory outcome.[70] He included six studies of steroids (one oral, five inhaled). One of these longitudinal studies found less wheeze and fewer hospitalizations after 16 weeks of therapy but at 1-year follow-up there was no difference in wheeze or asthma symptoms between groups.[71,72] The seven studies of anti-inflammatory therapies are summarized in Table 11.3. Only one RCT, which included 107 infants, showed fewer children on asthma medication at 2 years' follow-up, but this study was not blinded or placebo controlled.[73] One randomized double-blind placebo-controlled trial found more symptoms in the treatment group at 6 months' follow-up.[74] To summarize, there is evidence from five studies including 394 infants that steroids given in the acute and convalescent phase of hRSV bronchiolitis make no difference to long-term respiratory sequelae.

CONCLUSION

In 1965 Sir Austin Bradford Hill gave a landmark paper to the Royal Society of Medicine: 'The environment and disease: association or causation?', in which he discussed 'In what circumstances can we pass from this observed association to a verdict of causation?'[75] The criteria he set out for unraveling causation from association included strength, consistency, specificity, temporality, biological gradient, plausibility, coherence, experiment and analogy. These principles have been examined for the relationship between hRSV infection in infancy and wheeze in childhood using animal models and human studies. The jigsaw of data is incomplete but is it probable that hRSV infection in infancy causes wheeze in childhood.

hRSV disease in infancy heralds recurrent wheeze in childhood through common genetic mechanisms and probably direct causal mechanisms. Passive immunization appears to modulate acute disease and late sequelae in high-risk infants. Treatment in the acute or convalescent phase with current antiviral or anti-inflammatory drugs has no long-term benefits.

REFERENCES

1. National Asthma Campaign Asthma Audit 2002. Starting as we mean to go on: an audit of children's asthma in the UK. Asthma J 2002; 8: 1–4

2. Royal College of General Practitioners Birmingham Research Unit. Weekly Returns 1976–2000. Birmingham: Royal College of General Practitioners, 2000

3. Jartti T, Lehtinen P, Vuorinen T, et al. Respiratory picornaviruses and respiratory syncytial virus as causative agents of acute expiratory wheezing in children. Emerg Infect Dis 2004; 10: 1095–101

4. Stein RT, Holberg CJ, Morgan WJ, et al. Peak flow variability, methacholine responsiveness and atopy as markers for detecting different wheezing phenotypes in childhood. Thorax 1997; 52: 946–52

5. Stein RT, Martinez FD. Asthma phenotypes in childhood: lessons from an epidemiological approach. Paediatr Respir Rev 2004; 5: 155–61

6. Dodge R, Martinez FD, Cline MG, et al. Early childhood respiratory symptoms and the subsequent diagnosis of asthma. J Allergy Clin Immunol 1996; 98: 48–54

7. Halonen M, Stern D, Taussig LM, et al. The predictive relationship between serum IgE levels at birth and subsequent incidences of lower respiratory illnesses and eczema in infants. Am Rev Respir Dis 1992; 146: 866–70

8. World Health Organization. The World Health Report 2003: shaping the future. Geneva: World Health Organization, 2003

9. Maggon K, Barik S. New drugs and treatment for respiratory syncytial virus. Rev Med Virol 2004; 14: 149–68

10. Goodpasture EW, Auerbach SH, Swanson HS. Virus pneumonia of infants secondary to epidemic infections. Am J Dis Child 1939; 57: 997–1011

11. Adams JM. Primary virus pneumonitis with cytoplasmic inclusion bodies: study of an epidemic involving thirty-two infants with nine deaths. JAMA 1941; 116: 925–33

12. Chanock R, Roizman B, Myers R. Recovery from infants with respiratory illness of a virus related to

chimpanzee coryza agent (CCA) I: isolation, properties and characterization. Am J Hyg 1957; 66: 281–90

13. Beem M, Wright FH, Hamre D, et al. Association of the chimpanzee coryza agent with acute respiratory disease in children. N Engl J Med 1960; 263: 523–30

14. Chanock RM, Kim HW, Vargosko AJ. Respiratory syncytial virus. I. Virus recovery and other observations during 1960 outbreak of bronchiolitis, pneumonia, and minor respiratory diseases in children. JAMA 1961; 176: 647–53

15. Forbes JA, Bennett NM, Gray NJ. Epidemic bronchiolitis caused by a respiratory syncytial virus: clinical aspects. Med J Aust 1961; 48: 933–5

16. Hall CB, Douglas RG Jr. Respiratory syncytial virus and influenza. Practical community surveillance. Am J Dis Child 1976; 130: 615–20

17. Groothuis JR, Simoes EAF, Levin MJ, et al. Prophylactic administration of respiratory syncytial virus immune globulin to high-risk infants and young children. N Engl J Med 1993; 329: 1524–30

18. Bont L, Aalderen WM, Kimpen JL. Long-term consequences of respiratory syncytial virus (RSV) bronchiolitis. Paediatr Respir Rev 2000; 1: 221–7

19. McConnochie KM, Roghmann KJ. Bronchiolitis as a possible cause of wheezing in childhood: new evidence. Pediatrics 1984; 74: 1–10

20. Stein RT, Sherrill D, Morgan WJ, et al. Respiratory syncytial virus in early life and risk of wheeze and allergy by age 13 years. Lancet 1999; 354: 541–5

21. Sigurs N, Bjarnason R, Sigurbergsson F, Kjellman B. Respiratory syncytial virus bronchiolitis in infancy is an important risk factor for asthma and allergy at age 7. Am J Respir Crit Care Med 2000; 161: 1501–7

22. Forster J, Tacke U, Krebs H, et al. Respiratory syncytial virus infection: its role in aeroallergen sensitization during the first two years of life. Pediatr Allergy Immunol 1996; 7: 55–60

23. Schauer U, Hoffjan S, Bittscheidt J, et al. RSV bronchiolitis and risk of wheeze and allergic sensitization in the first year of life. Eur Respir J 2002; 20: 1277–83

24. Bont L, Steijn M, van Aalderen WM, et al. Seasonality of long term wheezing following respiratory syncytial virus lower respiratory tract infection. Thorax 2004; 59: 512–16

25. Kneyber MCJ, Steyerberg EW, De Groot R, Moll HA. Long-term effects of respiratory syncytial virus (RSV) bronchiolitis in infants and young children: a quantitative review. Acta Paediatr 2000; 89: 654–60

26. Pullan CR, Hey EN. Wheezing, asthma, and pulmonary dysfunction 10 years after infection with respiratory syncytial virus in infancy. BMJ (Clin Res Ed) 1982; 284: 1665–9

27. Sigurs N, Gustafsson PM, Bjarnason R, et al. Severe respiratory syncytial virus bronchiolitis in infancy and asthma and allergy at age 13. Am J Respir Crit Care Med 2005; 171: 137–41

28. Sigurs N. A cohort of children hospitalized with acute RSV bronchiolitis: impact on later respiratory disease. Paediatr Respir Rev 2002; 3: 177–83

29. Sigurs N, Bjarnason R, Sigurbergsson F, et al. Asthma and immunoglobulin E antibodies after respiratory syncytial virus bronchiolitis: a prospective cohort study with matched controls. Pediatrics 1995; 95: 500–5

30. Pattemore PK, Johnston SL, Bardin PG. Viruses as precipitants of asthma symptoms. I. Epidemiology. Clin Exp Allergy 1992; 22: 325–36

31. Falsey AR, Hennessey PA, Formica MA, et al. Respiratory syncytial virus infection in elderly and high-risk adults. N Engl J Med 2005; 352: 1749–59

32. Ebihara T, Endo R, Kikuta H, et al. Comparison of the seroprevalence of human metapneumovirus and human respiratory syncytial virus. J Med Virol 2004; 72: 304–6

33. Bhattarakosol P, Pancharoen C, Mungmee V, et al. Seroprevalence of anti-RSV IgG in Thai children aged 6 months to 5 years. Asian Pac J Allergy Immunol 2003; 21: 269–71

34. Openshaw PJ, Dean GS, Culley FJ. Links between respiratory syncytial virus bronchiolitis and childhood asthma: clinical and research approaches. Pediatr Infect Dis J 2003; 22: S58–S64

35. Legg JP, Hussain IR, Warner JA, et al. Type 1 and type 2 cytokine imbalance in acute respiratory syncytial virus bronchiolitis. Am J Respir Crit Care Med 2003; 168: 633–9

36. Mobbs KJ, Smyth RL, O'Hea U, et al. Cytokines in severe respiratory syncytial virus bronchiolitis. Pediatr Pulmonol 2002; 33: 449–52

37. Aberle JH, Aberle SW, Dworzak MN, et al. Reduced interferon-gamma expression in peripheral blood mononuclear cells of infants with severe respiratory syncytial virus disease. Am J Respir Crit Care Med 1999; 160: 1263–8

38. Bont L, Heijnen CJ, Kavelaars A, et al. Local interferon-gamma levels during respiratory syncytial virus lower respiratory tract infection are associated with disease severity. J Infect Dis 2001; 184: 355–8

39. Hull J, Thomson A, Kwiatkowski D. Association of respiratory syncytial virus bronchiolitis with the interleukin 8 gene region in UK families. Thorax 2000; 55: 1023–7

40. Choi EH, Lee HJ, Yoo T, Chanock SJ. A common haplotype of interleukin-4 gene IL4 is associated with severe respiratory syncytial virus disease in Korean children. J Infect Dis 2002; 186: 1207–11

41. Gentile DA, Doyle WJ, Zeevi A, et al. Cytokine gene polymorphisms moderate illness severity in infants with respiratory syncytial virus infection. Hum Immunol 2003; 64: 338–44

42. Hoebee B, Rietveld E, Bont L, et al. Association of severe respiratory syncytial virus bronchiolitis with interleukin-4 and interleukin-4 receptor alpha polymorphisms. J Infect Dis 2003; 187: 2–11

43. Tal G, Mandelberg A, Dalal I, et al. Association between common Toll-like receptor 4 mutations and severe respiratory syncytial virus disease. J Infect Dis 2004; 189: 2057–63

44. Lahti M, Lofgren J, Marttila R, et al. Surfactant protein D gene polymorphism associated with severe respiratory syncytial virus infection. Pediatr Res 2002; 51: 696–9

45. Lofgren J, Ramet M, Renko M, et al. Association between surfactant protein A gene locus and severe respiratory syncytial virus infection in infants. J Infect Dis 2002; 185: 283–9

46. Gentile DA, Doyle WJ, Zeevi A, et al. Cytokine gene polymorphisms moderate responses to respiratory syncytial virus in adults. Hum Immunol 2003; 64: 93–8

47. Culley FJ, Pollott J, Openshaw PJ. Age at first viral infection determines the pattern of T cell-mediated disease during reinfection in adulthood. J Exp Med 2002; 196: 1381–6

48. O'Donnell DR, Openshaw PJM. Anaphylactic sensitisation to aeroantigen during respiratory virus infection. Clin Exp Allergy 1998; 28: 1501–8

49. Barends M, van Oosten M, De Rond CG, et al. Timing of infection and prior immunization with respiratory syncytial virus (RSV) in RSV-enhanced allergic inflammation. J Infect Dis 2004; 189: 1866–72

50. Kim HW, Canchola JG, Brandt CD, et al. Respiratory syncytial virus disease in infants despite prior administration of antigenic inactivated vaccine. Am J Epidemiol 1969; 89: 422–34

51. Kapikian AZ, Mitchell RH, Chanock RM, et al. An epidemiologic study of altered clinical reactivity to respiratory syncytial (RS) virus infection in children previously vaccinated with an inactivated RS virus vaccine. Am J Epidemiol 1969; 89: 405–21

52. Schreiber P, Matheise JP, Dessy F, et al. High mortality rate associated with bovine respiratory syncytial virus (BRSV) infection in Belgian white blue calves previously vaccinated with an inactivated BRSV vaccine. J Vet Med B Infect Dis Vet Public Health 2000; 47: 535–50

53. Downham MA, Scott R, Sims DG, et al. Breast-feeding protects against respiratory syncytial virus infections. BMJ 1976; 2: 274–6

54. Groothuis JR, Simoes EA, Levin MJ, et al. Prophylactic administration of respiratory syncytial virus immune globulin to high-risk infants and young children. The Respiratory Syncytial Virus Immune Globulin Study Group [see comments]. N Engl J Med 1993; 329: 1524–30

55. The IMpact-RSV Study Group. Palivizumab, a humanized respiratory syncytial virus monoclonal antibody, reduces hospitalization from respiratory syncytial virus infection in high-risk infants. Pediatrics 1998; 102: 531–7

56. Wenzel SE, Gibbs RL, Lehr MV, Simoes EA. Respiratory outcomes in high-risk children 7 to 10 years after prophylaxis with respiratory syncytial virus immune globulin. Am J Med 2002; 112: 627–33

57. Reduction of respiratory syncytial virus hospitalization among premature infants and infants with bronchopulmonary dysplasia using respiratory syncytial virus immune globulin prophylaxis. The PREVENT Study Group. Pediatrics 1997; 99: 93–9

58. Simoes EAF, Carbonell-Estrany X, Kimpen J, et al. Palivizumab use decreases risk of recurrent wheezing in preterm children. Eur Respir J 2004; 24: 212

59. Mitchell I, Gillis L, Majaesic C, Tough S. Outcomes of two population-based approaches to prophylaxis with palivizumab. Eur Respir J 2004; 24: 23

60. Mejias A, Chavez-Bueno S, Rios AM, et al. Anti-respiratory syncytial virus (RSV) neutralizing antibody decreases lung inflammation, airway obstruction, and airway hyperresponsiveness in a murine RSV model. Antimicrob Agents Chemother 2004; 48: 1811–22

61. Piedimonte G, Rodriguez MM, King KA, et al. Respiratory syncytial virus upregulates expression of the substance P receptor in rat lungs. Am J Physiol 1999; 277: L831–L840

62. Inoue H, Aizawa H, Ikeda T, et al. [Nonadrenergic noncholinergic inhibitory nervous system in guinea pig airway]. Nihon Kyobu Shikkan Gakkai Zasshi 1992; 30: 248–55

63. Piedimonte G, King KA, Holmgren NL, et al. A humanized monoclonal antibody against respiratory syncytial virus (palivizumab) inhibits RSV-induced neurogenic-mediated inflammation in rat airways. Pediatr Res 2000; 47: 351–6

64. King KA, Hu C, Rodriguez MM, et al. Exaggerated neurogenic inflammation and substance P receptor upregulation in RSV-infected weanling rats. Am J Respir Cell Mol Biol 2001; 24: 101–7

65. Sabogal C, Auais A, Napchan G, et al. Effect of respiratory syncytial virus on apnea in weanling rats. Pediatr Res 2005; 57: 819–25

66. Kimpen JL. Prevention and treatment of respiratory syncytial virus bronchiolitis and postbronchiolitic wheezing. Respir Res 2002; 3 (Suppl 1): S40–S45

67. Ventre K, Randolph A. Ribavirin for respiratory syncytial virus infection of the lower respiratory tract in infants and young children. Cochrane Database Syst Rev 2004; 4: CD000181

68. Rodriguez WJ, Arrobio J, Fink R, et al. Prospective follow-up and pulmonary functions from a placebo-controlled randomized trial of ribavirin therapy in respiratory syncytial virus bronchiolitis. Ribavirin Study Group. Arch Pediatr Adolesc Med 1999; 153: 469–74

69. Bisgaard H. A randomized trial of montelukast in respiratory syncytial virus postbronchiolitis. Am J Respir Crit Care Med 2003; 167: 379–83

70. Simoes EA. Treatment and prevention of respiratory syncytial virus lower respiratory tract infection. Long-term effects on respiratory outcomes. Am J Respir Crit Care Med 2001; 163: S14–S17

71. Reijonen T, Korppi M, Kuikka L, Remes K. Anti-inflammatory therapy reduces wheezing after bronchiolitis. Arch Pediatr Adolesc Med 1996; 150: 512–17

72. Reijonen TM, Korppi M. One-year follow-up of young children hospitalized for wheezing: the influence of early anti-inflammatory therapy and risk factors for subsequent wheezing and asthma. Pediatr Pulmonol 1998; 26: 113–19

73. Kajosaari M, Syvanen P, Forars M, Juntunen-Backman K. Inhaled corticosteroids during and after respiratory syncytial virus-bronchiolitis may decrease subsequent asthma. Pediatr Allergy Immunol 2000; 11: 198–202

74. Richter H, Seddon P. Early nebulized budesonide in the treatment of bronchiolitis and the prevention of post-bronchiolitic wheezing. J Pediatr 1998; 132: 849–53

75. Hill AB. The environment and disease: association or causation? Proc R Soc Med 1965; 58: 295–300

76. Eisen AH, Bacal HL. The acute relationship of acute bronchiolitis to bronchial asthma – a 4-to-14 year follow up. Pediatrics 1963; 31: 859–61

77. Sims DG, Downham MAPS, Gardner PS, et al. Study of 8-year-old children with a history of respiratory syncytial virus bronchiolitis in infancy. BMJ 1978; 1: 11–14

78. Sims DG, Gardner PS, Weightman D, et al. Atopy does not predispose to RSV bronchiolitis or postbronchiolitic wheezing. BMJ (Clin Res Ed) 1981; 282: 2086–8

79. Mok JY, Simpson H. Outcome of acute lower respiratory tract infection in infants: preliminary report of seven-year follow-up study. BMJ (Clin Res Ed) 1982; 285: 333–7

80. Korppi M, Piippo-Savolainen E, Korhonen K, Remes S. Respiratory morbidity 20 years after RSV infection in infancy. Pediatr Pulmonol 2004; 38: 155–60

81. Gurwitz D, Mindorff C, Levison H. Increased incidence of bronchial reactivity in children with a history of bronchiolitis. J Pediatr 1981; 98: 551–5

82. Hall CB, Hall WJ, Gala CI, et al. Long-term prospective study in children after respiratory syncytial virus infection. J Pediatr 1984; 105: 358–64

83. Welliver RC, Duffy L. The relationship of RSV-specific immunoglobulin E antibody responses in infancy, recurrent wheezing, and pulmonary function at age 7–8 years. Pediatr Pulmonol 1993; 15: 19–27

84. Welliver RC, Sun M, Rinaldo D, Ogra PL. Predictive value of respiratory syncytial virus-specific IgE responses for recurrent wheezing following bronchiolitis. J Pediatr 1986; 109: 776–80

85. Sly PD, Hibbert ME. Childhood asthma following hospitalization with acute viral bronchiolitis in infancy. Pediatr Pulmonol 1989; 7: 153–8

86. Murray M, Webb MS, O'Callaghan C, et al. Respiratory status and allergy after bronchiolitis. Arch Dis Child 1992; 67: 482–7

87. Noble V, Murray M, Webb MS, et al. Respiratory status and allergy nine to 10 years after acute bronchiolitis. Arch Dis Child 1997; 76: 315–19

88. Osundwa VM, Dawod ST, Ehlayel M. Recurrent wheezing in children with respiratory syncytial virus (RSV) bronchiolitis in Qatar. Eur J Pediatr 1993; 152: 1001–3

89. Renzi PM, Turgeon JP, Yang JP, et al. Cellular immunity is activated and a TH-2 response is associated with early wheezing in infants after bronchiolitis. J Pediatr 1997; 130: 584–93

90. Bont L, Steijn M, van Aalderen WM, Kimpen JL. Impact of wheezing after respiratory syncytial virus infection on health-related quality of life. Pediatr Infect Dis J 2004; 23: 414–17

91. Bont L, Heijnen CJ, Kavelaars A, et al. Monocyte IL-10 production during respiratory syncytial virus bronchiolitis is associated with recurrent wheezing in a one-year follow-up study. Am J Respir Crit Care Med 2000; 161: 1518–23

92. Krilov LR, Mandel FS, Barone SR, Fagin JC. Follow-up of children with respiratory syncytial virus bronchiolitis in 1986 and 1987: potential effect of ribavirin on long term pulmonary function. The Bronchiolitis Study Group. Pediatr Infect Dis J 1997; 16: 273–6

93. Long CE, Voter KZ, Barker WH, Hall CB. Long term follow-up of children hospitalized with respiratory syncytial virus lower respiratory tract infection and randomly treated with ribavirin or placebo. Pediatr Infect Dis J 1997; 16: 1023–8

94. Edell D, Bruce E, Hale K, et al. Reduced long-term respiratory morbidity after treatment of respiratory syncytial virus bronchiolitis with ribavirin in previously healthy infants: a preliminary report. Pediatr Pulmonol 1998; 25: 154–8

95. Edell D, Khoshoo V, Ross G, Salter K. Early ribavarin treatment of bronchiolitis(*): effect on long-term respiratory morbidity. Chest 2002; 122: 935–9

96. Fox GF, Everard ML, Marsh MJ, Milner AD. Randomised controlled trial of budesonide for the prevention of post-bronchiolitis wheezing. Arch Dis Child 1999; 80: 343–7

97. van Woensel JB, Kimpen JL, Sprikkelman AB, et al. Long-term effects of prednisolone in the acute phase of bronchiolitis caused by respiratory syncytial virus. Pediatr Pulmonol 2000; 30: 92–6

98. Cade A, Brownlee KG, Conway SP, et al. Randomised placebo controlled trial of nebulised corticosteroids in acute respiratory syncytial viral bronchiolitis. Arch Dis Child 2000; 82: 126–30

PART III

In vitro experimental models of asthma exacerbations

CHAPTER 12

In vitro models of bronchial epithelial cell infection

Peter AB Wark, Donna E Davies and Stephen T Holgate

INTRODUCTION

The aim of *in vitro* models is to mimic the natural process of a disease in a framework that can be studied in depth and where the environment can be altered so as to investigate tissue responses. In terms of respiratory viral infections of humans, investigators are restricted in their ability to study the disease *in vivo*, particularly with respect to virus infection as a trigger of acute exacerbations of asthma. While this is a common cause of exacerbations in adults and children it is a challenging entity to study in terms of the inflammatory response of the airways from the time of initial infection, the subsequent immune response and the impact this has on asthma, both acutely and in the long term. Histological analysis of the lower airways is difficult and restricted to the proximal airways or by sampling airway secretions using induced sputum or bronchial lavage. The natural history of a virus-induced exacerbation of asthma is difficult to study, as this occurs several days after the initial virus infection and the pathological response is lost in the acute lower airway inflammation seen in acute asthma. For these reasons *in vitro* models have been developed to allow in-depth study of the mechanisms of epithelial cell infection and their response in terms of releasing proinflammatory mediators to recruit immune cells, wound repair and antiviral responses. Several respiratory viruses have

been associated with acute exacerbations of asthma, including human rhinoviruses (RVs), influenza viruses, respiratory syncytial virus (RSV), the parainfluenza viruses, coronaviruses and most recently human metapneumovirus. This chapter focuses on RVs and to a lesser extent RSV and influenza viruses, as these are the most common viruses associated with acute asthma and the viruses most extensively studied using *in vitro* models.

THE AIRWAY EPITHELIUM IN HEALTH AND IN ASTHMA

The airway epithelium is the initial interface between the environment and the lungs, acting as a protective barrier. In addition, it plays a central role in the immune response to inhaled stimuli and the repair response of the airways to damage that subsequently occurs. The epithelium is composed of several cell types, the most common being ciliated columnar cells, enriched with mitochondria and cilia to sweep mucus out of the lungs.[1] Interspersed among these ciliated cells are mucus-secreting goblet cells providing a protective mucus bilayer, co-operating with the ciliated cells to remove debris from the lungs.[1] These cells rest on a layer of basal epithelial cells that are firmly attached to the basement membrane and are thought to be the primary progenitors for the above cells.[2] In addition to the epithelial cells are a complex array of neuroendocrine cells, neurons and immune cells (lymphocytes, macrophages and dendritic cells).[3]

The airway epithelium is an important modulator of the immune response, capable of secreting proinflammatory cytokines and chemokines, lipid mediators, growth factors, bronchoconstricting peptides[4,5] and nitric oxide.[6] These effects are likely to impact upon surrounding cells such as (myo) fibroblasts[7] and airway smooth muscle with particular implications for asthma.

In asthma the epithelium appears to be in a permanent state of stress, with activation of proinflammatory transcription factors (NFκB, AP-1 and STAT1).[8] In addition, the repair response of the epithelium in asthma also appears to be impaired with overexpression of the epidermal growth factor (EGF) receptor[9] and the regulator of cell proliferation and apoptosis p21[waf].[10] If inherent differences exist in the asthmatic epithelium and associated cells, it makes it imperative that *in vitro* models reflect this heterogeneity of response in health and disease. In the case of respiratory virus infection where the clinical consequences in asthma differ from non-asthmatics so dramatically, a disease-specific response can be investigated using such models.

PATHOLOGY OF NATURAL RESPIRATORY VIRUS INFECTION

RVs are single-stranded RNA viruses, belonging to the picornavirus family, and are the viruses most frequently associated with the common cold as well as acute asthma.[11,12] RVs are transmitted by direct contact and via the respiratory route with inoculation and replication normally occurring in the epithelium of the upper airway.[13] Infection does not lead to widespread disruption of the epithelium, with minimal epithelial shedding along with a neutrophilic infiltrate[14] and evidence of increased vascular permeability.[15] In natural infection relatively few cells in the upper airway become infected[16] and the clinical effects of infection reflect predominately upper airway

involvement. In asthma, however, RVs have been associated with increased airway inflammation and worsened bronchial reactivity[17–19] and have been detected in the lower airways.[20,21]

As with RVs, the respiratory epithelium is the target of infection for both RSV and influenza viruses. In contrast to RVs, however, these infections result in widespread epithelial damage and predominately affect the lower airways. In RSV bronchiolitis there is epithelial necrosis, syncytial formation, mucus hypersecretion and a monocytic infiltrate.[22] In the case of influenza viruses, the lower airway is the site of most inflammatory change, with extensive loss of both ciliated and basal layers of the epithelium and an infiltrate of lymphocytes, neutrophils and histiocytes.[23] Both RSV and influenza viruses have been associated with increased airway inflammation and exacerbations of asthma.[11,24–26]

IN VITRO MODELS

In order to study virus infection of the distal lower airways, *in vitro* models of bronchial epithelial cells have been developed. These have included immortalized lines of airway epithelial cells or epithelial cells harvested from humans with the stock expanded under tissue culture conditions *in vitro*. The advantages and disadvantages of these approaches are summarized in Table 12.1.

Primary bronchial epithelial cells (BECs) are generally obtained in two ways. First, they can be obtained by bronchoscopy and brushing with cells, then expanded under tissue culture conditions[27] (Figure 12.1a). The advantage with this approach is that the epithelium can be obtained from a wide range of individuals with diseases of interest. In the case of asthma, bronchoscopy is possible in all but the severest chronic cases, or acute asthma (except in very mild exacerbations or where the individual has been intubated). Bronchoscopy can be performed in adult volunteers with mild sedation as an outpatient procedure, though in children this usually requires a

Table 12.1 Comparison of *in vitro* models of the airway epithelium

Cell type	Advantages	Disadvantages
Epithelial cell lines	Ready access to cells	Questionable how they reflect natural BEC responses
	Homogeneous response to stimuli	Unable to differentiate
	Response well characterized in the literature	Response to stimuli can vary with passage
Primary BECs	Able to differentiate to pseudostratified columnar epithelium	Cells are difficult to obtain
	Specimens can be obtained from individuals with diseases of interest	Differentiation of cells in culture conditions is time consuming
	Marked heterogeneity of response between individuals	Marked heterogeneity of response between individuals
		Limited ability to expand and passage in tissue culture

BEC, bronchial epithelial cell

general anesthetic. Nevertheless, volunteers are required to undergo an invasive procedure that is unpleasant and not without risk. Alternatively, cells can be obtained from resected lung tissue, dissociated from connective tissue and then grown under tissue culture conditions in a similar way to that above, including to a fully differentiated phenotype (Figure 12.1b). These cells can be obtained from postmortem human trachea[28] or the more distal airways from resected lung specimens.[29] The ability to grow cells to an undifferentiated or fully differentiated phenotype is as successful as the former method. Obtaining specimens, however, is obviously difficult and limited to postmortem or the surgical removal of lung tissue, the latter being limited to lung transplant donors or those undergoing surgery (the majority due to malignancies and the majority of those being smokers).

Access to the upper airway makes obtaining cells from here easier and nasal cells have been obtained by scrapings of the epithelium and by biopsy.[15,30] Cells have also been obtained from adenoidal tissue resected during surgery and grown out under culture conditions.[31] While access to the upper airway requires less invasive procedures, even obtaining nasal scrapings is unpleasant and usually limited to adults, while adenoidal tissue is more readily available from children postoperatively.

MODELS OF RHINOVIRUS INFECTION IN AIRWAY EPITHELIAL CELLS

Infectivity of airway epithelial cells

As RV is predominately an upper airway pathogen, it was unclear how infection would promote a lower airway response in asthma and other airway diseases. It is known that the optimum temperatures for RV replication occur at 33–34°C,[32] which was thought to be well below that of the airways. *In vitro* cell culture models of BEAS-2B cells, a cell line derived from lower airway BECs, demonstrated that RVs could infect and replicate in them[29,33] and in fact could replicate successfully at temperatures found in the lower airways.[34] These findings were then supported by the detection of RV in lower airway samples.[20,21] The difficulty found in isolating RV from the lower airways was consistent with the limited infection found in the upper airways, but made characterization of the infection complicated *in vivo*.

(a)

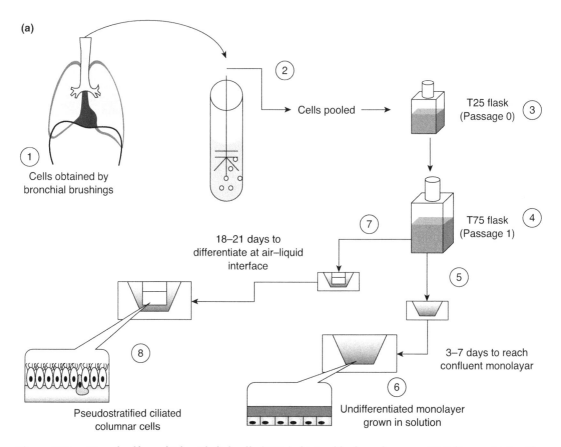

Figure 12.1a Growth of bronchial epithelial cells (BECs) obtained by bronchoscopy. (1) Cells are obtained by gently brushing the bronchial mucosa. (2) The cells are released by agitating in medium. (3) The medium is pooled and the cells plated into small (T25 cm) flasks and grown to approximately 80% confluence. (4) The cells are removed from the flask by trypsin and placed into a larger flask(s) to expand their numbers. (5) Cells can be plated in standard tissue culture plates and grown submerged in nutrient medium until confluence. (6) Cells then have formed an undifferentiated monolayer of cuboidal cells. (7) Alternatively, cells can be plated at high density onto porous wells, suspended in a tissue culture plate. Initially the cells are submerged in nutrient solution but when they have reached a confluent monolayer the medium in the transwell is removed. They derive their nutrients from the medium below and grow at the air–liquid interface. (8) Growth at the air–liquid interface encourages the cells to differentiate into pseudostratified columnar cells that are ciliated.

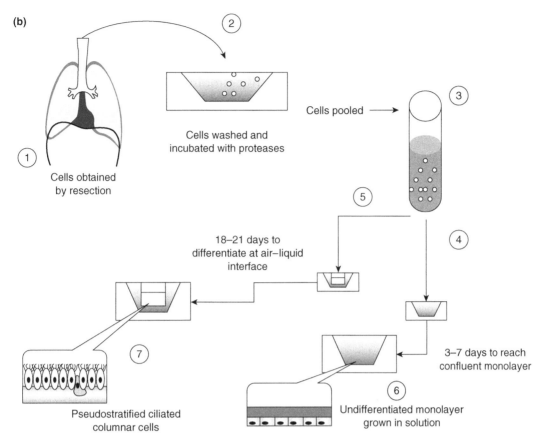

(b)

② Cells washed and
incubated with proteases

Cells pooled →

①
Cells obtained
by resection

③

⑤

④

18–21 days to
differentiate at air–liquid
interface

3–7 days to reach
confluent monolayer

⑦

Pseudostratified ciliated
columnar cells

⑥
Undifferentiated monolayer
grown in solution

Figure 12.1b Growth of BECs or human tracheal epithelial (HTE) cells from resected lung specimens. (1) Small airways or the trachea are obtained surgically. The tissue is rinsed with phosphate-buffered saline (PBS) to remove debris, mucus and inflammatory cells. (2) The resected tissue is mounted in a dissection tray. The surface epithelium is scored by longitudinal strips and pulled off the submucosa. These strips are rinsed in PBS and 5 mmol/l dithiothreitol and then PBS again. They are then incubated overnight in PBS and proteases. (3) The next day, enzymes are inactivated and the epithelial cells dislodged by agitation. Cells are pelleted and resuspended to the desired concentration before being plated down. Cells could be plated to tissue culture flasks to expand numbers or plated down for immediate growth. (4) Cells can be plated in standard tissue culture plates and grown submerged in nutrient medium until confluence. (5) Cells have now formed an undifferentiated monolayer of cuboidal cells. (6) Alternatively, cells can be plated in porous transwells and grown at the air–liquid interface encouraging differentiation to occur

Mosser et al.[35] directly compared RV infectivity in cells derived from an epithelial cell line, adenoidal tissue and non-differentiated human tracheal epithelium. Infectivity correlated closely with later viral yield, and marked differences were seen between yields from an epithelial cell line (Ohio HeLa cells) at 10^7 tissue culture infectivity dose $(TCID)_{50}$/ml compared to BECs at 10^3 $TCID_{50}$/ml. These findings were confirmed by immunohistochemical staining using a monoclonal antibody to RV-16, and demonstrated that this low yield in virus was reflected in relatively few infected cells. While an RV dose of 17 $TCID_{50}$/ml produced a typical cytopathic effect (CPE) and infection in 97% of HeLa cells, a dose up to 30 $TCID_{50}$/ml in adenoid-derived cells resulted in infection in only 0.74% of cells and, in BECs, 0.98% of cells. There was no difference seen in infectivity or viral yields from upper and lower airway epithelial cells and neither group demonstrated significant CPE.

Lopez-Souza et al. compared response and infectivity of human tracheal epithelial cells and nasal epithelial cells that were grown to an undifferentiated confluent monolayer or as fully differentiated ciliated cells.[36] Both groups of cells were incubated with RV-16 for 6 hours. Differentiated cells were significantly more resistant to infection with RV-16, with only 1.4% of cells positive for RV by fluorescent in situ hybridization compared to 9.6% of non-differentiated cells. This correlated with viral (v)RNA production that was 130-fold higher in non-differentiated cells compared to fully differentiated cells.

This low level of RV infection in airway-derived epithelial cells and the greater resistance again seen in fully differentiated ciliated cells appear reminiscent of in vivo pathological studies. This, however, should not discount work using cell lines or undifferentiated BECs. In fact, the low level of infectivity in fully differentiated models may make this too insensitive a tool to detect change in the limited culture environment and may not be as applicable to chronic airway diseases such as asthma and chronic obstructive pulmonary disease (COPD), where epithelial damage from inflammation leads to exposure of the basal BECs, which in itself may be a factor predisposing to lower airway infection with RV.

Inflammatory response to rhinovirus infection

Given the limited epithelial damage and the relatively few cells infected with RV it has been proposed that the main effects of infection are a consequence of the release of inflammatory cytokines and chemokines.

Infection of bronchial epithelial cell lines demonstrated that these cells would respond to infection with the release of inflammatory mediators that had been seen in vivo and were relevant to asthma. Infection of BEAS-2B cells with RV-14 demonstrated virus-specific release of IL-8, IL-6 and granulocyte–macrophage colony-stimulating factor (GM-CSF),[33] while infection of A549 cells also resulted in virus-specific release of interleukin (IL)-6.[37] Investigators have increasingly used cell lines to demonstrate mechanisms of response, confirming these findings in primary airway epithelial cells, for which inflammatory responses appear to be very similar. Epithelium derived from human tracheal epithelial (HTE) cells when infected with RV has also shown increased release of IL-6, IL-8, tumor necrosis factor (TNF)-α, and IL-1β[38] as well as RANTES and GM-CSF, with RANTES levels correlating with levels of virus replication.[29] Comparisons have been made between infection with several serotypes of RV, comparing major group RV-16, RV-14 and RV-39 as well as minor group HRV-1A. All viruses induced release of IL-8 and IL-6 in BEAS-2B cells and non-differentiated human tracheal epithelial cells, although RV-16 and RV-1A induced the most change.[39] Recently we have measured release of inflammatory mediators from BECs comparing cells from subjects with moderate asthma (requiring inhaled corticosteroids; ICS) mild asthma (ICS naive) and non-atopic healthy controls. Infection with RV-16 led to at least a 40-fold induction in RANTES, followed by a ten-fold increase in IL-6 and then much smaller increases in IL-8, TNF-α, IL-1β and MCP-1. There were no differences detected between any of the disease groups. Substantial differences, however, existed within groups, suggesting that there was significant heterogeneity between individuals in terms of response to RV infection. We then related the magnitude of the *in vitro* response of these BECs to severity of cold symptoms, as recorded by the common cold questionnaire, and found that RANTES correlated with more intense cold symptoms. These results suggest that the intensity of the initial epithelial response to infection is important in setting the tone of the subsequent inflammatory response and as a consequence cold symptoms.

Apart from the release of mediators that recruit inflammatory cells to the airways, the epithelium also produces mucus to protect itself and clear debris. Chronic inflammation such as in asthma and COPD may lead to mucus hypersecretion, which worsens airflow obstruction. Using undifferentiated BECs, infection with RV-16 has been shown to induce secretion of DBA mucin and MUC5AC.[40]

Induction of adhesion molecules

The receptor for major group RV is intercellular adhesion molecule (ICAM)-1, which is also an important adhesion molecule that leads to the recruitment of inflammatory cells to the airways. Susceptibility of epithelial cells to infection with major group RV was at least in part dependent on the level of baseline ICAM-1 expression.[35] The demonstration that inflammatory mediators that upregulate ICAM-1 enhance infectivity[41] suggested a link between susceptibility to RV infection and chronic inflammatory airway disease. In fact, RV-16 infection alone in BEC models has been shown to upregulate ICAM-1 expression directly by increasing ICAM-1 promoter activity through altering the intracellular redox potential, within 20 minutes of entering the cell.[42,43] This effect also appears to be specific to increased expression of membranous ICAM-1, which is responsible for RV binding and entry

into the cell. The release of soluble ICAM-1, that potentially would bind to extracellular virus and prevent entry into cells, was not increased.[44] Whether minor group RVs also enhance their own infectivity has yet to be investigated. In addition to ICAM-1, RV-16, RV-9 and RV-2 (minor group) induced expression of the vascular cell adhesion molecule (VCAM)-1 on epithelial cell lines and non-differentiated BECs.[45] VCAM-1 is an adhesion molecule expressed on epithelial and endothelial cells and is important in the migration of lymphocytes and eosinophils to the airways.[46,47] It also aids in activation of migrated eosinophils with the release of reactive oxidants[48] and thus can contribute to the inflammatory response seen in asthma.

Virus infection and replication initiates a specific response from the infected host cell. Attempts to modify this inflammatory response have also been made. Treatment of RV-infected cells with corticosteroid preparations was shown to have no significant effect on release of IL-6 and IL-8,[39] but successfully suppressed RANTES release.[29] Pre-treatment of A549 cells and HTE cells with interferon (IFN)-γ led to a massive upregulation of ICAM-1, enhanced binding of RV-16 and RV-49 (both major group viruses) to cells and significantly enhanced release of RANTES. Pre-treatment with TNF-α failed to show a similar effect.[41]

Antiviral responses of airway epithelial cells

As the epithelium is an important modulator of airway immune responses, it is reasonable to consider that it is capable of initiating antiviral responses of its own that may minimize the need for potentially damaging inflammatory responses. Nitric oxide (NO) is known to inhibit replication of picornaviruses in murine models[49] and levels are elevated in the exhaled air of individuals with viral upper respiratory tract infections.[39,50] In both airway epithelial cell lines and undifferentiated BECs, infection with RV-16 or the presence of dsRNA induced transcription of mRNA for nitric oxide synthase (NOS)-2.[39] In addition, treatment of cells with the NO donor NONOate inhibited virus replication and reduced the release of IL-6, IL-8[39] and GM-CSF.[39]

Type I IFNs are also an important component of the innate immune response, having a direct antiviral effect on infected and neighboring cells, while promoting acquired antiviral immune responses.[51] Recently they have been linked to apoptotic responses to virus infections in antiviral defence.[52] Thus, type I IFNs play critical roles in regulating apoptosis, as well as in innate and acquired immune responses in antiviral defence.

Pre-treatment of cells derived from HTE with IFN-α led to a significant reduction in virus replication of RV-16, RV-49 and parainfluenza III.[41] Using undifferentiated BECs from subjects with mild asthma who had never used ICS, moderate asthma using regular ICS and non-atopic healthy control subjects, we assessed the innate immune response. Infection with RV led to a significant increase in mRNA for ICAM-1 in all groups with no difference in ICAM expression at 24 hours. Cells from healthy controls demonstrated a 3.6 (interquartile range (IQR) 3.5–3.6)-fold increase in IFN-β mRNA, but there was no increase in asthmatic cells (0.25-fold; IQR 0.25–0.8; $p<0.01$). Impaired induction of IFN-β mRNA expression by RV-infected asthmatic BECs was also reflected by impaired protein production with IFN-β protein levels being >2-fold higher in supernatants from healthy control cells compared with those from asthmatic cells. There was significantly more RV viral (v)RNA, median 2.1×10^6 in asthmatic BECs compared to controls $(0.043 \times 10^6$; $p=0.01$). This was confirmed by live virus titration assays, where after 48 hours, significantly more viable virus was recovered from asthmatic epithelial cell cultures. There was a strong negative correlation between IFN-β release and virus release at 48 hours (TCID$_{50} \times 10^4$/ml, $r=-0.79$; $p=0.01$). Therefore, it appears that asthmatic BECs respond to RV infection with a deficient response in IFN-β, and this is associated with

increased virion production. This defect in the innate immune response to viral infection identifies a possible target for intervention.[53]

Intracellular signaling following rihinovirus infection

The induction and release of proinflammatory mediators from BECs occurs by virus-specific induction of intracellular signaling pathways. The use of cell culture has been central in understanding the replication cycle of picornaviruses and the subsequent inflammatory response. Picornavirus replication is summarized in Figure 12.2a. Briefly, RV enters the cell after attaching to its receptor (either ICAM-1 for major group RV or the low-density lipoprotein (LDL) receptor for minor group RV), the virus uncoats and the vRNA is released into the cell cytoplasm and binds to host ribosomes. The viral genome contains a sequence that initiates translation, leading to synthesis of viral polypeptides that are cleaved by viral proteinases. In the meantime, host cell protein synthesis is essentially switched off by disruption of the translation of mammalian mRNA. The vRNA and viral proteins are then assembled into virions and released from the cell by lysis, resulting phenotypically in the cytopathic effect.[32]

The binding of major group RV, as mentioned, initiates upregulation of cell-surface expression of ICAM-1. This occurs by activation of NFκB, which translocates to the nucleus and binds to the ICAM-1 promoter.[54] This has been shown to occur very rapidly after RV binding and is dependent on an increase in intracellular redox state, leading directly to the dissociation of inhibitory IκB, a process that is blocked by the administration of oxidized glutathione.[42] Activation of NFκB by reactive oxidants is well characterized as an important intracellular signaling pathway for cells under oxidative stress.[55] Other genes dependent on NFκB activation where production is induced by RV are IL-1, IL-6, IL-8 and GM-CSF,[33,37,39] while VCAM-1 depends also on GATA.[56] Therefore, early induction of an

(a)

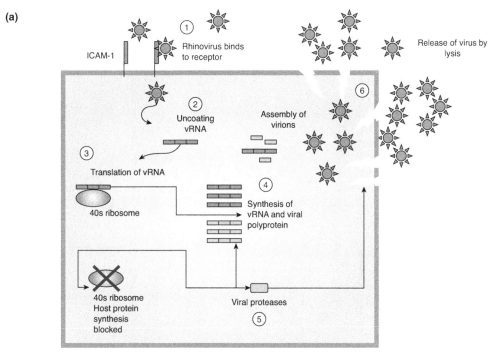

(b)

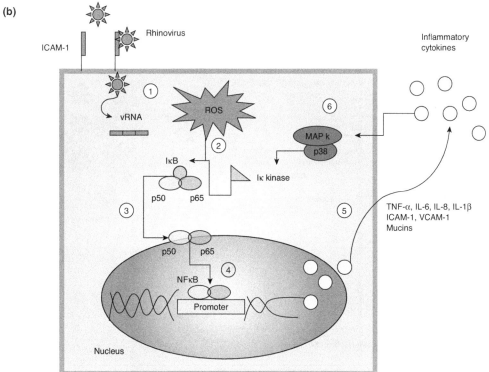

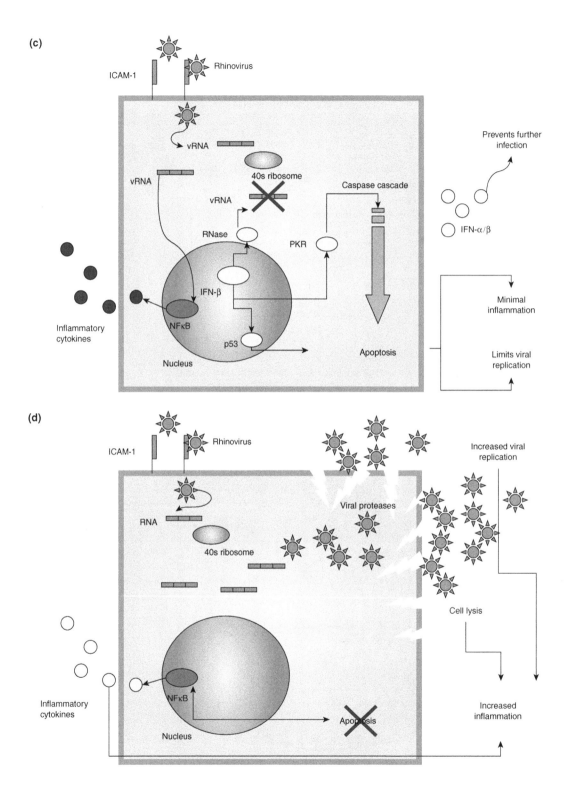

inflammatory response occurs following infection, leading to recruitment of inflammatory cells to the airways. However, these responses are likely to represent only a fraction of the events that may occur, and a proposed description of these is summarized in Figure 12.2b. Oxidant stress is known to regulate cell cycle events[57] and, when associated with NFκB activation, can influence cell viability. In alveolar epithelial cells, high levels of reactive oxidants can trigger apoptosis via Bax through induction of the tumor suppressor gene p53, though simultaneous activation of NFκB activates the anti-apoptotic factor Bcl-2,[58] thus preventing apoptosis. Apoptosis (programmed cell death) is an effective way of eliminating redundant or damaged cells without initiating an inflammatory response. It is a tightly controlled process with wide-ranging effects regulating inflammation and repair, and preventing the development of neoplastic change in cells. A detailed description of these processes is beyond the scope of this chapter and excellent reviews are available.[59–61] Briefly, apoptosis can be triggered externally by cells expressing Fas or TNF receptor-1 interacting with the cell-mediated immune system. Alternatively, internal events centered on the mitochondria and controlled by a balance of pro- and antiapoptotic members of the Bcl-2 family of proteins can initiate events. In both cases events are mediated by cysteine proteases collectively known as caspases, which play crucial roles in inducing a pro-apoptotic state.

Picornavirus infection (coxsackie B3 virus) of Ohio HeLa cells has been shown to lead to

Figure 12.2 (a) Rhinovirus (RV) replication in airway epithelial cells. (1) RV binds to its surface receptor (in the case of major group RV, intercellular adhesion molecule (ICAM)-1). It is then internalized. (2) The virus uncoats, releasing single-stranded vRNA. (3) Translation of vRNA then occurs. (4) This initiates synthesis of further vRNA and viral polyproteins. The polyprotein is cleaved to produce viral proteins. (5) Viral proteases work to cleave further viral polyprotein, inhibit capped host cell protein synthesis and may disrupt cytokeratins allowing cell lysis to occur and facilitate the release of virions. (6) Assembly of virions occurs. (7) Virions are released from the cell, probably by cell lysis.

(b) Intracellular signaling following RV infection. (1) RV binds to ICAM-1 and enters the cell; this triggers an increase in reactive oxidants (ROS). (2) This results in disassociation of IκB from p50 and p65. (3) Nuclear factor kappa B (NFκB) translocates to the nucleus. (4) In the nucleus NFκB binds to a promoter region, inducing transcription of genes. (5) The products of these genes are released. (6) These proteins can have far-reaching effects, to recruit inflammatory cells, enhance chemotaxis and act back on the cell which has produced them. TNF-α and IL-1β are known to activate pathways such as MAP kinase and enhance the inflammatory response from bronchial epithelial cells (BECs).

(c) In normal BECs RV adheres to its receptor ICAM-1. It is then internalized and uncoats, and single-stranded RNA replicates. If this were left unchecked, it would lead to the formation of vRNA and then virions. These events elicit activation of the NFκB that in turn leads to the production of proinflammatory cytokines. However, the presence of vRNA leads to the transcription of interferon (IFN)-β. IFN-α/β are known to induce the antiviral protein kinase (PKR), which represses host cell protein synthesis and induces apoptosis and RNases that lyse vRNA. Type I IFNs also induce activation of the tumor suppressor gene p53 in response to viral infection that leads to apoptosis. Infected cells are then induced to undergo apoptosis, limiting viral replication. In addition, released IFN-β reduces spread of infection to neighboring cells, in all limiting airway inflammation.

(d) Illustration of the proposed response in asthmatic BECs. The early events following infection proceed as described above. However, the asthmatic BEC is unable to mount an effective early IFN-β response. There is no early activation of apoptosis, even though there is a proinflammatory response. Viral replication proceeds and amplifies, resulting in the release of infectious virions and leading to proinflammatory cell lysis. Neighboring cells become infected, enhancing the release of proinflammatory cytokines and resulting in enormously enhanced airway inflammation activation of caspases, but this is independent of the eventual cell death that occurs, and results in lysis with the release of virions and the characteristic cytopathic effect on infected cells.[62] We therefore hypothesized that, if natural RV infection results in lysis and release of virions, early self-induction of apoptosis by infected BECs may limit infection and then also the inflammatory response. To investigate the underlying mechanisms of this increased susceptibility, we examined virus replication and innate responses to RV-16 infection of primary BEC cells from subjects with mild asthma who had never used ICS, subjects with moderate asthma using regular ICS and non-atopic healthy control subjects. Early viral RNA expression and late virus release into the supernatant was increased in asthmatic cells compared to healthy controls. Virus infection induced significant late cell lysis in asthmatic cells but minimal lysis in normal cells consistent with the differences seen in virus replication. Examination of the early cellular response to infection in healthy control cells indicated that there was induction of caspases and apoptosis following infection. This response was impaired in the asthmatic cultures. Apoptosis was triggered by cell treatment with dsRNA, suggesting that this response was specific to intracellular virus replication. Inhibition of apoptosis in healthy control cultures resulted in enhanced viral yield, comparable to that seen in infected asthmatic cultures. Examination of early innate immune responses revealed profound impairment of virus-induced IFN-β mRNA expression in asthmatic cultures and they produced >2.5 times less IFN-β protein. In infected asthmatic cells, exogenous IFN-β induced apoptosis and reduced virus replication, demonstrating a causal link between deficient IFN-β, impaired apoptosis and increased virus replication. Apoptosis and IFN-β production were impaired independently of corticosteroid therapy.[53] Using these results, we proposed a model to explain these differences seen in asthmatic cells that is summarized in Figure 12.2c. In non-asthmatic subjects, infection of bronchial

epithelial cells is limited by an innate antiviral response and induction of apoptosis in infected cells. A deficiency of IFN-β in asthma facilitates virus replication and cytolysis with increased infection of neighboring cells. Exaggerated inflammatory responses are likely to result in asthmatics *in vivo*, consequent upon the increased replication and the cytolytic effects of the virus infection. Crucially, this defect can be restored *in vitro* by provision of exogenous IFN-β that restores apoptotic responses and limits virus replication to levels observed in normal cells. These findings demonstrate that IFN-β may have therapeutic utility in preventing or treating virus-induced exacerbations of asthma.

MODELS OF RESPIRATORY SYNCYTIAL VIRUS INFECTION AND ASTHMA

RSV is an important lower respiratory pathogen, particularly in children, where it is the most frequent cause of bronchiolitis. Most investigators have concentrated on its role in bronchiolitis and much of this work has been developed in murine models of the disease. However, RSV has been implicated as a trigger for acute asthma[26] and COPD[63] though relatively less work has been done using cell culture models or considering its role in established asthma. Established models of RSV infection in both primary epithelial cells and epithelial cell lines exist and have made important contributions to the understanding of the disease.

Models of RSV infection using epithelial cell lines have determined that RSV binds and enters cells, dependent upon interactions with the viral F and G proteins. Using Hep2 cells (an epithelial cell line) it has been determined that the G protein binds to cell-surface glycosaminoglycans, which can be inhibited by heparins.[64] However, binding of the F protein is also required to allow RSV entry into the host cell and to lead to syncytial formation.[65] The F protein binds to the cell surface and interacts with a peptide called RhoA;[66] this peptide is activated by RSV and has the ability to induce the secretion of IL-1β, IL-6 and IL-8.[67]

Using an *in vitro* model of undifferentiated monolayers of BECs, low titer RSV infection led to reduced epithelial integrity with a fall in electrical resistance seen after 24 hours of infection. RSV enhanced expression of vascular endothelial growth factor (VEGF), while blockade of VEGF prevented the fall in electrical resistance. VEGF is known to enhance vascular leakage from endothelial and epithelial cells and thus could account for the loss of epithelial integrity and submucosal edema that is seen with RSV infection *in vivo* and is thought to contribute to airflow obstruction. In addition, infection of epithelial cell lines and undifferentiated BECs demonstrated that RSV induces release of RANTES and IL-8,[68,69] while murine models and *in vivo* studies have confirmed that infection is associated with the release of a wide range of inflammatory mediators that would contribute to the recruitment of neutrophils, lymphocytes and eosinophils to the airways.[70] RSV infection of BECs also leads to the release of IL-1β, and the auto-upregulation of ICAM-1 expression, which probably facilitates the binding of granulocytes to infected cells,[71] and would also increase their recruitment to the inflamed asthmatic airway. Apart from these inflammatory mediators, infection of A549 cells induced the release of fibrogenic growth factor (FGF).[72] FGF is known to be a potent regulator of fibroblast proliferation and migration, and induction by RSV could contribute to long-term airway wall remodeling in asthma.[7]

RSV appears to have the ability to evade innate immune responses of BECs. Infection of A549 cells was shown to lead to the induction of phosphotidyl inositol-3 kinase (PI-3K), which triggers NFκB transcription but also inhibits cellular apoptosis.[73] Infected cells underwent apoptosis, but this process was independent of RSV replication, and virus release was accompanied by cell lysis. However, when PI-3K was blocked, this resulted in early apoptosis with downregulation of NFκB gene transcription. These findings were suggestive that an early apoptotic response in infected epithelial cells may inhibit virus replication, reminiscent of the protective effect seen in RV-induced apoptosis. As previously stated, IFN-α/β exert autocrine and paracrine effects on infected and neighboring cells to induce an antiviral state.[74] Wild-type RSV infection of A549 cells leads to only limited production of IFN-α/β. It is known that RSV that lacks two proteins (NS1 or NS2) is less efficient in replicating *in vivo*. Recombinant RSV lacking either of these proteins, however, efficiently triggers an IFN response, suggesting that these viral proteins are directly involved in immune evasion by inhibiting the IFN-α/β response of infected BECs.[75] The use of these models to demonstrate how RSV evades BEC innate immunity is important, not only for our understanding of RSV infection but also for reinforcing the central role the epithelium must play in the innate immune response, in an effort to limit later cell-based immune activation.

MODELS OF INFLUENZA VIRUS INFECTION AND ASTHMA

While RVs can infect the lower airways, in the immunocompetent host infection is naturally limited to the upper airways. Like RSV, influenza virus has a greater tropism for the lower respiratory epithelium and can even infect distant organs, leading to a serious systemic illness if it is not contained by the immune system. When this occurs as a result of the emergence of a novel and highly pathogenic strain it may have fatal consequences. For this reason, much work has focused on the systemic immune response to influenza virus to understand how an effective immune response limits systemic infection. However, as with RV and RSV, influenza virus is a pathogen of the respiratory epithelium and this has a direct impact on airway inflammation in subjects with asthma. Influenza virus infection is known to worsen bronchial reactivity in asthmatics,[24] causes an increase in respiratory illnesses in children with asthma[76] and is associated with asthma exacerbations in children[11,77] and adults.[12,26] The mechanisms of how infection impacts on asthma and how asthma affects the course of infection are unclear.

Influenza virus infection of airway epithelial cells induces the release of proinflammatory mediators. There is virus-specific induction of RANTES, IL-1β and TNF-α from epithelial cell lines, nasal epithelial cells and BECs.[78,79] Infection of BECs enhances eosinophil chemotaxis, an effect that is suppressed by blocking RANTES.[79] Similar to the other respiratory viruses, influenza virus infection can directly activate NFκB, which is mediated by host expression of the viral hemagglutinin gene.[80]

Unlike RV, where few epithelial cells are infected, influenza virus efficiently infects nasal (85% infected at 12 hours) and airway epithelial cells (50% at 12 hours).[81] Also, in contrast to RV, infection with influenza virus leads to a widespread CPE evident 24 hours post-infection of cell lines (NCI-H292)[78] and within 48 hours post-infection of primary BECs.[82] The CPE is associated with necrosis or cell lysis, and coincides with the release of infective virions as well as the peak release of the proinflammatory mediator IL-8.[82] In primary BECs where CPE was relatively delayed compared to NCI-H292 cells, there was significantly more infectious virus produced.[82] Again, epithelial cell viability post-infection appears to be linked to successful viral replication. To address this relationship, Brydon et al. infected a human nasal cell line (RPMI 2650) and a lower airway epithelial cell line (NCI-H292) with influenza virus.[81] By 48 hours, 50% of the nasal cell line had become apoptotic and 100% of the NCI-H292 cells. Treatment of the cells with a pan-caspase inhibitor led to a 75% reduction in apoptosis, but had no effect on virus production, suggesting that this was already occurring at maximum efficiency. However, the cells where apoptosis was inhibited had a significant increase in the release of IL-6 and IL-8, suggesting that apoptosis may still exert some protection by minimizing the inflammatory response to infection. It remains unclear what consequences, if any, this may have on the clinical effects of infection, or how chronic inflammatory airway diseases such as asthma or COPD may influence this mechanism.

CONCLUSIONS

At the commencement of this chapter it was stated that the aim of in vitro models should be to allow the study of tissue responses to stimuli and relate this to known and unknown mechanisms of disease. In asthma the airway epithelium has come to be appreciated as more than just an inert barrier, but as an active tissue, interacting with the environment and responding to threats by recruiting inflammatory cells and initiating the subsequent process of wound repair. In the case of asthma the constantly assailed epithelium is closely related to the disease, both acutely and also chronically.

The central role that the epithelium plays in asthma is no more clearly seen than in respiratory virus infection, which remains the most important acute trigger for asthma exacerbations. In vitro epithelial cell models have demonstrated in detail the potent proinflammatory response of the epithelial cell to infection, leading to a rapid activation of the innate and cell-mediated immune system. In the case of asthma, where airway inflammation exists chronically, the implication is that there is a marked worsening of the pre-existing situation with further inflammatory cell recruitment and worsened inflammation. What remains unclear, however, is what if any effect this may have on the long-term inflammatory response in the airways or how this may impact on the epithelium's attempt to repair the damage, and whether there is a lasting effect that may lead to airway wall remodeling and worsening of fixed airflow obstruction. These remain important areas for future development.

In addition, these models have highlighted the previously under-appreciated antiviral responses of infected epithelial cells. Mechanisms of early cell apoptosis and the release of type I interferons have the potential to limit virus replication without invoking a potentially damaging immune response. A better understanding of these mechanisms and their operation in diseases such as asthma has the potential to identify potential therapeutic targets with substantial clinical benefits.

REFERENCES

1. Harkema JR, Mariassy A, St George J, et al. Epithelial cells of the conducting airways: a species comparison. In Farmer SG, Hay DWP, eds. The Airway Epithelium: Physiology, Pathophysiology and Pharmacology. New York: Marcel-Dekker, 1991: 3–39

2. Boers JE, den Brok JL, Koudstaal J, et al. Number and proliferation of neuroendocrine cells in normal human airway epithelium. Am J Respir Crit Care Med 1996; 154: 758–63

3. Knight DA, Holgate ST. The airway epithelium: structural and functional properties in health and disease. Respirology 2003; 8: 432–46

4. Chung KF, Barnes PJ. Cytokines in asthma. Thorax 1999; 54: 825–7

5. Barnes PJ. New concepts in the pathogenesis of bronchial hyperresponsiveness and asthma. J Allergy Clin Immunol 1989; 83: 1013–26

6. Gaston B, Drazen JM, Loscalzo J, Stamler JS. The biology of nitrogen oxides in the airways. Am J Respir Crit Care Med 1994; 149: 538–51

7. Holgate ST, Davies DE, Lackie PM, et al. Epithelial–mesenchymal interactions in the pathogenesis of asthma. J Allergy Clin Immunol 2000; 105: 193–204

8. Sampath D, Castro M, Look DC, Holtzman MJ. Constitutive activation of an epithelial signal transducer and activator of transcription (STAT) pathway in asthma. J Clin Invest 1999; 103: 1353–61

9. Puddicombe SM, Polosa R, Richter A, et al. Involvement of the epidermal growth factor receptor in epithelial repair in asthma. FASEB J 2000; 14: 1362–74

10. Puddicombe SM, Torres-Lozano C, Richter A, et al. Increased expression of p21waf cyclin-dependent kinase inhibitor in asthmatic bronchial epithelium. Am J Respir Cell Mol Biol 2003; 28: 61–8

11. Johnston SL, Pattemore PK, Sanderson G, et al. Community study of the role of viral infections in exacerbations of asthma in 9–11 year old children. BMJ 1995; 310: 1225–8

12. Nicholson KG, Kent J, Ireland DC. Respiratory viruses and exacerbations of asthma in adults. BMJ 1993; 307: 982–6

13. Winther B, Gwaltney JM, Mygind M, et al. Sites of rhinovirus recovery after point inoculation of the upper airway. J Am Med Assoc 1986; 256: 1763–7

14. Winther B, Farr B, Turner R, et al. Histopathological examination and enumeration of polymorphonuclear leukocytes in the nasal mucosa during experimental rhinovirus colds. Acta Otolayrngol 1984; 413 (Suppl): 19–24

15. Fraenkel DJ, Bardin P, Sanderson G, et al. Immunohistochemical analysis of nasal biopsies during rhinovirus experimental colds. Am J Respir Crit Care Med 1994; 150: 1130–6

16. Bardin PG, Johnston SL, Sanderson G, et al. Detection of rhinovirus infection of the nasal mucosa by oligonucleotide in situ hybridisation. Am J Respir Cell Mol Biol 1994; 10: 207–13

17. Lemanske RF, Dick EC, Swenson CA, et al. Rhinovirus upper respiratory tract infection increases airway reactivity and late asthmatic reactions. J Clin Invest 1989; 83: 1–10

18. Fraenkel DJ, Bardin P, Sanderson G, et al. Lower airway inflammation during rhinovirus colds in normal and in asthmatic subjects. Am J Respir Crit Care Med 1995; 151: 879–86

19. Grunberg K, Smits HH, Timmers MC, et al. Experimental rhinovirus 16 infection: effects on cell differentials and soluble markers in sputum in asthmatic subjects. Am J Respir Crit Care Med 1997; 156: 609–16

20. Gern JE, Galagan DM, Jarjour NN, et al. Detection of rhinovirus RNA in lower airway cells during experimentally induced infection. Am J Respir Crit Care Med 1997; 155: 1159–61

21. Papadopoulos NG, Bates PJ, Bardin PG, et al. Rhinoviruses infect the lower airways. J Infect Dis 2000; 181: 1875–84

22. Ahern W, Bird T, Court S, et al. Pathological changes in virus infections of the lower respiratory tract in children. J Clin Invest 1970; 23: 7–18

23. Walsh JJ, Dietlein LF, Low FN, et al. Bronchotracheal response in human influenza. Arch Intern Med 1961; 108: 376–88

24. Laitinen LA, Kava T. Bronchial reactivity following uncomplicated influenza A infection in healthy subjects and in asthmatic patients. Eur J Respir Dis 1980; 106: 51–8

25. Skoner DP, Doyle WJ, Seroky J, Fireman P. Lower airway responses to influenza A virus in healthy allergic and nonallergic subjects. Am J Respir Crit Care Med 1996; 154: 661–4

26. Wark PAB, Johnston SL, Moric I, et al. Neutrophil degranulation and cell lysis is associated with clinical severity in virus-induced asthma. Eur Respir J 2002; 19: 68–75

27. Puddicombe SM, Babu S, Thornber M, et al. Phenotypic characterization of severe asthmatic bronchial epithelial cells differentiated in vitro. Am J Respir Crit Care Med 2002; 165: A59

28. Yamaya M, Finkbeiner WE, Chun SY, Widdicombe JH. Differentiated structure and function of cultures from human tracheal epithelium. Am J Physiol Lung Cell Mol Physiol 1992; 262: L713–L724

29. Schroth MK, Grimm E, Frindt P, et al. Rhinovirus replication causes RANTES production in primary bronchial epithelial cells. Am J Respir Cell Mol Biol 1999; 20: 1220–8

30. Wu R, Yankaskas J, Cheng E, et al. Growth and differentiation of human nasal epithelial cells in culture. Am Rev Respir Dis 1985; 132: 311–20

31. Churchill L, Chilton FH, Resau JH, et al. Cyclooxygenase metabolism of endogenous arachidonic acid by cultured human tracheal epithelial cells. Am Rev Respir Dis 1989; 140: 449–53

32. Racianello VR. Picornaviridae: the viruses and their replication. In Fields BN, Knipe DM, eds. Virology, 2nd edn. New York: Raven Press, 1990: 685–722

33. Subauste MC, Jacoby DB, Richards SM, Proud D. Infection of human respiratory epithelial cell line with rhinovirus: induction of cytokine release and modulation of susceptibility to infection by cytokine exposure. J Clin Invest 1995; 96: 549–57

34. Papadopoulos NG, Sanderson G, Hunter J, Johnston SL. Rhinoviruses replicate effectively at lower airway temperatures. J Med Virol 1999; 58: 100–4

35. Mosser AG, Brockman-Schneider R, Amineva S, et al. Similar frequency of rhinovirus-infectible cells in upper and lower airway epithelium. J Infect Dis 2002; 185: 734–43

36. Lopez-Souza N, Dolganov G, Dubin R, et al. Resistance of differentiated human airway epithelium to infection by rhinovirus. Am J Physiol 2004; 286: L373–L381

37. Zhu Z, Tang W, Ray A, et al. Rhinovirus stimulation of interleukin-6 in vivo and in-vitro. Evidence for nuclear factor kappa B-dependent transcriptional activation. J Clin Invest 1996; 97: 421–30

38. Terajima M, Yamaya M, Sekizawa K, et al. Rhinovirus infection of primary cultures of human tracheal epithelium: role of ICAM-1 and IL-1beta. Am J Physiol 1997; 273: L749–L759

39. Sanders SP, Siekierski ES, Porter JD, et al. Nitric oxide inhibits rhinovirus-induced cytokine production and viral replication in a human respiratory epithelial cell line. J Virol 1998; 72: 934–42

40. He S, Zheng J, Duan M. Induction of mucin secretion from human bronchial tissue and epithelial cells by rhinovirus and lipopolysaccharide1. Acta Pharmacol Sin 2004; 25: 1176–81

41. Konno S, Grindle KA, Lee W-M, et al. Interferon-gamma enhances rhinovirus-induced RANTES secretion by airway epithelial cells. Am J Respir Cell Mol Biol 2002; 26: 594–601

42. Papi A, Papadopoulos N, Stanciu LA, et al. Reducing agents inhibit rhinovirus-induced up-regulation of the rhinovirus receptor intercellular adhesion molecule-1 (ICAM-1) in respiratory epithelial cells. FASEB J 2002; 16: 1934–6

43. Papi A, Johnston SL. Rhinovirus infection induces expression of its own receptor intracellular adhesion molecule 1 (ICAM-1) via increased NF-κB-mediated transcription. J Biol Chem 1999; 274: 9707–20

44. Whiteman SC, Bianco A, Knight RA, Spiteri MA. Human rhinovirus selectively modulates membranous and soluble forms of its intercellular adhesion molecule-1 (ICAM-1) receptor to promote epithelial cell infectivity. J Biol Chem 2003; 278: 11954–61

45. Papi A, Johnston SL. Respiratory epithelial cell expression of vascular cell adhesion molecule-1 and its up-regulation by rhinovirus infection via NF-kappa B and GATA transcription factors. J Biol Chem 1999; 274: 30041–51

46. Elices MJ, Osborn L, Takada Y, et al. VCAM-1 on activated endothelium interacts with the leukocyte integrin VLA-4 at a site distinct from the VLA-4/fibronectin binding site. Cell 1990; 23: 577–84

47. Bochner EM, Bochner BS, Georas SN, Schleimer RP. Eosinophil transendothelial migration induced by cytokines. I. Role of endothelial and eosinophil adhesion molecules in IL-1 beta-induced transendothelial migration. J Immunol 1992; 149: 4021–8

48. Nagata M, Sedgwick J, Busse W. Endothelial cells upregulate eosinophil superoxide generation via VCAM-1 expression. Clin Exp Allergy 1999; 29: 550–61

49. Lowenstein CJ, Hill SL, Lafond-Walker A, et al. Nitric oxide inhibits viral replication in murine myocarditis. J Clin Invest 1996; 97: 1837–43

50. Kharitonov S, Yates DH, Barnes PJ. Increased nitric oxide in exhaled air of normal human subjects with upper respiratory tract infections. Eur Respir J 1995; 8: 295–7

51. Parronchi P, De Carli M, Manetti R, et al. IL-4 and IFN (alpha and gamma) exert opposite regulatory effects on the development of cytolytic potential by Th1 or Th2 human T cell clones. J Immunol 1992; 149: 2977–83

52. Takaoka A, Hayakawa S, Hideyuki Y, et al. Integration of interferon-α/β signalling to p53 responses in tumour suppression and antiviral defence. Nature 2003; 424: 516–23

53. Wark PAB, Johnston SL, Bucchieri et al. Asthmatic bronchial epithelial cells have a deficient innate immune response to infection with rhinovirus. J Exp Med 2005; 201: 937–47

54. Papi A, Johnston SL. Rhinovirus infection induces expression of its own receptor intercellular adhesion molecule 1 (ICAM-1) via increased NF-kappa-B-mediated transcription. J Biol Chem 1999; 274: 9707–20

55. Hadad J. Oxygen-sensing mechanisms and the regulation of redox-responsive transcription factors in development and pathophysiology. Respir Res 2002; 3: 26–34

56. Papi A, Johnston SL. Respiratory epithelial cell expression of vascular cell adhesion molecule-1 and its upregulation by rhinovirus infection via NF-kappaB and GATA transcription factors. J Biol Chem 1999; 274: 30041–51

57. Shackleford RE, Kaufmann WK, Paules R. Oxidative stress and cell cycle checkpoint function. Free Radic Biol Med 2000; 28: 1387–404

58. Hadad J, Land SC. The differential expression of apoptosis factors in the alveolar epithelium is redox sensitive and requires NF-kB (RelA)-selective targeting. Biochem Biophysiol Res Comm 2000; 271: 257–67

59. Zimmermann K, Green D. How cells die: apoptosis pathways. J Allergy Clin Immunol 2001; 108: 99s–103s

60. Marsden VS, Strasser A. Control of apoptosis in the immune sytem: Bcl-2, BH3-only proteins and more. Annu Rev Immunol 2003; 21: 71–105

61. Vaux DL, Strasser A. The molecular biology of apoptosis. Proc Natl Acad Sci USA 1996; 93: 2239–44

62. Carthy CM, Granville DJ, Watson KA, et al. Caspase activation and specific cleavage of substrates after coxsackievirus B3-induced cytopathic effect in HeLa cells. J Virol 1998; 72: 7669–75

63. Seemungal T, Harper-Owen R, Bhowmik A, et al. Respiratory viruses, symptoms, and inflammatory markers in acute exacerbations and stable chronic obstructive pulmonary disease. Am J Respir Crit Care Med 2001; 164: 1618–23

64. Feldman SA, Hendry RM, Beeler JA. Identification of a linear heparin binding domain for human respiratory syncytial virus attachment glycoprotein G. J Virol 1999; 73: 6610–17

65. Collins PL, Mottet G. Post-translational processing and oligomerization of the fusion glycoprotein of human respiratory syncytial virus. J Gen Virol 1991; 72: 3095–101

66. Pastey MK, Gower TL, Spearman PW, et al. A RhoA derived peptide inhibits syncytium formation induced by respiratory syncytial virus and parainfluenza-3. Nat Med 2000; 6: 35–40.

67. Gower TL, Peeples ME, Collins PL, Graham BS. RhoA is activated during respiratory syncytial virus infection. Virology 2001; 283: 188–96

68. Fiedler M, Wernke-Dollries K, Stark J. Respiratory syncytial virus induced cytokine production of a human bronchial epithelial line. Am J Phsyiol 1995; 269: L865–L872

69. Becker S, Reed W, Henderson FW, Noah TL. RSV infection of human airway epithelial cells causes the production of the chemokine RANTES. Am J Physiol 1997; 269: L512–L520

70. Hacking D, Hull J. Respiratory syncytial virus–viral biology and the host response. J Infect 2002; 45: 18–24

71. Patel JA, Kunimoto M, Sim TC, et al. Interleukin-1a mediates the enhanced expression of intracellular adhesion molecule-1 in pulmonary epithelial cells infected with respiratory syncytial virus. Am J Respir Cell Mol Biol 1995; 13: 602–9

72. Dosanjh A, Rednam S, Martin M. Respiratory syncytial virus augments production of fibroblast growth factor basic in vitro: implications for a possible mechanism of prolonged wheezing after infection. Pediatr Allergy Immunol 2003; 14: 437–40

73. Thomas KW, Monick MM, Staber JM, et al. Respiratory syncytial virus inhibits apoptosis and induces NF-kappa B activity through a phosphatidylinositol 3-kinase-dependent pathway. J Biol Chem 2002; 277: 492–501

74. Kotenko SV, Gallagher G, Baurin VV, et al. IFN-λs mediate antiviral protection through a distinct class II cytokine receptor complex. Nat Immunol 2003; 4: 69–77

75. Spann KM, Tran K-C, Chi B, et al. Suppression of the induction of alpha, beta, and gamma interferons by the NS1 and NS2 proteins of human respiratory syncytial virus in human epithelial cells and macrophages. J Virol 2004; 78: 4363–9

76. Neuzil KM, Wright PF, Mitchel EF, Griffin MR. The burden of influenza illness in children with asthma and other chronic medical conditions. J Pediatr 2000; 137: 856–64

77. Minor TE, Dick EC, DeMeo AN, et al. Viruses as precipitants of asthmatic attacks in children. J Am Med Assoc 1974; 227: 292–8

78. Matsukura S, Kokubo F, Noda H, et al. Expression of IL-6, IL-8 and RANTES on human bronchial epithelial cells, NCI-H292, induced by influenza virus. J Allergy Clin Immunol 1996; 98: 1080–7

79. Matsukura S, Kokubu F, Kubo H, et al. Expression of RANTES by normal airway epithelial cells after influenza virus A infection. Am J Respir Cell Mol Biol 1998; 18: 255–64

80. Phal HL, Baeuerle PA. Expression of influenza virus hemagglutinin activates transcription factor NF-kappa B. J Virol 1995; 69: 1480–4

81. Brydon EWA, Smith H, Sweet C. Influenza A virus-induced apoptosis in bronchiolar epithelial (NCI-H292) cells limits pro-inflammatory cytokine release. J Gen Virol 2003; 84: 2389–400

82. Arndt U, Wennemuth G, Barth P, et al. Release of macrophage migration inhibitory factor and CXCL8/interleukin-8 from lung epithelial cells rendered necrotic by influenza A virus infection. J Virol 2002; 76: 9298–306

CHAPTER 13

In vitro models of macrophage infection

Vasile Laza-Stanca, Luminita A Stanciu and Sebastian L Johnston

OVERVIEW OF THE MONONUCLEAR PHAGOCYTE SYSTEM

On encounter with infectious agents, the first line of protection is the innate immune system.[1] This system has both humoral and cellular components and is ready to act as soon as pathogens enter an organism. Macrophages can be considered prototype cells of the innate immune system.[1] They are strategically placed in sites which have contact with the external environment (e.g. lung) or in organs to help clearance of already entered pathogens (e.g. spleen, liver, peritoneum). Classifications of macrophages have changed over time and now they are considered to be a part of the mononuclear phagocyte system (MPS) together with monoblasts, promonocytes and monocytes.[2] This classification has replaced the previous one (reticuloendothelial or reticulohistiocyte system) because of the lack of enough common features of cells classified in this system, such as fibroblasts or mesothelial cells, with macrophages.[2] Cells belonging to the MPS have in common morphological characteristics (detected by light and electron microscopy), express enzymes such as non-specific esterase, lysosomal hydrolases and ectoenzymes (detected by histochemical staining) and are capable of non-specific uptake of particles (latex or colloidal carbon). Also, they express specific receptors, especially for the Fc portion of immunoglobulin and for complement

system components, called opsonins.[3] Because none of the available methods and markers are optimal, classification of a cell population as mononuclear phagocytes must therefore be based on a combination of properties.

Another important step in establishing the affiliation of a cell population to the MPS is to ensure that it has its origin in monocytes or one of their precursors.[4] Differentiation of monoblasts to promonocytes and further to monocytes takes place in the bone marrow. Monocytes then migrate to the blood were their half-life is around 1 day in mice and 3 days in humans. From here they migrate into tissues and differentiate. Because there is no defined role for monocytes in blood, they are considered a form of transport from bone marrow to tissues.[4]

Dendritic cells and Langherhans cells also have many features in common with macrophages, such as cell-surface markers, and functions such as phagocytosis and antigen processing and presentation. However, these cells cannot be considered as authentic mononuclear phagocytes, because their derivation from monocytes has not yet been firmly established.

Heterogeneity of macrophages

Mononuclear phagocytes are known to exhibit marked heterogeneity. There is no study to investigate the heterogeneity of bone marrow precursors. However, there is strong evidence suggesting the existence of different populations of monocytes according to their surface markers. At least two populations can be distinguished: CD14++ CD16– DR+ or classical monocytes; and the CD14+ CD16+ DR++ or proinflammatory monocytes. The second population has characteristics closer to macrophages and/or dendritic cells, and they are able to produce significantly higher amounts of proinflammatory cytokines compared with classical monocytes.[5,6] Some studies have shown their involvement in inflammatory processes such as sepsis.[5]

In the case of macrophages, heterogeneity is a well-recognized fact. Macrophages exist in practically every tissue in the body. Despite a common origin in blood monocytes, macrophages from different tissues exhibit a wide range of phenotypes with regard to their morphology, cell-surface antigen expression and function.[7] This could be a reflection of the plasticity and versatility of macrophages when exposed to microenvironmental stimuli.[8,9] Two very well characterized, and somehow opposite, populations of macrophages are alveolar and peritoneal macrophages.[10] The exposure to two totally different environments: the lung/alveolar space (very well oxygenated, sterile and rich in granulocyte–macrophage colony-stimulating factor (GM-CSF)) and the peritoneal space (anaerobic metabolism, potential exposure to lipopolysaccharide (LPS)) will produce cells with marked differences not only in morphology but also in surface antigen expression and functional capabilities.[10]

The heterogeneity of macrophages is not reflected only in inter-tissue differences; differences are also present within the tissue. The best characterized are liver macrophages, Kupffer cells, peritoneal macrophages and lung macrophages. In the lung, at least two distinct populations can be identified, according to their histological localization: alveolar macrophages (AM) localized in the airway and interstitial macrophages (IM) localized in lung connective tissue.[11]

AM are the best studied of lung macrophages, because are they easily accessible by bronchoalveolar lavage (BAL). AM are strategically placed at the interface of the lung with the external environment, having a role in primary defense against inhaled particles, toxins and micro-organisms.[12,13] AM are considered the final stage of blood monocyte maturation. Several studies have suggested that, in the process of differentiation, IM are an intermediate step between monocytes and AM.[14,15] Morphologically, AM are larger cells, dissimilar in size, more mature and with an increased cytoplasm/nucleus ratio. IM are smaller with more uniform size and they have a more close similarity to the monocyte. Functionally, AM are more able to perform phagocytic and cytotoxic functions and to secrete larger amounts of proinflammatory cytokines. IM are still capable of proliferation. They have higher expression of surface intercellular adhesion molecule (ICAM)-1 and better immunoregulatory capacities.[10,14] Inside these two populations a further differentiation could be made, using density for classification. In general, AM or IM with higher density are less mature cells, smaller in size, while lower-density cells are more mature and larger.[16]

It was suggested that IM and AM are two different populations performing individual tasks, resulting from different pathways of differentiation from different precursors.[17] However, there are no definitive data to support this hypothesis and considering IM as an intermediate step between monocytes and AM, with a continuous differentiation rather than two well-defined populations, is more accepted.

ROLE OF MACROPHAGES IN VIRAL INFECTION

As noted above, macrophages are strategically located in organs to monitor physiological processes and contribute to homeostasis. Any local disturbance of tissue normality, ranging from abnormal cell turnover or wounding to infection or malignancy, will lead to a rapid recruitment of macrophages. The role of macrophages in bacterial infection and malignancy is well studied.[18] In case of viral infection, the best known is the role of macrophages in blood-borne viral infection, especially HIV.[19] In case of viruses infecting the airways, macrophages have been studied in influenza, respiratory syncytial virus (RSV) and more recently for SARS-virus infections.[13,20,21]

Macrophages can operate in three ways to stop viral infection: phagocytosis, release of soluble mediators and action as antigen-presenting cells.

Scavenging/phagocytosis takes place when a non-specific receptor is involved (e.g. scavenger receptor, mannose receptor, glucan receptor) and results in reduced viral load. This mechanism is potentially important for large viruses. This can be further enhanced by specific opsonization with antibody and complement, when smaller viruses can be retained and destroyed as well. This process is important mainly for blood-borne viral infection when macrophages from the spleen function as a filter.[22] Removal of necrotic or apoptotic cells, the result of viral replication, through phagocytosis is another important part played by macrophages in stopping viral spread. During phagocytosis viral particles are destroyed in the phagolysosome, therefore direct infection of macrophages does not take place after phagocytosis. However, viruses can directly infect macrophages as a result of attachment of the virus to a specific receptor on the cell surface. Endocytosis of viral particles and/or release of viral nucleic acid in the cytoplasm will lead to viral infection of macrophages.

Release of soluble mediators provides a second line of defense against viral infection. Following viral infection, macrophages are an important source of antiviral cytokines, such as type I interferons (IFNs).[23] Other secreted cytokines will lead to inflammation and/or activation of other antiviral mechanisms of the host (e.g. tumor necrosis factor (TNF)-α, interleukin (IL)-1β, IL-6, IL-15, IL-12, IL-18, IL-23) or will have immunoregulatory and/or anti-inflammatory effects (IL-10, IL-1R antagonist IL-1Ra).[1] Chemokines are known to be secreted from macrophages after viral infection and participate in attraction of neutrophils

(IL-8, extractable nuclear antigen (ENA)-78), natural killer (NK) cells, macrophage inflammatory protein (MIP)-1α and MIP-1β) or T cells (RANTES, interferon-γ-inducible protein (IP)-10, monokine induced by interferon-γ (MIG), macrophage-derived chemokine (MDC)).[1] Cytokine and chemokine production is the result of activation of several nuclear factors. One of the best studied is NFκB. During viral infections NFκB activation can be the result of several different events, including recognition of dsRNA or ssRNA, viral enzymes, stress induced by viral entry and/or replication. Also, by-products of cellular activation, such as cytokines produced after viral infection, could also contribute to NFκB activation.[24] Interferon regulatory factors (IRFs) are another group of transcription factors activated in macrophages during viral infections. IRF-3 and IRF-7 are recognized as crucial regulators of IFN-α/β but this is not the only function of IRFs.[23,25] They also control the transcription of the interferon-stimulated genes (e.g. MHC class I and II, inducible nitric oxide synthase (iNOS), RANTES, IP-10, double-stranded-RNA-associated protein kinase (PKR)).[25,26] The mechanisms of IRF activation are not clear. IRF-3 is recognized as the first to respond to viral infection. The main activation trigger is the presence of dsRNA recognized by retinoic acid inducible gene (RIG) or Toll-like receptor (TLR)-3 but recognition of ssRNA by TLR-7 or -8 is also recognized as an effective trigger of IRF-3 activation.[27]

However, these cytokines are produced by other cell types and it is not certain which is the important *in vivo* source of these cytokines. In the case of type I IFNs or IL-15, macrophages produce these cytokines more quickly in larger amounts, compared with epithelial cells, which make them a more plausible source in vivi.[28,29] On the other hand, the newly identified subtype of blood dendric cells (DCs), plasmocytoid DCs (pDCs), has been shown to be the major 'type I IFN-producing cell' *in vivo*.[30] If their role in blood-borne viral infection is evident, no clear role has been established for lung infection. Further, it has been shown that, in the case of

STAT1–/– mice, which have impaired IFN-α/β production capabilities from epithelial cells, fibroblasts and conventional DCs but not from pDCs, efficient protection during airway infection cannot be achieved and the function of pDCs is affected.[31] The exact identification of the cell type(s) other than pDCs that are responsible for producing type I IFNs *in vivo* is a difficult task, as many different cell types are likely to be involved, including conventional DCs and macrophages as well as non-hematopoietic cells (epithelial cells and fibroblasts).

Macrophages are considered as professional antigen-presenting cells. They express MHC class I and II as well as the co-stimulatory molecules necessary to induce antigen-specific activation of CD4+ and CD8+ T cells.[1] The antigen presented can result from direct infection of macrophages by the virus and from phagocytosed material (e.g. viral particles or apoptotic/necrotic epithelial cells). They are not capable of activating naive T cells, but they could be of decisive importance in secondary immune responses for inducing proliferation of memory T cells. Together with antigen presentation, macrophages secrete the chemokines required for T-cell migration (IP-10, MIG, MDC) and cytokines necessary to support and regulate generation of memory T cells in primary infection and proliferation and survival of memory effector cells during secondary infection (IL-7, IL-15).[32,33] However, in the lung, alveolar macrophages are considered poor antigen-presenting cells.[34]

Defects in macrophage function could therefore result in increased susceptibility to viral infection on the one hand and prolonged and uncontrolled release of proinflammatory mediators leading to chronic inflammation on the other hand.

Macrophage activation

For macrophages to function to their full capabilities it is necessary for them to become activated. The activation process occurs when inflammatory stimuli act directly upon the macrophages and change their functional state, or is mediated by cytokines secreted by lymphocytes or macrophages (i.e. an autocrine regulation), or by serum proteins such as immunoglobulins or complement.[9] The generic term 'macrophage activation' is commonly used to describe this process, but the nature of an 'activated macrophage' population depends on the nature of the stimulus and the anatomical location. The first population of macrophages to become activated is 'resident macrophages'. Because of the release of chemotactic factors, a population of newly recruited macrophages will also be present at the site of the inflammation. In the case of the lung, the newly recruited macrophages can be present in both the alveolar and the interstitial space. Recruited macrophages exhibit many phenotypic differences from resident tissue macrophages.[3]

Activation of macrophages by IFN-γ and LPS/TNF-α has long been recognized as classical activation. On the other hand, cytokines such as IL-4, IL-10 and IL-13 or glucocorticoid hormones were regarded as inhibitors/deactivator molecules. When analyzed more carefully it was revealed that only a subset of function was downregulated while others were upregulated. For example, IL-4 upregulates MHC class II antigen expression but inhibits inflammatory cytokine production by macrophages.[35] This is known as alternative activation resulting in type 2 macrophages (M2), opposite to classical activation via IFN-γ resulting in type 1 macrophages (M1).[36] Differential cytokine production is a key feature of polarized macrophages but also surface molecules and metabolic activities are affected. M1 macrophages secrete IL-12 and/or IL-23, TNF-α, IP-10 and MIG, upregulate surface expression of Fc-γR I, II and III and express high levels of iNOS, to name a few of the characteristics of classical activation. In M2 macrophages all the above characteristics are inhibited, different characteristics being upregulated: production of IL-10, IL-1 receptor antagonist (IL-1Ra), eotaxin and MDC, upregulation of surface

Fc-εRII and predominance of the arginase pathway in arginine metabolism.[9,37] Interestingly, human monocytes differentiated with GM-CSF or macrophage colony-stimulating factor (M-CSF) have M1 and M2 properties, respectively.[38] M1 macrophages present potent killing capability (micro-organisms and tumor cells) and produce proinflammatory cytokines in large amounts. In contrast, M2 cells tune inflammatory responses and adaptive Th1 immunity, scavenge debris, promote angiogenesis, tissue remodeling and repair by using the arginase pathway in arginine metabolism and promote collagen production and fibroblast proliferation.[9] Because of the differences in molecules stimulated/inhibited by IL-10 on the one hand and IL-4/IL-13 on the other hand, and identification of M2 variants following stimulation through immune complexes and IL-1R stimulation, three different sub-phenotypes of M2 have also been described.[37,39] However, the above classification makes no reference to macrophage activation during innate immune responses to infections. A more expanded and complete classification was proposed by Gordon.[36] Along with classical activation (IFN-γ and TNF-α) and alternative activation (IL-4 or IL-13), a humoral activation phenotype is introduced which is the result of Fc receptor and/or complement receptor cross-linking and an innate activation phenotype as a result of microbial stimulation. The hallmark of innate activation is the production of type I IFNs. This is not specific for viral infection, as TLR ligation is also known to induce IFN-α/β production. As a result of innate activation, macrophages secrete cytokines and chemokines with roles in inflammation and in anti-infectious responses, upregulate co-stimulatory molecules to enhance antigen presentation and release low molecular-weight metabolites such as reactive oxygen species and nitric oxide with strong antimicrobial activities. Gordon also proposed a 'deactivated' phenotype, which can result from innate or acquired mechanisms. The uptake of apoptotic cells, scavenger receptor stimulation and stimulation through cytokines such as IL-10 and TGF-β are known to induce anti-inflammatory responses (Figure 13.1).

Macrophage polarization following activation should not be regarded as a fixed process. During inflammation macrophages are exposed to opposing signals *in vivo* at different times and therefore different profiles of activation will be present. In viral infection it is proposed that innate activation of macrophages, followed by classical activation, will help to stop viral replication and spread of the infection. This process is followed by alternative activation and deactivation, which reduce the inflammation and take part in the healing process.

MACROPHAGES AND ASTHMA

Macrophages are the most numerous immune effector cells in the airway. They have a central role in protecting the airway against infective and non-infective aggression.[13] The same cell participates in two opposite processes: inflammation and anti-inflammation/healing. A delayed response to aggression as well as an excessive and/or prolonged inflammatory response could lead to damage to the airways. AM are one of the most well studied cells of the lung. However, despite overwhelming evidence suggesting an important function in pulmonary defense there is little interest in the role of macrophages in asthma compared with any other cell type involved in allergic inflammation of the airways.[40]

Macrophages have a well-established role in immune-mediated disease. Abundance and activation of macrophages in the inflamed synovial membrane/pannus significantly correlates with the severity of rheumatoid arthritis (RA), an autoimmune disease which is considered a prototype of Th1-mediated diseases.[41] Also, cytokines that are products of classically activated macrophages, such as TNF-α, are a target for treatment in RA. TNF-α has multiple biological effects relevant to the pathogenesis of exacerbations of airway disease, including the

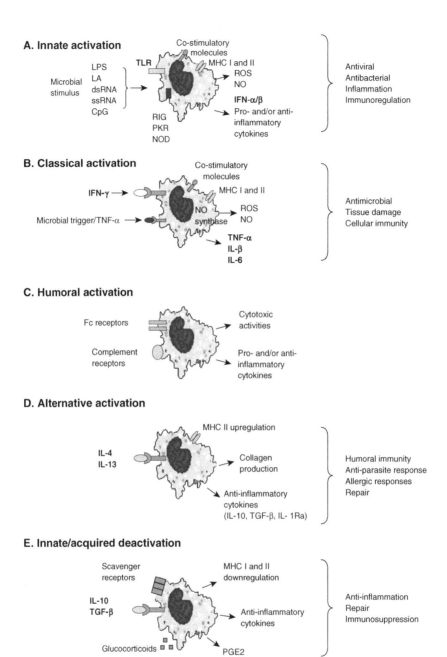

Figure 13.1 Macrophage activation – inducers and selected functional proprieties. A. Innate activation is the result of microbial recognition by pattern-recognition receptors and leads to increased antimicrobial activity, inflammation and activation of other components of the immune response. B. Classical activation is the result of IFN-γ stimulation of macrophages together with a TNF-α-inducing stimulus, leading to strong proinflammatory activity and tissue damage, and promoting cellular immunity.

enhanced release of other proinflammatory/ chemotactic mediators, upregulation of adhesion molecules, enhanced migration of eosinophils and neutrophils and induction of hyper-contractile airway smooth muscle, emphasizing the context dependence of TNF-α roles.[42]

Animal models are providing important clues in establishing the role of macrophages in asthma. The rat is one of the most well-characterized models for lung macrophages. The difference in susceptibility to ovalbumin (OVA)-induced airway hyperresponsiveness between the Brown Norway and Sprague Dawley rat strains makes them a good model of allergic inflammation of the airway. Brown Norway rats resemble atopic humans and develop antigen-specific IgE, Th2 cytokine production, eosinophilic inflammation and early- and late-phase bronchoconstrictor responses.[43] Along with rats, other small animals such as BALBc mice and guinea-pigs are also used. Important evidence is coming from studies using depletion and/or adoptive transfer of alveolar macrophages. Depletion is carried out by intratracheal instillation of liposome-encapsulated chloromethylene diphosphonate, which induces macrophage apoptosis.[44] By this method depletion of up to 85% of alveolar macrophages can be achieved. Adoptive transfer involves using genetically engineered macrophages or macrophages from a donor animal with or without previous depletion of resident macrophages.

Several studies have shown the immuno-suppressive effect of alveolar macrophages, in vivo depletion leading to increased antibody production in the lung to inhaled allergen in mice.[44] One of the targets of immunosupression by macrophages has been shown to be pulmonary DCs, by downregulating their antigen-presenting function in vivo and in vitro.[45]

Other studies had shown the role of macrophages in preventing allergic inflammation. Airway macrophage depletion in OVA-sensitized mice resulted in T cells with a Th2 phenotype (producing less IFN-γ and more IL-4 and IL-5) leading to more severe airway hyperreactivity and inflammation after intranasal antigen challenge. Adoptive transfer of macrophages promoted a Th1 response in antigen-sensitized recipients and did not induce pulmonary eosinophilia, while the transfer of a lung cell preparation (DCs, B cells and macrophages) promoted a Th2 response. However, in this study a mixture of lung macrophages (alveolar, interstitial and vascular) with low purity was used.[46] Experiments using depletion followed by transfer of macrophages in OVA-sensitized rats give more evidence supporting the protective role of macrophages in allergic inflammation. Transfer of alveolar macrophages from Sprague Dawley allergy-resistant rats into Brown Norway allergy-susceptible rats abrogated the airway hyperresponsiveness of the latter. Because cells obtained from BAL were used (containing more than 98% macrophages) this study points towards a direct role of alveolar macrophages and raises the question of whether a defect in macrophage activation in asthmatics could be responsible, at least partially, for allergic airway inflammation.[47]

A recent study showed a harmful role of macrophages in airway hyperresponsiveness induced by virus infections, in contradiction

---

Figure 13.1   (Continued)

C. Humoral activation is mediated mainly by Fc and complement receptors and leads to activation of cytotoxic functions. D. Alternative activation is the result of IL-4/IL-13 stimulation and leads to anti-parasitic immunity and promotes humoral immunity, allergic inflammation and tissue repair. E. Innate/acquired deactivation is the result of apoptotic cell uptake, TGF-β/IL-10 stimulation (produced by T cells) or glucocorticoid hormones and reduces inflammation through production of anti-inflammatory products and decreased antigen presentation. Modified from reference 36 with the protective role in allergen-induced inflammation. By depleting alveolar macrophages in guinea-pigs infected with parainfluenza virus, hyperactivity following electrical stimulation of the vagus was reduced.[48]

How macrophages modulate allergic inflammation in asthmatics is not clear. However, production of mediators such as type 1-inducing cytokines (IL-12, IL-18), immunomodulatory molecules (IL-10, prostaglandin (PG)E2) or anti-cytokines (IL-1R antagonist) produced by macrophages is likely to suppress allergic inflammation. IL-10 is known to regulate excessive inflammation and is produced mainly by T regulatory cells, but other leukocytes, including macrophages, can release this cytokine as well. During the early/innate phase of immune responses, macrophages could be the main source of IL-10. Macrophages can also be a target for IL-10. It has been reported that epithelial cells do not express IL-10 or IL-10R, which is expressed by alveolar macrophages.[49] Deficient production of IL-10 by macrophages could lead to excessive activation of T cells and prolonged classical activation of macrophages, both events leading to increased inflammation. PGE2 is another possible regulatory candidate but contradictory results about its role have been reported. PGE2 is recognized as an inducer of Th2 cytokines from lymphocytes and promotes eosinophil survival *in vitro*. However, there is evidence for a protective role of PGE2 through a bronchodilatory effect, inhibitory effects on airway smooth muscle and fibroblasts and possible suppression of type 2 cytokine production *in vivo*.[50] Cytokine decoy receptors and receptor antagonists are recognized to have anti-inflammatory proprieties.[51] A defect in IL-1R production by lung macrophages in asthmatics could also participate in generation of allergic inflammation of the airways. Macrophage stimulation through IgE or CD23 (low-affinity IgE receptor) cross-linking induces both pro- and anti-inflammatory responses (TNF-α, IL-1β, IL-8, MCP-1, MIP-1α and IL-10) with no significant differences

between controls and asthmatics. However, IL-1Ra was significantly increased only in controls, suggesting a preferential upregulation of proinflammatory responses by macrophages during allergic inflammation.[52]

MODELS OF MACROPHAGES USED FOR *IN VITRO* STUDIES

Several models of macrophages are used, each one with its advantages and disadvantages. We review the models of human macrophages for *in vitro* and *ex vivo* studies, as it is very difficult to obtain *in vivo* findings about macrophages.

Cell lines

Human cells lines are easy to obtain and grow in large amounts. Therefore, extensive experiments or experiments which require an increased number of cells can be performed, especially when molecular mechanisms are investigated. The main disadvantage is their tumoral origin, and therefore differences when compared with normal cells are likely to be present. Also, it will always provide the same phenotype as opposed to the heterogeneity encountered in macrophages. Confirmatory experiments have to be carried out, using one of the other models in order to confirm the results obtained in cell lines.

THP-1 is a human monocytic cell line (promonocytic leukemia) which has been used extensively as a model of monocytes. Treatment with phorbol-esters (PMA) or vitamin D induces the last stages of differentiation into monocyte/macrophage. PMA treatment is one of the most well-established protocols of monocyte maturation.[53] After an exposure of 24–72 hours to PMA these cells become adherent, substantially reduce their proliferative rate and increase their phagocytic and antigen-presenting capabilities. They have been used extensively in experiments investigating the mechanisms of cytokine production following different stimuli (including viral infection) and monocyte to macrophage differentiation.[54,55]

U937 is a human cell line derived from a histiocytic lymphoma and was used extensively for HIV studies and less for other viruses. Differentiation can also be induced by PMA but also using vitamin D3, IFN-γ, TNF-α and retinoic acid.

MonoMac is a human cell line established more recently and is used less than the other two cell lines mentioned above. MonoMac cells have morphology, surface markers and intracellular enzymes very similar to those of normal monocytes.[56] LPS can induce their maturation but there is no established protocol.

Peripheral blood mononuclear cells and monocytes

Peripheral blood mononuclear cells (PBMC) consist of a mixture of lymphocytes, monocytes and DCs. The separation of PBMC from total blood is usually obtained by gradient centrifugation. Because they are very easy to obtain they are frequently used as a model of monocytes/ macrophages. One disadvantage of using this model is that it provides a mixture of different cells, so it is difficult to interpret how much is the effect of stimulus on monocytes and how much is the effect of by-products of lymphocyte or DC stimulation. To obtain clearer results, purification of monocytes can be employed.

Purified monocytes can be obtained following purification by adherence or after positive or negative selection using magnetic beads. The most often employed method is adherence purification, which is simple and inexpensive, and relies on the monocyte property to adhere quickly to plastic surfaces. However, the yield and purity are difficult to control. Positive selection gives a very good purity and yield, but the cells can become activated after bead attachment. CD14 positive selection using MACS is the most usually employed method to obtain pure monocytes. Negative selection has the advantage of providing 'untouched' cells

but the purity and the yield are worse than with positive selection. Another issue for negative selection could be the use of anti-CD16 beads for depletion of NK cells, which can lead to the depletion of CD16+ monocytes as well.

Short-term growth and experiments with monocytes can be performed in media containing bovine serum; however, a degree of non-specific stimulation due to components in serum and batch-to-batch variation of serum can raise technical difficulties.

Monocytes have many similarities with macrophages; however, many differences have been reported as well. Differential responses to IL-4 and IL-13 due to reduced expression of the gamma chain receptor on macrophages, reduced CD14 in alveolar macrophages, differential regulation of eotaxin production after IL-4 or LPS stimulation and reduced expression of IL-1β and IL-18 after virus infection in monocytes are some of the differences reported.[57–60]

Monocyte-derived macrophages

Monocyte-derived macrophages (MDM) provide further enhancement compared with monocytes as the differentiation process will bring them closer to tissue macrophages. Several protocols are used, all of them employing monocytes separated by adherence or positive or negative selection. As expected, positive selection provides a better yield and the activation induced during the separation seems not to influence the differentiation process. Otherwise, there is no other advantage over protocols using adherence. Cells are grown for 5–14 days in order to obtain macrophages.

The simplest way is to use bovine serum-containing media (10–20%), but again batch-to-batch variation of serum can lead to inconsistency. Some protocols use human serum, from donors with the AB blood group, in concentrations of 10–20%. It has been shown that M-CSF and/or GM-CSF are the stimulating factors in sera which lead to the differentiation process. Protocols using recombinant M-CSF or GM-CSF

Table 13.1   Characteristics of M-CSF and GM-CSF MDM compared with peritoneal and alveolar macrophages

	M-CSF MDM	Peritoneal macrophages	GM-CSF MDM	Alveolar macrophages
Surface molecules				
CD11b/CD11c	++	++	++	++
CD14	++	++	–	–
MHC II	+	+++	++	++
FcγR I/II	+	++	+	+
FcγR III	+	NA	–	+
Scavenger R type A	+	NA	+	+
Functions				
Phagocytosis (Fcγ)	Strong	Strong	Very weak	Weak
H_2O_2 production	Strong	Strong	Weak	Weak
Catalase activity	Low	Low	High	High
HIV-1 susceptibility	Susceptible	Susceptible	Resistant	Resistant
M. tb. susceptibility	Resistant	Resistant	Susceptible	Susceptible
IL-10 production	Strong	Very strong	Weak	Weak

–, absent; +, minimal levels; ++, high levels; +++, maximal levels; NA, data not available; MDM, monocyte-derived macrophages; *M. tb.*, *Mycobacterium tuberculosis*

have also been developed, and can use serum-containing media or special supplemented serum-free media (i.e. macrophage serum-free-media from Invitrogen®).

The use of M-CSF will render macrophages similar to peritoneal macrophages, while macrophages obtained using GM-CSF are similar to alveolar macrophages. M-CSF-derived macrophages are larger, have a higher phagocytic capacity and are highly resistant to infection by vesicular stomatitis virus compared to GM-CSF MDM. Conversely, GM-CSF MDM are more cytotoxic, more efficiently kill *Listeria monocytogenes* and constitutively secrete more PGE2.[61] Other differences, together with the similarities with alveolar and peritoneal macrophages, are summarized in Table 13.1.

Different structures and signal transduction mechanisms of the receptors for M-CSF and GM-CSF which initiate activation of different pathways could account for the differences between macrophages obtained using one or other growth factor.

GM-CSF and M-CSF MDM have been shown to play opposing roles in cellular immunity. GM-CSF MDM produce IL-23 rather than IL-12

(which is produced mainly by DC) as the primary type 1 cytokine. Unlike IL-12, the expression of IL-23 in response to microbial stimulation seems to be less dependent on IFN-γ. IL-12 was produced in response to LPS or mycobacterial stimulation only with the addition of exogenous IFN-γ. A similar dependence on IFN-γ was observed in the production of IL-12 by DCs in response to microbial stimulation. Interestingly, the addition of IFN-γ only slightly enhanced IL-23 expression in GM-CSF MDM and it was not required for monocyte-derived DCs to produce IL-23 in response to microbial stimulation. Unlike GM-CSF MDM, M-CSF MDM were unable to produce either IL-12 or IL-23 in response to microbial stimulation and instead produced IL-10.[38]

Lung/alveolar macrophages

A large part of the knowledge about human lung macrophages is the result of studies performed on AM, collected by BAL. Following the BAL procedure, the cells obtained are over 90% macrophages. To enhance purity further, a 2–24-hour adherence step can be used. One of the advantages of this procedure is that it does not require complicated purification procedures or further maturation steps. The AM can be used immediately and provide the best model of lung macrophages available.

Despite obvious advantages, this approach has some drawbacks. During the procedure of collecting these cells, only the less adherent cells are harvested. Also, no information about IM, which constitute around 40% of total lung macrophages, is obtained. However, the main limitation is the BAL procedure itself. BAL is an invasive procedure which may produce discomfort and could have adverse effects such as hypoxemia, fever and very rarely bleeding.

VIRAL INFECTION OF LUNG MACROPHAGES

It is well established now that the majority of asthma exacerbations are caused by respiratory viral infection. Most viral exacerbations are due to either RSV (~5–10%), coronaviruses (~10–15%), influenza viruses (~5–10%) or human rhinoviruses (RVs) (~60–80%).[62] The mechanisms by which viruses exacerbate asthma are not yet known. Along with respiratory epithelial cells, macrophages are believed to play an important role. However, very few studies directly addressed the role of macrophages in virus-induced asthma exacerbation. Most of the available information to date is on RSV and influenza virus, both acknowledged as important pathogens of the lower airways.[13,20] RVs were considered as pathogens of the upper respiratory tract (common cold agents). Only after their association with asthma exacerbations became apparent has the interaction with monocytes/ macrophages been studied. Except SARS coronavirus, there is almost no information available about the effect of coronaviruses on lung macrophages. Therefore, we focused on influenza, RSV and RV infection of macrophages, and how this can contribute to the inflammatory and immune response generated by viral infections.

Influenza

Influenza viruses cause an acute respiratory infection of lower and upper airways that is accompanied by systemic symptoms. The disease is more severe in children, the elderly and immunocompromised individuals. Influenza is an important human pathogen and is recognized as an important cause of epidemic and pandemic infections.[63] However, they account for only a minority of asthma exacerbations in children and adults.

The viral infection will usually start in the upper airway but also invades the lower airway, affecting the bronchial and alveolar spaces. Infection of respiratory epithelium will lead to productive infection and is probably the most important source of virus *in vivo*. Macrophages and other types of leukocyte can be infected, but this is usually a non-productive infection. Several transcription factors are activated with subsequent production of chemokines and cytokines. In addition, antigen presentation machinery and apoptotic pathways are also activated.[28]

Virus can enter macrophages and in some studies the proportion of infected cells can reach 90%, as assessed by the presence of the hemagglutinin and nucleoprotein viral antigens. However, productive replication could not be detected in most of the studies.[64] Replication of influenza virus in macrophages is probably limited as a result of immediate and vigorous antiviral responses.

Epithelial cells are the primary site of virus replication for influenza virus. However, they are poor producers of type I IFNs, TNF-α or IL-1β after influenza infection. By contrast, macrophages produce large amounts of these cytokines in response to influenza infection.[28,65] They also produce IL-15 and IL-18 and to a lesser extent IL-10, but they fail to produce IL-12.[65] Type I IFNs were proved to be an important component of anti-influenza immunity through induction of antiviral proteins, especially MxA.[66] The lack of STAT1 in mice led to fulminant systemic influenza virus infection following intranasal inoculation, while in wild-type animals influenza replicated only in the lungs.[67] Along with antiviral effects, type I IFNs modulate innate and specific anti-influenza immunity. Macrophages from mice lacking type I IFN receptor or STAT1 failed to upregulate IL-15 and IL-10 mRNA, while IL-6 production was unaffected.[68] Because type I IFNs are so efficient in preventing viral replication, it is no surprise that influenza viruses developed mechanisms that subvert production and activity of type I IFNs. A nonstructural influenza protein NS1 has been proved to block IRF-3 translocation – one of the main events in initiation of IFN-β promoter activation. NS1 also counterattacks antiviral activity of type I IFNs by interfering with PKR-mediated inhibition of viral replication.[69–71]

Macrophages also produce large amounts of chemokines as a result of influenza virus infection, participating in this way in the recruitment of immune effector cells (e.g. memory T cells, NK cells). MIP-1α, MIP-1β, RANTES, MCP-1, MCP-3, MIP-3α and IP-10 are secreted in large amounts, whereas the production of IL-8 appears to be limited. Interestingly, epithelial cells produce IL-8 after influenza infection (influenza A) but lower amounts of IP-10 compared with macrophages, suggesting activation of different signaling pathways in epithelial cells compared to macrophages during influenza infection.[20]

It appears that macrophages, probably in conjunction with dendritic cells, are the major players in the antiviral immune responses against influenza virus. They also participate in the general inflammatory response responsible for the local cellular infiltrate and systemic manifestations during influenza infection.

Respiratory syncytial virus

RSV is the most common cause of hospitalization for severe lower respiratory tract infection in infants, and it causes severe respiratory tract illness in older immunodeficient children and the elderly. Bronchiolitis caused by RSV during infancy is associated with the later development of asthma, and RSV is implicated in exacerbations of asthma.[72]

RSV preferentially infects and replicates in the epithelium of the upper and lower respiratory tracts. A direct cytopathic effect on lung epithelial cells has been demonstrated, leading to loss of specialized functions such as cilial motility and sometimes to epithelial destruction.[73] In human macrophages RSV replication is limited. AM exposed to RSV demonstrate a time-dependent increased expression of RSV fusion gene and viral glycoproteins in a limited number of infected cells. These cells can release infectious virus over a long period of time (up to 10 days).[74,75] BAL macrophages from naturally occurring RSV infections in children demonstrated expression of viral protein and productive replication. Co-expression of viral antigens and IL-1β and TNF-α in AM demonstrated a direct effect of RSV on macrophages. After in vitro exposure of PBMC to RSV, both lymphocytes and monocytes expressed viral antigens. Further, circulating mononuclear leukocytes obtained from symptomatic children infected with RSV frequently expressed viral antigens, showing that RSV can infect circulating immune cells.[76,77]

Most studies in mouse macrophages report abortive/non-productive replication. Viral RNA and proteins can be detected intracellularly but no release of infective virus could be demonstrated.[78] This difference could be explained by the fact that RSV exhibits a degree of species specificity, mice being less susceptible to infection with strains of human RSV.

In vitro/ex vivo studies showed differential requirement for the presence of replicative virus in order to induce cytokine/chemokine production in macrophages. Alveolar macrophages upregulate RANTES and macrophage inflammatory protein (MIP)-2 after RSV infection and viral replication is necessary for optimal chemokine production.[79] Ultraviolet (UV)-inactivated virus failed to induce IL-1β mRNA and protein, but was effective in triggering IL-6 production by mouse alveolar macrophages.[78] Similar observations have been made in human macrophages where RSV replication was required for TNF-α upregulation but not for IL-6 and IL-8.[80]

NFκB is a major transcription factor involved in cytokine/chemokine production after RSV infection. Using a mouse model of RSV infection, Haeberle et al. investigated the requirement for RSV replication in NFκB activation and showed the existence of distinct but sequentially integrated RSV-inducible early NFκB responses in the lung.[81] The first response occurred early (day 1) after RSV inoculation, was dependent on AM and was viral replication independent, depletion of AM significantly decreasing NFκB activation. The second response (days 5–7) involved epithelial cells and/or inflammatory cells. The early response, but not the late response, was abolished when TLR4–/– mice were used, establishing TLR4 as a critical regulator of RSV-induced NFκB activation during the innate immune response by AM.[81]

Chemokine production follows the same pattern as NFκB activation: an early peak, at 24 hours after infection followed by a second one during days 5–8 post-infection.[79]

RSV is known to subvert the immune response (innate and adaptive) and lead to incomplete or short protective immunity.[82] Suppressing production of early immunoregulatory cytokines could be one of the mechanisms responsible for the immune evasion. RSV infection of human macrophages has been shown to induce secretion of IL-10, IL-11 and PGE2, all known to have immunosuppressive effects.[83,84] Another possible mechanism is inhibition of the type I IFN system through NS1 and NS2, nonstructural proteins present during viral replication. By using RSV with deletion of NS1 and NS2 viral titers were greatly decreased in epithelial cells and type I IFN expression was increased in epithelial cells and MDM.[85] NS1/NS2 act mainly by inhibiting STAT2, thus interfering with type I IFN signaling.[86]

In conclusion, macrophages are important components of the antiviral and proinflammatory response against RSV and are involved in both early and delayed phases of the process.

Rhinovirus

RVs are the most common trigger of acute exacerbations; however, the mechanisms by which RVs provoke exacerbations are not well understood.[62] An important advance in the understanding of the mechanisms of exacerbations was confirming infection of the lower airway by RV.[87] The airway epithelium is thought to be the site of RV replication and many studies have observed RV induction of proinflammatory cytokines, chemokines and adhesion molecules in epithelial cells.[88–90] During RV infection the number of epithelial cells infected with virus is low, both in vitro and in vivo. Nonetheless, it is currently believed that inflammatory cytokine production from RV-infected epithelial cells is an important mechanism contributing to the pathogenesis of exacerbations of asthma.[91] Cytokines such as TNF-α or IL-1β detected in the airway during exacerbations are reported not to be produced in significant quantities by epithelial cells after RV infection in vitro.[92] On the other hand, lung macrophages are a very well-documented source for TNF-α and also of many other cytokines and chemokines.[93]

Relatively few studies have investigated interactions between RV and cells of macrophage or monocytic origin. One of the focuses of these studies was to investigate whether RV can replicate in macrophages. When evidence for RV replication in macrophages was specifically investigated, attachment and entry of virus was detected, but no further evidence of replication was detected, as RV titers in supernatants decreased over time and RV RNA synthesis was not observed.[94] However, when the THP-1 monocytic cell line was used, a low-grade replication could be detected, suggesting that RV is capable of replication in cells of monocytic origin, but replication in macrophages/monocytes is limited by the strong antiviral response mounted by these cells following RV infection.[95]

The mechanisms responsible for this monocyte/macrophage activation are unclear. Induction of IL-8, IL-10, IL-12, TNF-α and MCP-1 and alteration of surface expression of CD14, CD80 and CD69 in PBMCs, monocytes or macrophages have all been reported after exposure to RV. Production of IL-10, TNF-α and MCP-1 was reported to be replication independent, while IL-8 secretion and CD69 upregulation appeared in part replication dependent as UV-inactivated RV had a significantly reduced effect compared to live virus.[94–99]

The molecular mechanisms regulating RV induction of inflammatory cytokines in macrophages are poorly understood, although RV induction of MCP-1 in monocytes and macrophages is reported to be dependent on the p38 MAPK/AP-1 pathway. The same study showed transient degradation of IκB (a kinase involved in NFκB regulation) and suggested that NFκB was important also for MCP-1 production.[97] Studies of RV infection of respiratory epithelial cells indicate a central role for NFκB in upregulation of several proinflammatory molecules.[88,100] NFκB plays an important role in the activation of several genes during viral infection (e.g. TNF-α, IFN-α/β, IL-8) and it is likely that its activation in macrophages will be important during RV infection.

Recently, we assessed the degree of replication of RV in macrophages using THP-1-derived macrophages and MDM. We showed that rhinovirus replication was productive in THP-1 macrophages, leading to release of infectious virus into supernatants, but was limited in MDM, probably due to type I IFN production which was robust in monocyte-derived but deficient in THP-1-derived macrophages.[101] Similar to bronchial epithelial cells, only small numbers of cells supported complete virus replication leading to the release of infective virus. We also demonstrated RV-induced activation of NFκB and co-localization of NFκB nuclear translocation with virus replication in both macrophage types, indicating that the major stimulus for NFκB activation in a cell was virus infection of the same cell. The infection strongly induced TNF-α release, which was dependent upon virus replication and required NFκB.[101] Work carried out in our department also showed induction of type III IFNs in MDM and AM by RV infection. The induction was deficient in AM from asthmatics compared with normal individuals, providing the first evidence to support a deficient response of macrophages to viral infections in asthmatics (see also Chapter 10).

A role of macrophages in RV infection of the lower airways *in vivo* has not been firmly established. Further studies are necessary to establish to what extent activation of macrophages occurs during *in vivo* RV infection.

CLOSING REMARKS

Macrophages have an important but complex role in viral infections. Along with a direct antiviral role, macrophages have multiple roles from sensing the infection and triggering early innate responses to activation of other components of the antiviral immune response (Figure 13.2a). Also, they play an important part in the reduction of inflammation and healing processes once virus replication has been stopped (Figure 13.2b).

The role of macrophages in asthma is not clear. Some rodent evidence suggests a beneficial role for macrophages in suppressing allergic inflammation of the lung, but there is no clear evidence that this occurs in humans and, if so, how this occurs. However, a role for macrophages in virus-induced asthma exacerbation is highly plausible. Defects in asthmatics in production of antiviral cytokines during viral infection could lead to increased viral load and failure to clear virus as rapidly, which in turn can induce excessive and prolonged inflammatory responses. Also, delays in switching from activated to deactivated/alternative activation phenotypes will lead to

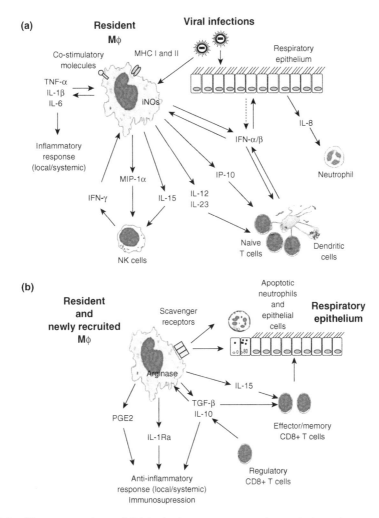

Figure 13.2   Role of lung macrophages (Mφ) in the immune response to respiratory viruses.

(a) In the early stages, respiratory viruses infect resident macrophages which will become activated (innate activation), produce proinflammatory cytokines (TNF-α, IL-1β, IL-6) and antiviral cytokines IFN-α/β. They also secrete chemokines (IP-10, MIP-1α) and cytokines (IL-15, IL-12, IL-23) which modulate other components of the antiviral immune response, including NK cells, DCs and T cells. IFN-γ produced by NK and T cells in turn modulates macrophage function (classical activation). Macrophage infection also upregulates the antigen-presenting molecules (MHC class I and II, co-stimulatory molecules) and will use the iNOS pathway for arginine metabolism, generating reactive nitrogen intermediates with antiviral function. In this way macrophages are participating in a co-ordinated effort to stop viral infection.

(b) Later during viral infection macrophages phagocytose apoptotic/necrotic cells and participate in the mainte-nance of effector and memory CD8 T cells, through IL-15 production, helping the further clearing of virus or virus-induced pathology. When viral infection is cleared, macrophages undergo deactivation/alternative activation and participate in reduction of inflammation and healing processes through secreting anti-inflammatory and/or immunoregulatory (PGE2, IL-1Ra, IL-10, TGF-β) molecules. Also, macrophages participate in the repair process by using the arginase pathway in arginine metabolism and promoting collagen production and fibroblast proliferation prolonged inflammation. Because of the close interrelations between macrophages and other components of lung defense it is likely that defects in macrophage function will also be reflected in alterations in functional responses of other cell types.

Models of macrophages for *in vitro/ex vivo* studies are already available. These models have been used to study the mechanisms of macrophage activation after influenza virus, RSV and to a lesser extent RV infection. However, only a minority of these studies address this issue in the context of asthma exacerbation and we believe that more studies (*in vitro/ex vivo* and *in vivo*) are necessary to firmly establish the involvement of macrophages in virus-induced asthma exacerbations.

REFERENCES

1. Janeway CA Jr, Travers P, Walport M, et al. Innate immunity. In Immunobiology – The Immune System in Health and Disease. New York: Churchill Livingstone, 2001: 35–91

2. van Furth R, Cohn ZA, Hirsch JG, et al. The mononuclear phagocyte system: a new classification of macrophages, monocytes, and their precursor cells. Bull World Health Organ 1972; 46: 845–52

3. Hume DA, Ross IL, Himes SR, et al. The mononuclear phagocyte system revisited. J Leukoc Biol 2002; 72: 621–7

4. van Furth R. Production and migration of monocytes and kinetics of macrophages. In van Furth R, ed. Mononuclear Phagocytes. Dordrecht: Kluwer Academic Publishers, 1992; 3–12

5. Fingerle G, Pforte A, Passlick B, et al. The novel subset of CD14+/CD16+ blood monocytes is expanded in sepsis patients. Blood 1993; 82: 3170–6

6. Belge KU, Dayyani F, Horelt A, et al. The proinflammatory CD14+CD16+DR++ monocytes are a major source of TNF. J Immunol 2002; 168: 3536–42

7. van Furth R. Current view on the mononuclear phagocyte system. Immunobiology 1982; 161: 178–85

8. Kennedy DW, Abkowitz JL. Mature monocytic cells enter tissues and engraft. Proc Natl Acad Sci USA 1998; 95: 14944–9

9. Mantovani A, Sozzani S, Locati M, et al. Macrophage polarization: tumor-associated macrophages as a paradigm for polarized M2 mononuclear phagocytes. Trends Immunol 2002; 23: 549–55

10. Laskin DL, Weinberger B, Laskin JD. Functional heterogeneity in liver and lung macrophages. J Leukoc Biol 2001; 70: 163–70

11. Lehnert BE. Pulmonary and thoracic macrophage subpopulations and clearance of particles from the lung. Environ Health Perspect 1992; 97: 17–46

12. Zhang P, Summer WR, Bagby GJ, Nelson S. Innate immunity and pulmonary host defense. Immunol Rev 2000; 173: 39–51

13. Gordon SB, Read RC. Macrophage defences against respiratory tract infections: the immunology of childhood respiratory infections. Br Med Bull 2002; 61: 45–61

14. Holt PG, Warner LA, Papadimitriou JM. Alveolar macrophages: functional heterogeneity within macrophage populations from rat lung. Aust J Exp Biol Med Sci 1982; 60: 607–18

15. Blusse van Oud Alblas A, van Furth R. The origin of pulmonary macrophages. Immunobiology 1982; 161: 186–92

16. Zwilling BS, Campolito LB, Reiches NA. Alveolar macrophage subpopulations identified by differential centrifugation on a discontinuous albumin density gradient. Am Rev Respir Dis 1982; 125: 448–52

17. Chandler DB, Bayles G, Fuller WC. Prostaglandin synthesis and release by subpopulations of rat interstitial macrophages. Am Rev Respir Dis 1988; 138: 901–7

18. Mantovani A, Bottazzi B, Colotta F, et al. The origin and function of tumor-associated macrophages. Immunol Today 1992; 13: 265–70

19. Verani A, Gras G, Pancino G. Macrophages and HIV-1: dangerous liaisons. Mol Immunol 2005; 42: 195–212

20. Julkunen I, Melen K, Nuqvist M, et al. Inflammatory responses in influenza A virus infection. Vaccine 2000; 19 (Suppl 1): S32–7

21. Perlman S, Dandekar AA. Immunopathogenesis of coronavirus infections: implications for SARS. Nat Rev Immunol 2005; 5: 917–27

22. Mims CA. Aspects of the pathogenesis of virus diseases. Bacteriol Rev 1964; 28: 30–71

23. Malmgaard L. Induction and regulation of IFNs during viral infections. J Interferon Cytokine Res 2004; 24: 439–54

24. Mogensen TH, Paludan SR. Molecular pathways in virus-induced cytokine production. Microbiol Mol Biol Rev 2001; 65: 131–50

25. Taniguchi T, Takaoka A. The interferon-alpha/beta system in antiviral responses: a multimodal machinery of gene regulation by the IRF family of transcription factors. Curr Opin Immunol 2002; 14: 111–16

26. Taniguchi T, Ogasawara K, Takaoka A, et al. IRF family of transcription factors as regulators of host defense. Annu Rev Immunol 2001; 19: 623–55

27. Schroder M, Bowie AG. TLR3 in antiviral immunity: key player or bystander? Trends Immunol 2005; 26: 462–8

28. Ronni T, Matikainen S, Sareneva T, et al. Regulation of IFN-alpha/beta, MxA, 2',5'-oligoadenylate synthetase and HLA gene expression in influenza A-infected human lung epithelial cells. J Immunol 1997; 158: 2363–74

29. Liew FY. The role of innate cytokines in inflammatory response. Immunol Lett 2003; 85: 131–4

30. Barchet W, Cella M, Colonna M. Plasmacytoid dendritic cells – virus experts of innate immunity. Semin Immunol 2005; 17: 253–61

31. Prakash A, Smith E, Lee CK, Levy DE. Tissue-specific positive feedback requirements for production of type I interferon following virus infection. J Biol Chem 2005; 280: 18651–7

32. Schluns KS, Lefrancois L. Cytokine control of memory T-cell development and survival. Nat Rev Immunol 2003; 3: 269–79

33. Bisset LR, Schmid-Grendelmeier P. Chemokines and their receptors in the pathogenesis of allergic asthma: progress and perspective. Curr Opin Pulmon Med 2005; 11: 35–42

34. Blumenthal RL, Campbell DE, Hwang P, et al. Human alveolar macrophages induce functional inactivation in antigen-specific CD4 T cells. J Allergy Clin Immunol 2001; 107: 258–64

35. Stein M, Keshav S, Harris N, et al. Interleukin 4 potently enhances murine macrophage mannose receptor activity: a marker of alternative immunologic macrophage activation. J Exp Med 1992; 176: 287–92

36. Gordon S. Alternative activation of macrophages. Nat Rev Immunol 2003; 3: 23–35

37. Mantovani A, Sica A, Sozzani S, et al. The chemokine system in diverse forms of macrophage activation and polarization. Trends Immunol 2004; 25: 677–86

38. Verreck FA, deBoer T, Langenberg DM, et al. Human IL-23-producing type 1 macrophages promote but IL-10-producing type 2 macrophages subvert immunity to (myco)bacteria. Proc Natl Acad Sci USA 2004; 101: 4560–5

39. Mosser DM. The many faces of macrophage activation. J Leukoc Biol 2003; 73: 209–12

40. Peters-Golden M. The alveolar macrophage: the forgotten cell in asthma. Am J Respir Cell Mol Biol 2004; 31: 3–7

41. Kinne RW, Braver R, Stuhlmuller B, et al. Macrophages in rheumatoid arthritis. Arthritis Res 2000; 2: 189–202

42. Thomas PS. Tumour necrosis factor: the role of this multifunctional cytokine in asthma. Immunol Cell Biol 2001; 79: 132–40

43. Hylkema MN, Hoekstra MO, Luinge M, et al. The strength of the OVA-induced airway inflammation in rats is strain dependent. Clin Exp Immunol 2002; 129: 390–6

44. Thepen T, Van Rooijen N, Kraal G. Alveolar macrophage elimination in vivo is associated with an increase in pulmonary immune response in mice. J Exp Med 1989; 170: 499–509

45. Strickland DH, Thepen T, Kees UR, et al. Regulation of T-cell function in lung tissue by pulmonary alveolar macrophages. Immunology 1993; 80: 266–72

46. Tang C, Inman MD, Van Rooijen N, et al. Th type 1-stimulating activity of lung macrophages inhibits Th2-mediated allergic airway inflammation by an IFN-gamma-dependent mechanism. J Immunol 2001; 166: 1471–81

47. Careau E, Bissonnette EY. Adoptive transfer of alveolar macrophages abrogates bronchial hyperresponsiveness. Am J Respir Cell Mol Biol 2004; 31: 22–7

48. Lee AM, Fryer AD, van Rooijen N, et al. Role of macrophages in virus-induced airway hyperresponsiveness and neuronal M2 muscarinic receptor dysfunction. Am J Physiol 2004; 286: L1255–9

49. Lim S, Caramori G, Tomita K, et al. Differential expression of IL-10 receptor by epithelial cells and alveolar macrophages. Allergy 2004; 59: 505–14

50. Vancheri C, Mastruzzo C, Sortino MA, et al. The lung as a privileged site for the beneficial actions of PGE2. Trends Immunol 2004; 25: 40–6

51. Mantovani A, Locati M, Vecchi A, et al. Decoy receptors: a strategy to regulate inflammatory cytokines and chemokines. Trends Immunol 2001; 22: 328–36

52. Gosset P, Tillie-Leblond I, Oudin S, et al. Production of chemokines and proinflammatory and antiinflammatory cytokines by human alveolar macrophages activated by IgE receptors. J Allergy Clin Immunol 1999; 103: 289–97

53. Tsuchiya S, Kobayashi Y, Goto Y, et al. Induction of maturation in cultured human monocytic leukemia cells by a phorbol diester. Cancer Res 1982; 42: 1530–6

54. Takashiba S, Van Dyke TE, Amar S, et al. Differentiation of monocytes to macrophages primes cells for lipopolysaccharide stimulation via accumulation of cytoplasmic nuclear factor kappa B. Infect Immun 1999; 67: 5573–8

55. Auwerx J. The human leukemia-cell line, THP-1 – a multifaceted model for the study of monocyte–macrophage differentiation. Experientia 1991; 47: 22–31

56. Ziegler-Heitbrock HW, Thiel E, Futterer A, et al. Establishment of a human cell line (Mono Mac 6) with characteristics of mature monocytes. Int J Cancer 1988; 41: 456–61

57. Pirhonen J, Sareneva T, Kurimoto M, et al. Virus infection activates IL-1 beta and IL-18 production in human macrophages by a caspase-1-dependent pathway. J Immunol 1999; 162: 7322–9

58. Hart PH, Bonder CS, Balogh J, et al. Differential responses of human monocytes and macrophages to IL-4 and IL-13. J Leukoc Biol 1999; 66: 575–8

59. Watanabe K, Jose PJ, Rankin SM. Eotaxin-2 generation is differentially regulated by lipopolysaccharide and IL-4 in monocytes and macrophages. J Immunol 2002; 168: 1911–18

60. Haugen TS, Nakstad B, Skjonsberg OH, et al. CD14 expression and binding of lipopolysaccharide to alveolar macrophages and monocytes. Inflammation 1998; 22: 521–32

61. Akagawa KS. Functional heterogeneity of colony-stimulating factor-induced human monocyte-derived macrophages. Int J Hematol 2002; 76: 27–34

62. Johnston SL, Pattemore PK, Sanderson G, et al. Community study of role of viral infections in exacerbations of asthma in 9–11 year old children. BMJ 1995; 310: 1225–9

63. Cox NJ, Subbarao K. Influenza. Lancet 1999; 354: 1277–82

64. Rodgers BC, Mims CA. Influenza virus replication in human alveolar macrophages. J Med Virol 1982; 9: 177–84

65. Sareneva T, Matikainen S, Kurimoto M, et al. Influenza A virus-induced IFN-alpha/beta and IL-18 synergistically enhance IFN-gamma gene expression in human T cells. J Immunol 1998; 160: 6032–8

66. Horisberger MA. Interferons, Mx genes, and resistance to influenza virus. Am J Respir Crit Care Med 1995; 152: S67–71

67. Garcia-Sastre A, Durbin RK, Zheng H, et al. The role of interferon in influenza virus tissue tropism. J Virol 1998; 72: 8550–8

68. Durbin JE, Fernandez-Sesma A, Lee CK, et al. Type I IFN modulates innate and specific antiviral immunity. J Immunol 2000; 164: 4220–8

69. Bergmann M, Garcia-Sastre A, Carnero E, et al. Influenza virus NS1 protein counteracts PKR-mediated inhibition of replication. J Virol 2000; 74: 6203–6

70. Donelan NR, Dauber B, Wang X, et al. The N- and C-terminal domains of the NS1 protein of influenza B virus can independently inhibit IRF-3 and beta interferon promoter activation. J Virol 2004; 78: 11574–82

71. Talon J, Salvatore M, O'Neill RE, et al. Influenza A and B viruses expressing altered NS1 proteins: a vaccine approach. Proc Natl Acad Sci USA 2000; 97: 4309–14

72. Sigurs N, Gustafsson PM, Bjarnason R, et al. Severe respiratory syncytial virus bronchiolitis in infancy and asthma and allergy at age 13. Am J Respir Crit Care Med 2005; 171: 137–41

73. Aherne W, Bird T, Court SD, et al. Pathological changes in virus infections of the lower respiratory tract in children. J Clin Pathol 1970; 23: 7–18

74. Panuska JR, Cirino NM, Midulla F, et al. Productive infection of isolated human alveolar macrophages by respiratory syncytial virus. J Clin Invest 1990; 86: 113–19

75. Cirino NM, Panuska JR, Villani A, et al. Restricted replication of respiratory syncytial virus in human alveolar macrophages. J Gen Virol 1993; 74: 1527–37

76. Domurat F, Robert NJ Jr, Walsh EE, et al. Respiratory syncytial virus infection of human mononuclear leukocytes in vitro and in vivo. J Infect Dis 1985; 152: 895–902

77. Yui I, Hoshi, A, Shigeta Y, et al. Detection of human respiratory syncytial virus sequences in peripheral blood mononuclear cells. J Med Virol 2003; 70: 481–9

78. Stadnyk AW, Gillan TL, Anderson R. Respiratory syncytial virus triggers synthesis of IL-6 in BALB/c mouse alveolar macrophages in the absence of virus replication. Cell Immunol 1997; 176: 122–6

79. Miller AL, Bowlin TL, Lukacs NW. Respiratory syncytial virus-induced chemokine production: linking viral replication to chemokine production in vitro and in vivo. J Infect Dis 2004; 189: 1419–30

80. Becker S, Quay J, Soukup J. Cytokine (tumor necrosis factor IL-6, and IL-8) production by respiratory syncytial virus-infected human alveolar macrophages. J Immunol 1991; 147: 4307–12

81. Haeberle HA, Takizawa R, Casola A, et al. Respiratory syncytial virus-induced activation of nuclear factor-kappaB in the lung involves alveolar macrophages and toll-like receptor 4-dependent pathways. J Infect Dis 2002; 186: 1199–206

82. Hall CB, Walsh EE, Long CE, et al. Immunity to and frequency of reinfection with respiratory syncytial virus. J Infect Dis 1991; 163: 693–8

83. Bartz H, Buning-Pfaue F, Turkel O, et al. Respiratory syncytial virus induces prostaglandin E2, IL-10 and IL-11 generation in antigen presenting cells. Clin Exp Immunol 2002; 129: 438–45

84. Panuska JR, Merolla R, Rebert NA, et al. Respiratory syncytial virus induces interleukin-10 by human alveolar macrophages. Suppression of early cytokine production and implications for incomplete immunity. J Clin Invest 1995; 96: 2445–53

85. Spann KM, Tran KC, Chi B, et al. Suppression of the induction of alpha, beta, and lambda interferons by the NS1 and NS2 proteins of human respiratory syncytial virus in human epithelial cells and macrophages [corrected]. J Virol 2004; 78: 4363–9

86. Lo MS, Brazas RM, Holtzman MJ. Respiratory syncytial virus nonstructural proteins NS1 and NS2 mediate inhibition of Stat2 expression and alpha/beta interferon responsiveness. J Virol 2005; 79: 9315–19

87. Papadopoulos NG, Bates PJ, Bardin PG, et al. Rhinoviruses infect the lower airways. J Infect Dis 2000; 181: 1875–84

88. Papi A, Johnston SL. Rhinovirus infection induces expression of its own receptor intercellular adhesion molecule 1 (ICAM-1) via increased NF-kappaB-mediated transcription. J Biol Chem 1999; 274: 9707–20

89. Terajima M, Yamaya M, Sekizawa K, et al. Rhinovirus infection of primary cultures of human tracheal epithelium: role of ICAM-1 and IL-1beta. Am J Physiol 1997; 273: L749–59

90. Schroth MK, Grimm E, Frindt P, et al. Rhinovirus replication causes RANTES production in primary bronchial epithelial cells. Am J Respir Cell Mol Biol 1999; 20: 1220–8

91. Message SD, Johnston SL. Host defense function of the airway epithelium in health and disease: clinical background. J Leukoc Biol 2004; 75: 5–17

92. Calhoun WJ, Dick EC, Schwartz LB, et al. A common cold virus, rhinovirus 16, potentiates airway inflammation after segmental antigen bronchoprovocation in allergic subjects. J Clin Invest 1994; 94: 2200–8

93. Tracey KJ, Cerami A. Tumor necrosis factor, other cytokines and disease. Annu Rev Cell Biol 1993; 9: 317–43

94. Gern JE, Dick EC, Lee WM, et al. Rhinovirus enters but does not replicate inside monocytes and airway macrophages. J Immunol 1996; 156: 621–7

95. Johnston SL, Papi A, Monick MM, et al. Rhinoviruses induce interleukin-8 mRNA and protein production in human monocytes. J Infect Dis 1997; 175: 323–9

96. Gern JE, Vrtis R, Kelly EA, et al. Rhinovirus produces nonspecific activation of lymphocytes through a monocyte-dependent mechanism. J Immunol 1996; 157: 1605–12

97. Hall DJ, Bates ME, Guar L, et al. The role of p38 MAPK in rhinovirus-induced monocyte chemoattractant protein-1 production by monocytic-lineage cells. J Immunol 2005; 174: 8056–63

98. Papadopoulos NG, Stanciu LA, Papi A, et al. A defective type 1 response to rhinovirus in atopic asthma. Thorax 2002; 57: 328–32

99. Papadopoulos NG, Stanciu LA, Papi A, et al. Rhinovirus-induced alterations on peripheral blood mononuclear cell phenotype and costimulatory molecule expression in normal and atopic asthmatic subjects. Clin Exp Allergy 2002; 32: 537–42

100. Zhu Z, Tang W, Ray A, et al. Rhinovirus stimulation of interleukin-6 in vivo and in vitro. Evidence for nuclear factor kappa B-dependent transcriptional activation. J Clin Invest 1996; 97: 421–30

101. Laza-Stanca V, et al. Rhinovirus replication in human macrophages induces NF-kappaB dependent TNF-alpha production. J Immunol 2006; 80: in press

PART IV

In vivo experimental models of asthma exacerbations

CHAPTER 14

Murine models of allergen exposure and virus infection

Azzeddine Dakhama and Erwin W Gelfand

INTRODUCTION

Asthma is a chronic disease of the airways characterized by reversible airflow obstruction, airway hyperresponsiveness (AHR) and persistent airway inflammation. Most patients with asthma can trace the origin of their disease to early childhood. While the etiological factors responsible for the onset of asthma remain largely unknown, considerable progress has been made towards identifying potential mechanisms involved in the maintenance or exacerbation of the disease. A variety of environmental factors can influence the activity of the disease in susceptible individuals. Among these factors, allergens and respiratory viruses are the best-known triggers of asthma exacerbations both in children and in adults.

Most commonly, asthma is described as being the result of an imbalanced T helper type 1 (Th1)–Th2 immune regulation, resulting in increased production of Th2 cytokines associated with increased immunoglobulin E (IgE) levels and development of airway eosinophilia. This response is driven for the most part by allergen-specific CD4+ T helper cells. Apparently, allergen exposure via mucosal surfaces such as the respiratory epithelium favors immune responses associated with the development of Th2 cells.[1,2] However, the airway mucosa is also the portal of entry for common respiratory pathogens such as viruses, which are known to induce a predominant Th1 response in the lung. Based on the

conventional dogma that Th1 and Th2 immune responses can be cross-regulated by their respective characteristic cytokines,[3] viral respiratory infections have been regarded in a generalized fashion as an opposing factor to the development of allergic airway diseases, although they are known to exacerbate asthma symptoms.

Geographically, there is no evidence of differences in the prevalence of viral respiratory infections. However, in most developed countries, the prevalence of Th2-associated allergic airway disorders, including asthma, has increased at an alarming rate over the past decades.[4] Because such increases cannot simply be explained by genetic factors, with natural mutations occurring at very low rates in humans, altered environmental/lifestyle conditions have been considered as potential factors to explain the increased prevalence of asthma worldwide.

Epidemiological studies have indeed provided evidence that suggests a possible link between the increasing incidence of allergic asthma and the lack of individual and natural exposure to microbial pathogens including viruses, which are considered to be the prototypic inducers of Th1-biased immune responses.[5] The 'hygiene' hypothesis thus proposes that early exposure of children to microbial pathogens (viruses and bacteria) or their products (endotoxin, CpG-DNA, dsRNA) may protect against the development of asthma and other allergic disorders.[6–8] However, this notion is challenged by clinical as well as experimental data supporting a role for respiratory viruses not only as promoters of allergic sensitization and asthma,[9–11] but also as triggers of asthma exacerbations both in children and in adults.[12,13]

Nonetheless, the difficulty in human studies remains: how to relate the onset of a disease or an exacerbation of established airway disease to an associated respiratory pathogen? Respiratory pathogens can be found ubiquitously in the human respiratory tract and hence might be considered 'guilty' by association only. Viruses in particular are highly opportunistic pathogens as they are absolutely dependent on the host for survival. A difference in the prevalence of viral infection between healthy subjects and individuals with established airway disease could be related to differences in host response, the latter individuals being more permissive towards developing such infections.

To establish pathogen causation in disease, one must satisfy Koch's postulates by demonstrating that the causative pathogen (a) is frequently associated with the disease; (b) is isolated from the affected tissue or organ; (c) initiates the disease when introduced to a host; and (d) is recovered again from the affected tissue or organ of the host. For the most part, due to a number of ethical issues, not all of these postulates can be satisfied in human studies. In addition, the heterogeneity of the disease and variability in host response make it difficult to establish a consensus on basic underlying mechanisms. To overcome some of these limitations, experimental animal models become very useful for investigating potential mechanisms of complex human airway diseases such as asthma and can help provide proof of concept for rational therapy.

MURINE MODELS OF AIRWAY ALLERGEN EXPOSURE

A hallmark of reactive airway diseases such as asthma is AHR. In humans, this altered airway function is best assessed by measuring the extent of bronchoconstriction produced after inhalation challenge of the airways with pharmacological stimuli such as methacholine (MCh), a cholinergic agonist which induces airway smooth muscle contraction. Classically, the pathophysiology of asthma is thought to be driven by a Th2-dominated inflammatory airway response, leading to the development of airway tissue eosinophilia and AHR. Several animal species have been used to model these aspects of the pathophysiology of bronchial asthma, with the ultimate goal of defining potential mechanisms underlying the human disease. Mice are the most widely used animal species because of numerous advantages including a well-described genome, fully characterized immune system, and the availability of immunological reagents and genetically modified strains to study a particular pathway or function. However, like many laboratory animals, mice do not spontaneously develop asthma. Asthma is a human disease and it is well recognized that 'man is the best model of human disease'.[14] Nonetheless, studies in humans are limited and murine models provide unique opportunities to study several aspects of the disease owing to the availability of selective immunological and pharmacological reagents, and genetically modified strains. In addition, these murine models allow for more thorough assessments of morphological, immunological and physiological changes in the airways that can mimic some of the characteristic features of human asthma pathophysiology. Most importantly, assessment of airway function in mice is no longer a challenge, owing to considerable technological advances recently achieved in animal physiology.[15]

The usefulness of murine models to study allergic asthma has recently been reviewed and discussed.[16] Often, allergen-sensitized and airway-challenged animals are described as models of 'asthma'. At most, and more precisely, these models mimic and should be referred to as models of allergic airway inflammation and AHR, emphasizing the two major components of allergic asthma. These pathophysiological responses are generally induced in mice by sensitization to an allergen, which elicits an allergen-specific T-cell response accompanied by the development of an allergen-specific IgE antibody response. Sensitization can be carried out in various ways, most often systemically, by intraperitoneal or subcutaneous administration of the allergen pre-mixed with an adjuvant (e.g. aluminum hydroxide). Sensitized animals are then exposed to the allergen, which is introduced to the airways by inhalation (as an aerosol), intranasally, or by intratracheal routes. Similar to the response seen in human allergic asthma, airway allergen challenge can elicit allergen-specific early- and late-phase responses in sensitized mice.[17] In this system, the early-phase response, which develops during the first 30 minutes, peaking at around 15 minutes following airway allergen challenge, is blocked by cromoglycate and albuterol. This response is followed by a late-phase response, which peaks at about 6 hours following allergen challenge, and is preventable by anti-inflammatory steroids.

Also, similar to the response elicited by segmental airway allergen challenge in asthma patients, an early but transient neutrophilic airway response can be observed following allergen challenge in sensitized mice.[18] This response is allergen-specific and appears to be mediated by allergen-specific IgG antibodies in an FcγIII receptor-dependent manner.

Interestingly, although an allergen-specific late-phase response can occur during the same period of time following allergen challenge, the recruited neutrophils do not seem to be required for the development of AHR in this allergen challenge model.[19] Temporally, when followed after a single intranasal allergen challenge, AHR developed following the decline of the neutrophilic response, peaking at 48 hours, and was paralleled by a concomitant accumulation of eosinophils in the airways.[20] Although bronchoalveolar lavage (BAL) eosinophilia persisted for up to 1 week after the single intranasal allergen challenge, airway tissue eosinophilia

followed a similar pattern of resolution as seen for AHR (Figure 14.1). Importantly, eosinophil activation, as detected by increased BAL levels of eosinophil peroxidase, was maximal at 48 hours after intranasal challenge, when AHR was also maximal. Although the appearance of lymphocytes was delayed in the BAL, their accumulation and activation in tissue probably occurred much earlier, as indicated by increased BAL levels of the predominantly T-cell cytokines interleukin (IL)-4 and IL-13, which peaked at 24 hours and 48 hours, respectively, after intranasal allergen challenge. Most remarkably, mucus production as reflected by the number of goblet cells increased to maximum levels by 96 hours and was maintained for up to 8 days after allergen challenge, while AHR began to decline and ultimately resolved during this period. These findings illustrate the dissociation between mucus production and AHR and support the notion that it is not necessarily the quantity (amount), but the quality (type and activation) of the cellular inflammatory response that determines the pathophysiology of AHR.

It is noteworthy that, although allergen-specific IgE antibodies are a major component of the allergic airway response in the murine model, neither IgE,[21] nor B cells[22] or mast cells,[23] are required for the development of a Th2 response in the lung or AHR if the mice are systemically sensitized to allergen with the use of an adjuvant such as alum. However, in the absence of systemic sensitization, repeated airway allergen challenge leads to the development of a rather modest airway inflammatory response, low levels of allergen-specific IgE and altered airway function that can best be detected by monitoring contractile responses of isolated tracheal smooth muscle segments to electrical field stimulation *in vitro*.[24] This altered airway responsiveness is dependent on IgE and is caused by increased acetylcholine release from stimulated airway cholinergic nerve fibers, which is due to altered muscarinic M2 acetylcholine receptor function.[25] Moreover, CD8+ T cells appear to be the major T-cell subset mediating this altered response following allergic

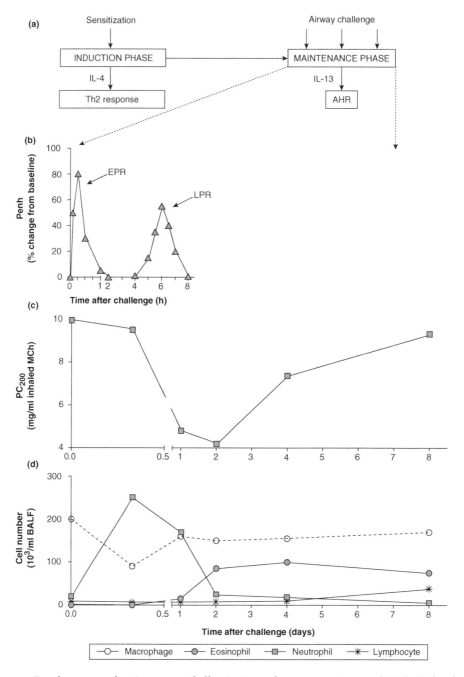

Figure 14.1 Development and maintenance of allergic airway hyperresponsiveness (AHR). Under the influence of genetic and environmental factors, allergic sensitization occurs during the induction phase leading to interleukin (IL)-4-dependent development of a Th2 response (a). This response is subsequently established in the lung, leading to IL-13-dependent development of AHR following airway allergen challenge. This challenge phase triggers early (EPR) and late (LPR) phase responses (b), which are antigen-specific and occur during the

248

sensitization through the airways.[26] Further characterization of this allergen challenge model has led to the uncovering of an IgE-mediated, mast cell- and IL-13-dependent mechanism of allergen-induced airway dysfunction.[27] Thus, following repeated allergen airway exposure without systemic sensitization, interaction of allergen-specific IgE with its high-affinity receptor FcεRI on mast cells leads to the development of altered airway function in an IL-13-dependent manner. Unpredictably, although mast cells have the capacity to produce IL-13, the data suggested that another cellular source of IL-13 was essential to the response. These findings implied that a mast cell mediator(s) was required in the response leading to IL-13 production and AHR in this model. This mediator could be required for the activation of CD8+ T cells, which were shown to be involved in the response using the same allergen challenge model.[26]

T cells play an important, if not essential, role in the development of allergic immune responses. Murine models have been pivotal in defining the role of T cells in allergic airway responsiveness. The importance of αβ CD4+ T cells in the development of these responses is now well established. These cells initiate an inflammatory response after recognition of antigen determinants that are presented by MHC class II molecules on the surface of antigen-presenting cells. In the context of an allergic response, these T cells differentiate into a type-2 cytokine-producing phenotype characterized by secretion of IL-4, IL-5, IL-9 and IL-13.[28] IL-4 is required for the development of a Th2 response,[29] at least during the induction phase

(i.e. initial sensitization), whereas IL-5 and IL-13, but not IL-4, appear to be required for the maintenance phase (i.e. airway challenge) of allergic airway disease.[30–33] In addition to promoting mucus production, IL-13 plays a downstream role in AHR by affecting airway smooth muscle function.[34] In addition to Th2-differentiated CD4+ T cells, CD8+ T cells,[35] natural killer (NK) T cells,[36] mast cells, basophils and eosinophils[37] are all potential sources of IL-13 in vivo.

Because of these distinct requirements for IL-4 and IL-13 and the emerging data that CD4+ T cells are more involved in the induction phase and less so during the maintenance phase,[38] this suggests that other cell types may be involved in the maintenance or progression phase of continuing AHR and structural alterations of the airways. αβ CD8+ T cells have been defined as suppressor T cells, capable of reducing airway inflammation and hyperresponsiveness.[39] Classically, αβ CD8+ T cells recognize antigens presented in the context of MHC class I molecules and are mostly known for their defensive role during infection. However, similar to CD4+ T cells, CD8+ T cells can develop into type-1 cytokine (interferon (IFN)-γ-producing (Tc1) or type-2 cytokine (IL-4, IL-5, IL-13)-producing (Tc2) subsets. Recent observations suggested that in vivo primed antigen-specific CD8+ T cells are required for the full development of allergic AHR.[35] Indeed, CD8-deficient mice develop lower airway eosinophilia, IL-13 levels and AHR following sensitization and airway allergen challenge. Full responsiveness can be restored in these mice by adoptive transfer of antigen-primed

Figure 14.1 (Continued)

first hours of airway allergen exposure, followed by the development of AHR to non-specific stimuli such as the cholinergic agonist methacholine (MCh), which develops 24–48 hours later (c). AHR is best determined by measuring changes in lung resistance, reflecting increased sensitivity and reactivity of the lower airways to MCh. Analyses of inflammatory cells recovered in bronchoalveolar lavage fluid (BALF) show an early but transient influx of neutrophils, peaking at 8 hours after airway challenge, followed by the appearance of eosinophils and lymphocytes at later time points (d). In tissue, however, eosinophils and lymphocytes are both recruited and activated at earlier time points (24 hours after airway allergen challenge). Penh, enhanced pause; PC_{200}, dose of inhaled MCh causing 200% increase in lung resistance over baseline values

CD8+ T cells. In the lung, these cells are capable of producing IL-13 and promoting airway eosinophilia. Once primed, antigen-specific CD8+ T cells can develop into one of two memory phenotypes: central memory (T_{CM}) and effector memory (T_{EFF}) CD8 T cells. T_{CM} are CD44^{hi}/CD62L^{hi}/CCR7^{hi} and preferentially home to the lymph nodes, whereas T_{EFF} are CD44^{hi}/CD62L^{lo}/CCR7^{lo} and are efficiently recruited to non-lymphoid tissues and accumulate at sites of inflammation. Antigen-specific T_{CM} and T_{EFF} can be induced to differentiate *in vitro* by culture with IL-15 or IL-2, respectively. Interestingly, both subsets can produce large amounts of IFN-γ *in vitro*, but when adoptively transferred into allergen-sensitized CD8-deficient mice, T_{EFF} but not T_{CM} are recruited to the airways and shift their function to IL-13 production, resulting in enhanced AHR and eosinophilic inflammation following airway allergen challenge.[40] Factors involved in the selective recruitment of these T_{EFF} into the airways are not fully identified, but leukotriene B4 appears to be a major candidate as its high-affinity receptor BLT1 is preferentially expressed on T_{EFF}.[41] Importantly, mast cells can be a considerable source of leukotriene B_4 (LTB_4), which they release in an IgE-dependent and allergen-specific manner. *In vitro* studies have shown that IgE-mediated mast cell activation can initiate T_{EFF} cell migration in culture. These findings establish a functional link between mast cells, allergen-specific IgE, LTB_4 and its high-affinity receptor BLT1, and T_{EFF} in the development of allergic AHR (Figure 14.2).

MURINE MODELS OF VIRAL RESPIRATORY INFECTION

Viral respiratory tract infections are common to all ages. Respiratory viruses are usually shed through respiratory secretions and transmitted from one host to the next by fomites (hand-to-nose) or by inhalation of aerosols generated by sneeze or cough. The stability of respiratory viruses in aerosols is influenced by environmental factors such as temperature and humidity. Once transmitted to an exposed host, these viruses accomplish their first rounds of replication in the nasopharynx before spreading to the lower airways, where they first come in contact with the epithelium, the main portal of entry and site of replication in the lung. Generally, epithelial cells do not survive an acute viral infection but they are capable of signaling local (resident) and central immune systems through release of a variety of mediators. Inflammatory cells are then recruited to the site of infection and mount an antiviral response, which ultimately leads to clearance of the pathogen followed by recovery of normal airway structure and function. Incidentally, the lower respiratory tract is also the major site of airway inflammation and remodeling in asthma and chronic obstructive pulmonary disease (COPD), which are frequently exacerbated by viral respiratory tract infections. These infections can cause airway epithelial damage, airway inflammation and AHR. The extent and duration of these induced alterations, however, depend on the susceptibility of the host, the type and virulence of the virus and a variety of environmental factors.

Several animal species have been utilized to model viral respiratory tract infections in order to define immunological and pathophysiological aspects relevant to human disease. Accordingly, the choice of the virus is important and is generally based on its prevalence in human disease. On the other hand, the animal species is selected on the basis of its permissiveness to infection with the specific virus and its ability to reproduce characteristic aspects of the human disease. As with allergen exposure, mice offer numerous advantages that make them useful models on which to study the pathogenesis of viral respiratory infections. Infection of mice is generally carried out by intranasal instillation of the virus, which is then aspirated to the lower airways as the mice recover from light anesthesia. This inoculation procedure results in a viral lung infection

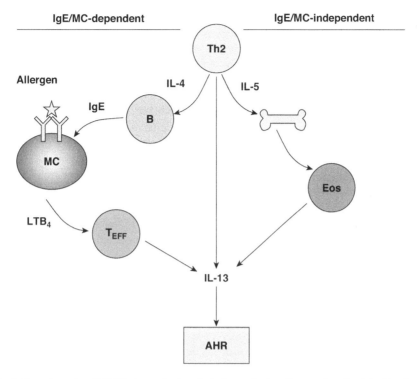

Figure 14.2 IgE- and mast cell (MC)-dependent and -independent pathways involved in the development of allergic airway hyperresponsiveness (AHR). Following active sensitization with use of adjuvant and subsequent airway allergen challenge, a strong T-cell-dependent AHR develops without a requirement for IgE or MCs. This IgE- and MC-independent development of allergic AHR is critically dependent on interleukin (IL)-13 and is associated with IL-5-dependent airway eosinophilia (Eos). In the absence of systemic sensitization with adjuvant, repeated airway exposure to allergen leads to local production of specific IgE antibodies, which sensitize airway MCs. Interaction of allergen with IgE on the surface of sensitized mast cells leads to degranulation of these cells and release of leukotriene B4 (LTB$_4$), which mediates the recruitment of antigen-specific memory CD8 T effector (T$_{EFF}$) cells. T$_{EFF}$ expressing the high-affinity receptor of LTB$_4$ (BLT1) are preferentially recruited to sites of airway tissue inflammation and are activated to produce IL-13, thereby contributing to the development of IgE- and MC-dependent AHR

that mimics an acute lower respiratory tract infection in humans. Following infection, the animals develop a response that can be evaluated at the cellular, biochemical and molecular levels in different anatomic locations and at different time points after infection. In addition, the precise pathways, mediators and potential therapeutic targets involved in the pathophysiology of the induced disease can be defined, depending on the availability of selective immunological reagents and genetic tools.

A variety of respiratory viruses have been used to study the pathogenesis and consequences of respiratory tract infections in mice. These include human viruses such as adenovirus,[42,43] respiratory syncytial virus (RSV)[44] and influenza virus,[45] and murine viruses such as Sendai virus (mouse parainfluenza type-1 virus) and pneumovirus (mouse equivalent of human respiratory syncytial virus). However, murine viruses can cause severe disease with significant mortality in immunocompetent mice,[46,47] an event that is rarely seen in humans infected with common human respiratory viruses. In addition, certain antiviral therapies directed more specifically against human respiratory viruses cannot be tested in these models using murine viruses. On the other hand, unlike natural hosts (i.e. humans) where they can replicate to high titers, not all human respiratory viruses can replicate in the mouse lung, and large doses of virus may be required to produce infection and initiate an immune response in mice. This is the case with human adenovirus (serotype 5), which failed to replicate in the lung of various strains of mice inoculated with up to 10^{10} plaque-forming units (PFUs), yet this high dose was required to produce a characteristic inflammatory cellular response (mainly pneumonia) in the lungs of these animals.[42] Such a non-permissive mouse model is nonetheless helpful to investigate early host response events to adenovirus infection and to define molecular mechanisms of adenovirus-mediated pneumonia that are independent of viral replication. By contrast with human adenovirus, human RSV is capable of actively replicating in the mouse lung[48] and an inflammatory cellular response can be initiated with as low as 10^5 PFUs without visible signs of clinical disease.[49]

However, the extent and duration of lung histopathology may vary with the dose, type and virulence of the virus. In mice, a high dose of RSV inoculum (e.g. 10^7–10^8 PFUs) may cause severe alveolitis with pneumonia,[50] whereas a lower dose (10^5–10^6 PFUs) mainly causes bronchiolitis with no alveolitis or pneumonia.[51] In children, RSV is known to cause most cases of bronchiolitis but pneumonia can also be associated with RSV infection. The latter could be related to viral load and to the ability of the host's antiviral response to restrict viral replication and spreading to the alveolar compartments of the lung. Therefore, the dose of viral inoculation should be taken into consideration in modeling aspects of human pathophysiology in animal models. In addition, the virus preparation needs to be purified free of culture-derived factors (cytokines, chemokines, etc.) that could potentially influence the host lung response when inoculated into the animals.

Respiratory viruses that enter the airways interact primarily with the airway epithelium, the primary site of viral replication, but it is also the source of a variety of mediators that initiate both innate and adaptive immune responses. Following viral infection, airway epithelial cells secrete type-I interferons (IFN-α/β), pro-inflammatory cytokines (tumor necrosis factor (TNF)-α, IL-1β) and various CC and CXC chemokines. Type-I IFNs act via autocrine mechanisms to inhibit viral replication in infected cells, but also by paracrine mechanisms to prevent the propagation of the virus to adjacent cells. These cytokines trigger intracellular antiviral pathways that lead to the degradation of viral RNA and inhibit viral replication in infected cells without the contribution of the immune system during the early time points of infection.

In parallel, the infected airway epithelial cells secrete IL-1β and TNF-α, which induce the expression of adhesion molecules on the surface of endothelial cells in adjacent blood vessels to allow for adhesion and transmigration of inflammatory cells to the sites of airway tissue infection. TNF-α also has cytocidal activities and can mediate lysis of infected cells to expose intracellular viral particles to the immune system. Under a co-ordinated action of chemokines secreted by infected epithelial cells, phagocytes (macrophages and neutrophils) and NK cells are attracted to the site of infection, where they recognize and kill infected target cells.

However, most viruses can escape this innate immune response, which is transient and antigen non-specific. For the host to remember a pathogen, an antigen-specific immune response follows after the innate response. This adaptive memory response is initiated by antigen-presenting cells which capture and select immunologically relevant viral antigens and present them to CD4 and CD8 T cells in the context of class II and class I major histocompatibility complex (MHC) molecules, respectively. Antigen presentation is further promoted by IFN-γ produced during the innate response by activated NK cells. During antigen presentation, T cells are instructed via a complex program involving cytokines and cognate interactions that lead to the development and establishment of antigen-specific T-cell responses. After a few rounds of clonal expansion, these T cells differentiate into cytokine-producing effector CD4 T cells and cytolytic CD8 T cells. The latter are specialized in killing of infected cells in an antigen-specific manner, via secretion of perforin and granzymes A and B.

In parallel, upon recognition of the appropriate viral antigen presented by B lymphocytes, antigen-specific CD4 T cells produce cognate help driving the proliferation and differentiation of antigen-specific naive B cells into memory B cells and antibody-forming plasma B cells. Depending on the nature of the antigen and cognate T-cell help, B cells produce antibodies that contribute to the antiviral response by neutralizing the virus, preventing it from propagating and infecting other cells, and by promoting antibody-dependent cell-mediated cytotoxicity and phagocytosis that play a role in removal of infected cells.

In general, viral replication peaks on days 3–4 after infection in the mouse lung, and clearance of the pathogen is usually achieved within 2 weeks after intranasal inoculation.[52–54] Studies in the guinea-pig suggested that RSV could establish a persistent lung infection; both viral RNA and proteins can be detected in the lung for up to 60 days after intranasal inoculation and low levels of replicating RSV can be recovered by culture at this same time point.[55,56] Using a polymerase chain reaction (PCR)-based detection method, recent studies in mice have shown that both genomic and messenger RNA encoding the G and F glycoproteins of RSV can be detected in the lung for at least 100 days after intranasal inoculation despite the presence of RSV-specific T cells;[57] however, replicating virus could not be recovered by culture from the lungs

of these animals unless T cells were depleted. These findings further suggest that RSV can persist in the mouse lung, but replication is restricted by the antiviral T-cell responses. Similar observations of persistent or latent viral infection have recently been reported in a mouse model of respiratory infection with human metapneumovirus.[58] In this study, replicating virus was recovered by culture from the lungs up to 60 days after intranasal inoculation, whereas genomic viral RNA could be detected in lung tissue (not in other organs) for at least 180 days after inoculation despite the presence of a sustained neutralizing antibody response. The mechanisms for this persistence are not known, but they may involve immune evasion via interference of non-structural NS1 and NS2 proteins with type I IFNs[59] or conformational changes to surface viral proteins making them less susceptible to binding of neutralizing antibodies.[60] The biological significance of virus persistence remains unknown and there is no current evidence to suggest that low-level replicating, persistent virus can cause chronic disease, even though virus-specific memory T cells can be present. Unless the virus persists in 'immunologically privileged' sites that may not be reached by inflammatory cells,[61] it might simply be ignored, because larger amounts of viral antigens could be necessary to induce signals that are required for recruitment and reactivation of memory T cells and induction of disease. On the other hand, viral persistence could play a role in the maintenance of T-cell memory to infection.[62]

During acute viral lung infection, disease can be abrogated by depletion of T cells despite prolonged viral replication, indicating that disease is caused by host response factors, which mainly involve the adaptive immune response. In this context, both CD4 and CD8 T cells have been implicated in the development of disease after viral respiratory infection in murine models. However, both cell types are also important in recovery from viral disease.[63] CD4 T cells orchestrate cellular and humoral immune responses associated with the production of antibodies that are involved in neutralization of the virus and in recognition and removal of infected target cells by phagocytes via antibody-dependent mechanisms. CD8 T cells play a critical role in direct killing of infected cells by exocytosis of cytotoxic granules and release of perforin and granzymes. This process involves recognition by clonally expressed T-cell receptors to a viral peptide presented in the context of MHC class I on the surface of infected cells. The common impression is that both CD4+ (Th1) and CD8+ (cytotoxic) T cells are needed for the development of an optimal immune response to viral infection. In the absence of either CD4 or CD8 T cells, mice infected with influenza or RSV can clear the virus and recover, although with delayed kinetics, suggesting the contribution of compensatory mechanisms involving host innate immunity.[52,64] Similarly, without antibodies mice can also clear the virus and recover after infection, with delayed kinetics.[65] Thus, a successful antiviral host response may rely on both innate and adaptive immune responses to clear the virus in an appropriate time frame, providing immunoprotection without causing significant immunopathology. In some cases immunopathology may persist longer after clearance of the pathogen as shown by studies of Sendai virus infection in mice.[66] Following infection with RSV there is no long-lasting immunity and re-infection can occur at all ages, even within the same RSV season and in each following season.

A recent study has shown that the pattern of BAL T-cell response to re-infection of adult mice varies depending on age at first infection by RSV.[67] Indeed, when mice were infected as newborns, but not at later ages, they developed a Th2-biased T-cell response associated with eosinophilia, a rarely seen event after primary RSV infection. Our recent studies have further demonstrated that neonatal RSV infection predisposes mice to an asthma-like phenotype with severe lung immunopathology when re-infected by this virus.[68] This response to RSV reinfection was characterized by the development of

enhanced AHR in association with increased IL-13 production, airway eosinophilia and mucus hyperproduction. By contrast, mice infected for the first time at weaning developed protective airway responses on re-infection with RSV, and no significant IL-13 production, eosinophilia, mucus or AHR could be detected in this age group. Thus, re-infection may have different outcomes depending on whether the host has mounted the appropriate primary response or not. In the case of RSV infection, age at initial RSV infection emerges as a major host factor in the development of altered airway responses and function at re-infection.

The development of altered airway function is perhaps the most serious complication of lower respiratory tract viral infection; it is a physiological reflection of virus-induced or host response-induced pathology. In murine models, airway function can be assessed in many different ways: (1) by measuring respiratory rates in unrestrained, spontaneously breathing animals using whole body plethysmography;[69] (2) by measuring airway smooth muscle responses to pharmacological agonists or to electrical field stimulation of isolated segments of mouse airways in vitro;[70] or (3) by measuring changes in lung resistance and dynamic compliance in response to cholinergic agonists, such as MCh, in anesthetized mechanically ventilated animals.[71] Each of these methods is linked to a particular experimental approach. Respiratory rates are controlled by neural mechanisms, but they can be influenced by nasal obstruction and are not directly related to airway mechanics. Assessment of airway function in vitro can reveal alterations in neurogenic control of airway smooth muscle function, detected for example after electrical stimulation, whereas in vivo assessment of airway responsiveness to MCh is most commonly used as a standard for detection of non-specific AHR, a hallmark of reactive airway diseases such as asthma. The inception of asthma is believed to take place during early childhood, at a time when lower respiratory tract viral infections play an important role.[72] At this age, RSV is known to be the major cause of bronchiolitis, which shares many similarities with asthma. Moreover, there is a potential link between RSV bronchiolitis and the subsequent development of asthma as suggested by several epidemiological and clinical studies.[73] This intriguing relationship is not well understood but a number of reasons have been proposed to explain the association. These include persistent viral infection, chronic airway inflammation and tissue remodeling and/or persistent AHR. As emphasized above, AHR is ultimately the most reliable marker of asthma. Using whole body plethysmography, a recent study monitored RSV-induced changes in Penh (enhanced pause) values at baseline and after a single dose of MCh challenge to evaluate airway obstruction and AHR, respectively, in unrestrained, spontaneously breathing mice.[74] The study reported that airway obstruction could last for up to 42 days, but AHR persisted for up to 154 days following a single infection with RSV. However, these findings need to be confirmed using standard invasive physiology measurements to determine whether these changes in Penh values are paralleled by similar changes in lung resistance, that is they occur in the lower airways of the infected animals. In addition, a full MCh dose–response curve needs to be established to support the notion of AHR, documenting changes in airway sensitivity and reactivity to the cholinergic agonist. Therefore, further studies paralleled by appropriate physiology assessments are required to determine whether persistent RSV infection is associated with persistent AHR.

AHR is usually detected at the peak of airway inflammation, i.e. on days 6–7 after infection, as documented in mouse studies of RSV infection by whole-body plethysmography, measuring changes in Penh,[49] or by invasive methods, measuring changes in lung resistance in response to inhaled MCh.[70] Both methods provided concordant results demonstrating that AHR and airway inflammation subsided by 3 weeks after RSV

infection in BALB/c mice. The mechanisms involved in the development of virus-induced AHR in mice are not fully understood. However, both neurogenic and inflammatory mechanisms could be involved.[75] We have recently shown that RSV infection alters the expression of airway sensory neuropeptides, causing significant increases in substance P but decreases in calcitonin gene-related peptide (CGRP) levels in the lungs of infected mice.[70] Using a selective antagonist of neurokinin-1, the high-affinity receptor of substance P, we showed that substance P contributes to the development of AHR following RSV infection in this model. Most remarkably, not only did AHR not develop in mice that received prophylactic administration of exogenous CGRP (before infection), AHR was completely abrogated by therapeutic administration of CGRP (post-infection) to RSV-infected mice, despite established airway inflammation and increased substance P levels. Thus, viral infection of the lower airways contributes to the development of AHR by altering airway neurogenic responses. Other mechanisms of virus-induced AHR may involve inflammatory cells and their mediators. T cells play important roles in viral infection. To examine the role of CD4 and CD8 T cells in the development of RSV-induced AHR, we used an antibody-mediated depletion approach. CD4 T cells were depleted using a rat antimouse CD4 monoclonal antibody. For CD8 T-cell depletion we used a rat monoclonal antibody directed against the CD8 β chain, because anti-CD8 α chain antibodies may also deplete other cells that express the CD8 α chain such as dendritic cells. Depletion of either T-cell subset produced only marginal effects on AHR during primary RSV infection in newborn and weanling mice: in both age groups, depletion of CD4 T cells attenuated whereas depletion of CD8 T cells exacerbated RSV-induced AHR. However, when T cells were depleted during primary RSV infection the effects on airway responses to re-infection were markedly enhanced.[76] In particular, depletion of CD4 T cells during primary neonatal RSV infection prevented the development of the asthma-like phenotype that develops following re-infection of the newborn. On the other hand, if CD4 T cells were depleted during primary infection of weanling mice, the animals were no longer protected against re-infection. Instead, they developed AHR, mucus hyperproduction and airway eosinophilia. Depletion of CD8 T cells during primary infection did not alter the outcome of airway responses to re-infection in both age groups. These new findings further establish the crucial role of CD4 T cells in the development or prevention of an asthma-like phenotype after re-infection with RSV. In the newborn, the asthma-like phenotype is initiated during primary RSV infection by CD4 T cells. At a later age, however, CD4 T cells are essential to the development of protective airway responses against re-infection.

CD8+ T cells play a crucial role in defense mechanisms against intracellular pathogens.[63] After encountering antigen, these cells differentiate into long-lived (memory) effector CD8+ T cells, which are retained preferentially in tissue for immediate protective responses against re-infection with the same pathogen.[77] Also, recent studies have suggested that pre-existing virus-specific memory CD8+ T cells can contribute to protective immunity against unrelated viral infections,[78] a mechanism termed 'heterologous' antiviral immunity. This can be a beneficial protective mechanism for the host, given the enormous diversity of viral pathogens. In addition, under the influence of an IL-4-rich Th2 environment, CD8 T cells can differentiate into type-2 cytokine (IL-5)-producing Tc2 cells that can mediate eosinophilia and contribute to an asthma-like response.[79] Under these particular circumstances, heterologous reactivation of memory T cells may also result in severe immunopathological responses, especially if these cells are biased in their response to express or exhibit unwanted/deleterious functions.

The role of Th2 cytokines in the development of AHR is well established for allergen exposure models. Among these cytokines, IL-13 plays a central role in mucus production by airway goblet cells and in the development of AHR.[80] Although RSV can induce IL-13 among other Th2 cytokines, IL-13 is not required for the development of AHR during primary RSV infection in mice.[81] This is in contrast to the requirement for IL-13 in the development of enhanced AHR, mucus hyperproduction and airway eosinophilia following re-infection of the newborn with RSV.[68] Virus-specific IgE antibodies can also contribute to the development of AHR,[82] further emphasizing the link between RSV bronchiolitis, wheezing and asthma (Figure 14.3). Further studies are necessary to fully define the mechanisms of virus-mediated AHR in these models.

In reality, humans are of a complex genetic background and differences in susceptibilities to viral infection may exist. In addition, humans are often exposed to multiple respiratory pathogens as well as innocuous allergens. The latter are of particular clinical importance because they can elicit long-lasting effects in sensitized hosts. For this reason, interactions between allergen and respiratory viruses have been the subject of numerous studies aimed at defining the mechanisms and consequences of such interactions on airway inflammation and airway function.

MURINE MODELS COMBINING ALLERGEN EXPOSURE AND VIRAL INFECTION

Murine models have also been developed to investigate the effects of combined, concomitant or sequential airway exposures to allergens and respiratory viruses on airway function and lung inflammation. Despite some disparities between the models, most studies demonstrated that viral respiratory infections enhanced allergen-induced AHR, establishing useful approaches to define mechanisms of virus-induced 'asthma' exacerbations. Several mechanisms have been proposed based on these studies to explain how viral infections

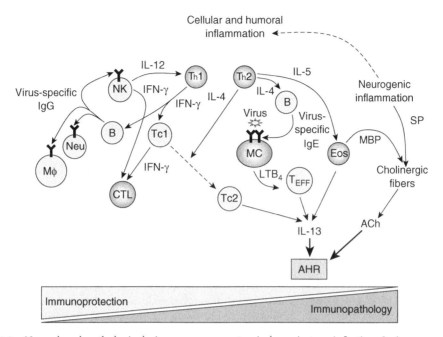

Figure 14.3 Normal and pathological airway responses to viral respiratory infection. In immunocompetent hosts, viral respiratory infections usually trigger a Th1-dominated airway inflammatory response associated with interferon (IFN)-γ-producing (Tc1) CD8 T cells, potent cytolytic T lymphocytes (CTL) and IgG neutralizing antibody-producing B cells. With concurrent activation of phagocytes (macrophages (Mφ), neutrophils (Neu)) and natural killer (NK) cells, these cells contribute to clearance of the virus and provide immunoprotection to the host without damaging the structure or function of the airways. Depending on the type and virulence of the virus and a number of host factors (age, genetic susceptibilities, etc.), altered airway responses may develop. These responses can be biased towards a Th2 phenotype that orchestrates the development of airway eosinophilia (Eos) and virus-specific IgE, which are capable of sensitizing mast cells (MC) to release mediators responsible for recruitment and activation of T_{EFF}. Under the influence of interleukin (IL)-4, a skewed Tc2 CD8 T-cell response may also develop. These cells are a potent source of IL-13, a central mediator of airway hyper-responsiveness (AHR) and a major regulator of mucus hyperproduction in the airways. These pathways are further amplified by a neurogenic inflammatory response also triggered by viral infection. Mediators of neurogenic inflammation, such as substance P (SP), and eosinophil-derived cationic proteins, such as major basic protein (MBP), also contribute to the development of virus-induced AHR by activating airway cholinergic fibers to release more acetylcholine (ACh). This asthma-like phenotype can persist following development of these type-2 (Th2/Tc2, IgE)-biased immune responses, potentially linking early-life viral respiratory tract infection to the development of childhood asthma in susceptible individuals

can mediate exacerbations.[10,83] The general impression is that inflammatory cellular responses, which develop during viral respiratory infection or allergen exposure, can be amplified via non-specific recruitment and activation of cells leading to excess inflammatory cell activation and enhanced AHR (Figure 14.4). In this context, chemokines may play important roles.[84–86] However, these interactions can be more complex and, depending on the type of virus and timing of infection and allergen exposure, enhancement or inhibition could be observed.[87–91]

Studies with RSV have shown that even after complete recovery from prior viral infection, AHR can be enhanced during subsequent

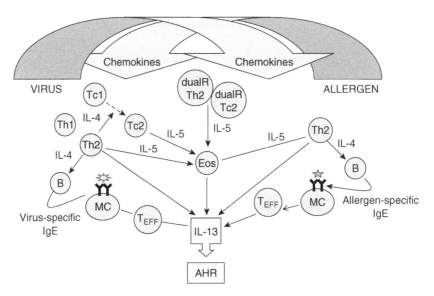

Figure 14.4 Virus-mediated triggering and exacerbation of allergic airway hyperresponsiveness (AHR). Depending on the type of virus, timing of infection and predisposing host factors, viral respiratory infections can trigger exacerbations of allergic AHR via induction of chemokines, type-2 cytokines and other inflammatory mediators leading to the development of enhanced AHR. In turn, airway allergen exposure can also lead to non-specific recruitment and bystander activation of Th2/Tc2-biased virus-specific cells, further augmenting the effects of allergen exposure in sensitized hosts. These altered airway responses could be further enhanced in the presence of dualR Th2 or Tc2 cells, which can be re-activated during viral infection or allergen exposure by both antigen-specific and non-specific (bystander) mechanisms. As a result, the 'dual' effects of virus infection and allergen exposure can lead to excessive generation of pro-asthma inflammatory mediators despite or in the presence of 'putatively protective' virus-mediated Th1 immune responses

exposure to allergen via a mechanism that appears to involve type-2 cytokine-producing CD8 T (Tc2) cells.[49,92,93] This was not the case in one study with influenza A virus, in which CD8 T cells retained in the lung after infection, or adoptively transferred, mediated suppression of allergic airway inflammation and AHR in the recipients, apparently through non-specific activation and IFN-γ secretion during allergen airway challenge.[94] However, other studies have shown that concurrent influenza A infection abrogates tolerance induced by intranasal exposure of sensitized mice to allergen.[95] Timing of allergen exposure appears to be critical in determining the effect of influenza A on the allergic response. Allergic airway inflammation is exacerbated and correlates with increased

recruitment of allergen-specific Th2 cells in mice exposed to allergen during acute influenza infection, whereas mice exposed to allergen after recovery from infection were protected against the development of airway eosinophilia.[96] Perhaps more surprising, allergic inflammation appeared to be enhanced by IFN-γ generated during Th1 responses to acute influenza A virus infection in mice,[97] a finding that challenges the 'hygiene' hypothesis of allergic airway disease.

It is generally believed that antigen-specific memory T cells are reactivated upon engagement of their T-cell receptor (TCR), usually with a single antigen. However, due to inefficient allelic exclusion of the TCRα chain, a proportion of mature T cells may express dual TCR and are potentially capable of responding to two (or more) unrelated antigens. This ability is thought to be beneficial for expanding the immune repertoire of TCRs specific for foreign antigens.[98] A model in which T cells express a dual TCR capable of recognizing two unrelated antigens with two specificities, one for a virus and one for an allergen, and which can undergo repetitive expansion and activation, has been proposed as a potential mechanism whereby viral infections influence the pathogenesis of allergic asthma.[99] In this study, dual TCR-expressing (dualR) T cells were isolated from spleen and lymph nodes of double TCR transgenic BALB/c mice obtained by crossing DO-11.10 BALB/c mice (transgenic for a TCR recognizing the I-A^d-restricted ovalbumin peptide 323–339) with influenza A hemagglutinin (HNT) BALB/c mice (transgenic for a TCR recognizing an I-A^d-restricted HNT peptide). The cells were activated with influenza A HNT and differentiated under polarizing conditions into dualR Th1 or Th2 phenotypes. When adoptively transferred into recipient BALB/c mice before sensitization to an allergen (e.g. ovalbumin), dualR Th1 cells but not Th2 cells inhibited the development of allergic airway inflammation and AHR in these mice following allergen inhalation. By contrast, when transferred into non-sensitized recipient mice, dualR Th2 but not Th1 cells mediated allergic airway inflammation and AHR following either viral infection or inhalation of ovalbumin. Thus, reactivation of virus-primed dualR Th2 cells through the allergen-specific TCR may lead to exaggerated allergic airway responses during allergen exposure. The counterpart is also true as, when allergen-primed dualR Th2 cells were reactivated through the virus-specific TCR, this resulted in the exacerbation of airway disease during viral infection.

THERAPEUTIC AVENUES BASED ON MURINE MODELS

Various therapeutic agents are now available for use either as intervention (reliever) or maintenance (controller) therapies for asthma. These include β_2-adrenergic receptor agonists with long-acting duration, inhaled and oral corticosteroids, theophylline, cromolyn and leukotriene modifiers. Specific immunotherapy and anti-IgE are also helpful therapies for allergic asthma. Because of the inflammatory nature of the disease, corticosteroids are considered to be the most effective medication recommended for persistent asthma. At conventional maintenance doses, however, inhaled corticosteroids usually fail to prevent exacerbations of asthma due to viral respiratory infections.[100,101]

Therefore, there is an important unmet need for the development of more effective therapies, without side-effects, for the prevention of these virus-induced episodes. Murine models offer unique opportunities to identify potential therapeutic targets based on advances gained from experimental studies of cellular and molecular mechanisms of virus- and/or allergen-mediated airway pathophysiology. In addition to developing and testing specific therapies (vaccines, specific antibodies, antiviral drugs, etc.) applicable to individual viruses or groups of viruses and other pathogens, a variety of immune cells (e.g. T cells) and inflammatory mediators (e.g. cytokines, chemokines, neuropeptides, leukotrienes, lipid mediators, etc.) or their receptors can be targeted for therapy. Once identified, the relevant targets could be evaluated for their potential as an interventional strategy. These strategies necessarily must be selective and specific without compromising the protective responses of the host or its vital lung functions.

ACKNOWLEDGMENTS

This work was supported by National Institutes of Health Grants HL-61005, HL-36577, AI-42246 and Environmental Protection Agency Grant R825702.

REFERENCES

1. Bochner BS, Undem BJ, Lichtenstein LM. Immunological aspects of allergic asthma. Annu Rev Immunol 1994; 12: 295–335

2. Constant SL, Lee KS, Bottomly K. Site of antigen delivery can influence T cell priming: pulmonary environment promotes preferential Th2-type differentiation. Eur J Immunol 2000; 30: 840–7

3. Morel PA, Oriss TB. Crossregulation between Th1 and Th2 cells. Crit Rev Immunol 1998; 18: 275–303

4. Redd SC. Asthma in the United States: burden and current theories. Environ Health Perspect 2002; 110: 557–60

5. Erb KJ. Atopic disorders: a default pathway in the absence of infection? Immunol Today 1999; 20: 317–22

6. Strachan DP. Hay fever, hygiene, and household size. BMJ 1989; 299: 1259–60

7. Illi S, von Mutius E, Lau S, et al. Early childhood infectious diseases and the development of asthma up to school age: a birth cohort study. BMJ 2001; 322: 390–5

8. Wills-Karp M, Santeliz J, Karp CL. The germless theory of allergic disease: revisiting the hygiene hypothesis. Nat Rev Immunol 2001; 1: 69–75

9. Gern JE, Busse WW. Relationship of viral infections to wheezing illnesses and asthma. Nat Rev Immunol 2002; 2: 132–8

10. Schwarze J, Gelfand EW. Respiratory viral infections as promoters of allergic sensitization and asthma in animal models. Eur Respir J 2002; 19: 341–9

11. Holtzman MJ, Shornick LP, Grayson MH, et al. 'Hit-and-run' effects of paramyxoviruses as a basis for chronic respiratory disease. Pediatr Infect Dis J 2004; 23: S235–45

12. Nicholson KG, Kent J, Ireland DC. Respiratory viruses and exacerbations of asthma in adults. BMJ 1993; 307: 982–6

13. Johnston SL, Pattemore PK, Sanderson G, et al. Community study of role of viral infections in exacerbations of asthma in 9–11 year old children. BMJ 1995; 310: 1225–9

14. Gelfand EW. Pro: mice are a good model of human airway disease. Am J Respir Crit Care Med 2002; 166: 5–6

15. Irvin CG, Bates JH. Measuring the lung function in the mouse: the challenge of size. Respir Res 2003; 4: 4

16. Taube C, Dakhama A, Gelfand EW. Insights into the pathogenesis of asthma utilizing murine models. Int Arch Allergy Immunol 2004; 135: 173–86

17. Cieslewicz G, Tomkinson A, Adler A, et al. The late, but not early, asthmatic response is dependent on IL-5 and correlates with eosinophil infiltration. J Clin Invest 1999; 104: 301–8

18. Taube C, Dakhama A, Rha YH, et al. Transient neutrophil infiltration after allergen challenge is dependent on specific antibodies and Fc gamma III receptors. J Immunol 2003; 170: 4301–9

19. Taube C, Nick JA, Siegmund B, et al. Inhibition of early airway neutrophilia does not affect development of airway hyperresponsiveness. Am J Respir Cell Mol Biol 2004; 30: 837–43

20. Tomkinson A, Cieslewicz G, Duez C, et al. Temporal association between airway hyperresponsiveness and airway eosinophilia in ovalbumin-sensitized mice. Am J Respir Crit Care Med 2001; 163: 721–30

21. Mehlhop PD, van de Rijn M, Goldberg AB, et al. Allergen-induced bronchial hyperreactivity and eosinophilic inflammation occur in the absence of IgE in a mouse model of asthma. Proc Natl Acad Sci USA 1997; 94: 1344–9

22. Hamelmann E, Takeda K, Schwarze J, et al. Development of eosinophilic airway inflammation and airway hyperresponsiveness requires interleukin-5 but not immunoglobulin E or B lymphocytes. Am J Respir Cell Mol Biol 1999; 21: 480–9

23. Takeda K, Hamelmann E, Joetham A, et al. Development of eosinophilic airway inflammation and airway hyperresponsiveness in mast cell-deficient mice. J Exp Med 1997; 186: 449–54

24. Hamelmann E, Tadeda K, Oshiba A, et al. Role of IgE in the development of allergic airway inflammation and airway hyperresponsiveness in a murine model. Allergy 1999; 54: 297–305

25. Larsen GL, Fame TM, Renz H, et al. Increased acetylcholine release in tracheas from allergen-exposed IgE-immune mice. Am J Physiol 1994; 266: L263–70

26. Hamelmann E, Oshiba A, Paluh J, et al. Requirement for CD8+ T cells in the development of airway hyperresponsiveness in a murine model of airway sensitization. J Exp Med 1996; 183: 1719–29

27. Taube C, Wei X, Swasey CH, et al. Mast cells, Fc epsilon RI, and IL-13 are required for development of airway hyperresponsiveness after aerosolized allergen exposure in the absence of adjuvant. J Immunol 2004; 172: 6398–406

28. Romagnani S. Cytokines and chemoattractants in allergic inflammation. Mol Immunol 2002; 38: 881–5

29. Kopf M, Le Gros G, Bachmann M, et al. Disruption of the murine IL-4 gene blocks Th2 cytokine responses. Nature 1993; 362: 245–8

30. Cohn L, Tepper JS, Bottomly K. IL-4-independent induction of airway hyperresponsiveness by Th2, but not Th1, cells. J Immunol 1998; 161: 3813–16

31. Tomkinson A, Kanehiro A, Rabinovitch N, et al. The failure of STAT6-deficient mice to develop airway eosinophilia and airway hyperresponsiveness is overcome by interleukin-5. Am J Respir Crit Care Med 1999; 160: 1283–91

32. Grunig G, Warnock M, Wakil AE, et al. Requirement for IL-13 independently of IL-4 in experimental asthma. Science 1998; 282: 2261–3

33. Taube C, Duez C, Cui ZH, et al. The role of IL-13 in established allergic airway disease. J Immunol 2002; 169: 6482–9

34. Wills-Karp M, Luyimbazi J, Xu X, et al. Interleukin-13: central mediator of allergic asthma. Science 1998; 282: 2258–61

35. Miyahara N, Takeda K, Kodama T, et al. Contribution of antigen-primed CD8+ T cells to the development of airway hyperresponsiveness and inflammation is associated with IL-13. J Immunol 2004; 172: 2549–58

36. Akbari O, Stock P, Meyer E, et al. Essential role of NKT cells producing IL-4 and IL-13 in the development of allergen-induced airway hyperreactivity. Nat Med 2003; 9: 582–8

37. Gessner A, Mohrs K, Mohrs M. Mast cells, basophils, and eosinophils acquire constitutive IL-4 and IL-13 transcripts during lineage differentiation that are sufficient for rapid cytokine production. J Immunol 2005; 174: 1063–72

38. Joetham A, Takeda K, Taube C, et al. Airway hyperresponsiveness in the absence of CD4+ T cells after primary but not secondary challenge. Am J Respir Cell Mol Biol 2005; 33: 89–96

39. Huang TJ, MacAry PA, Wilke T, et al. Inhibitory effects of endogenous and exogenous interferon-gamma on bronchial hyperresponsiveness, allergic inflammation and T-helper 2 cytokines in Brown-Norway rats. Immunology 1999; 98: 280–8

40. Miyahara N, Swanson BJ, Takeda K, et al. Effector CD8+ T cells mediate inflammation and airway hyper-responsiveness. Nat Med 2004; 10: 865–9

41. Miyahara N, Takeda K, Miyahara S, et al. Leukotriene B4 receptor-1 is essential for allergen-mediated recruitment of CD8+ T cells and airway hyperresponsiveness. J Immunol 2005; 174: 4979–84

42. Ginsberg HS, Moldawer LL, Sehgal PB, et al. A mouse model for investigating the molecular pathogenesis of adenovirus pneumonia. Proc Natl Acad Sci USA 1991; 88: 1651–5

43. Kajon AE, Gigliotti AP, Harrod KS. Acute inflammatory response and remodeling of airway epithelium after subspecies B1 human adenovirus infection of the mouse lower respiratory tract. J Med Virol 2003; 71: 233–44

44. Openshaw PJ. Immunity and immunopathology to respiratory syncytial virus. The mouse model. Am J Respir Crit Care Med 1995; 152: S59–62

45. Doherty PC, Hou S, Tripp RA. CD8+ T-cell memory to viruses. Curr Opin Immunol 1994; 6: 545–52

46. Lee HJ, Moody CT, Reiss CS, et al. Sendai virus infection of normal and protein malnourished mice: response of airway leukocytes to infection. Microb Pathog 1991; 11: 149–57

47. Bonville CA, Easton AJ, Rosenberg HF, et al. Altered pathogenesis of severe pneumovirus infection in response to combined antiviral and specific immunomodulatory agents. J Virol 2003; 77: 1237–44

48. Cook PM, Eglin RP, Easton AJ. Pathogenesis of pneumovirus infections in mice: detection of pneumonia virus of mice and human respiratory syncytial virus mRNA in lungs of infected mice by in situ hybridization. J Gen Virol 1998; 79: 2411–17

49. Schwarze J, Hamelmann E, Bradley KL, et al. Respiratory syncytial virus infection results in airway hyperresponsiveness and enhanced airway sensitization to allergen. J Clin Invest 1997; 100: 226–33

50. Bolger G, Lapeyre N, Dansereau N, et al. Primary infection of mice with high titer inoculum respiratory syncytial virus: characterization and response to antiviral therapy. Can J Physiol Pharmacol 2005; 83: 198–213

51. Makela MJ, Tripp R, Dakhama A, et al. Prior airway exposure to allergen increases virus-induced airway hyperresponsiveness. J Allergy Clin Immunol 2003; 112: 861–9

52. Wells MA, Albrecht P, Ennis FA. Recovery from a viral respiratory infection. I. Influenza pneumonia in normal and T-deficient mice. J Immunol 1981; 126: 1036–41

53. Graham BS, Perkins MD, Wright PF, et al. Primary respiratory syncytial virus infection in mice. J Med Virol 1988; 26: 153–62

54. Price GE, Gaszewska-Mastarlarz A, Moskophidis D. The role of alpha/beta and gamma interferons in development of immunity to influenza A virus in mice. J Virol 2000; 74: 3996–4003

55. Hegele RG, Hayashi S, Bramley AM, et al. Persistence of respiratory syncytial virus genome and protein after acute bronchiolitis in guinea pigs. Chest 1994; 105: 1848–54

56. Dakhama A, Vitalis TZ, Hegele RG. Persistence of respiratory syncytial virus (RSV) infection and development of RSV-specific IgG1 response in a guinea-pig model of acute bronchiolitis. Eur Respir J 1997; 10: 20–6

57. Schwarze J, O'Donnell DR, Rohwedder A, et al. Latency and persistence of respiratory syncytial virus despite T cell immunity. Am J Respir Crit Care Med 2004; 169: 801–5

58. Alvarez R, Harrod KS, Shieh WJ, et al. Human metapneumovirus persists in BALB/c mice despite the presence of neutralizing antibodies. J Virol 2004; 78: 14003–11

59. Spann KM, Tran KC, Chi B, et al. Suppression of the induction of alpha, beta, and lambda interferons by the NS1 and NS2 proteins of human respiratory syncytial virus in human epithelial cells and macrophages [corrected]. J Virol 2004; 78: 4363–9

60. Parren PW, Poignard P, Ditzel HJ, et al. Antibodies in human infectious disease. Immunol Res 2000; 21: 265–78

61. Ahmed R, Morrison LA, Knipe DM. Persistence of viruses. In Fields BN, Knipe DM, Howley PM, eds. Fields Virology. Philadelphia: Lippincott-Raven, 1996: 219–49

62. Doherty PC, Allan W, Eichelberger M, et al. Roles of alpha beta and gamma delta T cell subsets in viral immunity. Annu Rev Immunol 1992; 10: 123–51

63. Doherty PC, Topham DJ, Tripp RA, et al. Effector CD4+ and CD8+ T-cell mechanisms in the control of respiratory virus infections. Immunol Rev 1997; 159: 105–17

64. Graham BS, Bunton LA, Wright PF, et al. Role of T lymphocyte subsets in the pathogenesis of primary infection and rechallenge with respiratory syncytial virus in mice. J Clin Invest 1991; 88: 1026–33

65. Epstein SL, Lo CY, Misplon JA, et al. Mechanism of protective immunity against influenza virus infection in mice without antibodies. J Immunol 1998; 160: 322–7

66. Walter MJ, Morton JD, Kajiwara N, et al. Viral induction of a chronic asthma phenotype and genetic segregation from the acute response. J Clin Invest 2002; 110: 165–75

67. Culley FJ, Pollott J, Openshaw PJ. Age at first viral infection determines the pattern of T cell-mediated disease during reinfection in adulthood. J Exp Med 2002; 196: 1381–6

68. Dakhama A, Park JW, Taube C, et al. The enhancement or prevention of airway hyperresponsiveness during reinfection with respiratory syncytial virus is critically dependent on the age at first infection and IL-13 production. J Immunol 2005; 175: 1876–83

69. Tripp RA, Dakhama A, Jones LP, et al. The G glycoprotein of respiratory syncytial virus depresses respiratory rates through the CX3C motif and substance P. J Virol 2003; 77: 6580–4

70. Dakhama A, Park JW, Taube C, et al. Alteration of airway neuropeptide expression and development of airway hyperresponsiveness following respiratory syncytial virus infection. Am J Physiol 2005; 288: L761–70

71. Dakhama A, Kanehiro A, Makela MJ, et al. Regulation of airway hyperresponsiveness by calcitonin generelated peptide in allergen sensitized and challenged mice. Am J Respir Crit Care Med 2002; 165: 1137–44

72. Lemanske RF. Viral infections and asthma inception. J Allergy Clin Immunol 2004; 114: 1023–6

73. Sigurs N. Epidemiologic and clinical evidence of a respiratory syncytial virus-reactive airway disease link. Am J Respir Crit Care Med 2001; 163: S2–6

74. Jafri HS, Chavez-Bueno S, Mejias A, et al. Respiratory syncytial virus induces pneumonia, cytokine response, airway obstruction, and chronic inflammatory infiltrates associated with long-term airway hyperresponsiveness in mice. J Infect Dis 2004; 189: 1856–65

75. Jacoby DB. Virus-induced asthma attacks. J Am Med Assoc 2002; 287: 755–61

76. Dakhama A, El-Gazzar M, Joetham A, et al. Role of CD4 and CD8 T cells in the enhancement and prevention of airway hyperresponsiveness following reinfection with respiratory syncytial virus. Am J Respir Crit Care Med 2005; 2: A602

77. Masopust D, Vezys V, Marzo AL, et al. Preferential localization of effector memory cells in nonlymphoid tissue. Science 2001; 291: 2413–17

78. Chen HD, Fraire AE, Joris I, et al. Memory CD8+ T cells in heterologous antiviral immunity and immunopathology in the lung. Nat Immunol 2001; 2: 1067–76

79. Coyle AJ, Erard F, Bertrand C, et al. Virus-specific CD8+ cells can switch to interleukin 5 production and induce airway eosinophilia. J Exp Med 1995; 181: 1229–33

80. Wills-Karp M. Interleukin-13 in asthma pathogenesis. Immunol Rev 2004; 202: 175–90

81. Park JW, Taube C, Yang ES, et al. Respiratory syncytial virus-induced airway hyperresponsiveness is independent of IL-13 compared with that induced by allergen. J Allergy Clin Immunol 2003; 112: 1078–87

82. Dakhama A, Park JW, Taube C, et al. The role of virus-specific immunoglobulin E in airway hyperresponsiveness. Am J Respir Crit Care Med 2004; 170: 952–9

83. Herz U, Lacy P, Renz H, et al. The influence of infections on the development and severity of allergic disorders. Curr Opin Immunol 2000; 12: 632–40

84. Lett-Brown MA, Aelvoet M, Hooks JJ, et al. Enhancement of basophil chemotaxis in vitro by virus-induced interferon. J Clin Invest 1981; 67: 547–52

85. Stephens R, Randolph DA, Huang G, et al. Antigen-nonspecific recruitment of Th2 cells to the lung as a mechanism for viral infection-induced allergic asthma. J Immunol 2002; 169: 5458–67

86. John AE, Berlin AA, Lukacs NW. Respiratory syncytial virus-induced CCL5/RANTES contributes to exacerbation of allergic airway inflammation. Eur J Immunol 2003; 33: 1677–85

87. Matsuse H, Behera AK, Kumar M, et al. Recurrent respiratory syncytial virus infections in allergen-sensitized mice lead to persistent airway inflammation and hyperresponsiveness. J Immunol 2000; 164: 6583–92

88. Peebles RS Jr, Sheller JR, Collins RD, et al. Respiratory syncytial virus infection does not increase allergen-induced type 2 cytokine production, yet increases airway hyperresponsiveness in mice. J Med Virol 2001; 63: 178–88

89. Wohlleben G, Muller J, Tatsch U, et al. Influenza A virus infection inhibits the efficient recruitment of Th2 cells into the airways and the development of airway eosinophilia. J Immunol 2003; 170: 4601–11

90. Barends M, de Rond LG, Dormans J, et al. Respiratory syncytial virus, pneumonia virus of mice, and influenza A virus differently affect respiratory allergy in mice. Clin Exp Allergy 2004; 34: 488–96

91. Barends M, Van Oosten M, De Rond CG, et al. Timing of infection and prior immunization with respiratory syncytial virus (RSV) in RSV-enhanced allergic inflammation. J Infect Dis 2004; 189: 1866–72

92. Schwarze J, Makela M, Cieslewicz G, et al. Transfer of the enhancing effect of respiratory syncytial virus infection on subsequent allergic airway sensitization by T lymphocytes. J Immunol 1999; 163: 5729–34

93. Schwarze J, Cieslewicz G, Joetham A, et al. Critical roles for interleukin-4 and interleukin-5 during respiratory syncytial virus infection in the development of airway hyperresponsiveness after airway sensitization. Am J Respir Crit Care Med 2000; 162: 380–6

94. Marsland BJ, Harris NL, Camberis M, et al. Bystander suppression of allergic airway inflammation by lung resident memory CD8+ T cells. Proc Natl Acad Sci USA 2004; 101: 6116–21

95. Tsitoura DC, Kim S, Dabbagh K, et al. Respiratory infection with influenza A virus interferes with the induction of tolerance to aeroallergens. J Immunol 2000; 165: 3484–91

96. Marsland BJ, Scanga CB, Kopf M, et al. Allergic airway inflammation is exacerbated during acute influenza infection and correlates with increased allergen presentation and recruitment of allergen-specific T-helper type 2 cells. Clin Exp Allergy 2004; 34: 1299–306

97. Dahl ME, Dabbagh K, Liggitt D, et al. Viral-induced T helper type 1 responses enhance allergic disease by effects on lung dendritic cells. Nat Immunol 2004; 5: 337–43

98. He X, Janeway CA Jr, Levine M, et al. Dual receptor T cells extend the immune repertoire for foreign antigens. Nat Immunol 2002; 3: 127–34

99. Aronica MA, Swaidani S, Zhang YH, et al. Susceptibility to allergic lung disease regulated by recall responses of dual-receptor memory T cells. J Allergy Clin Immunol 2004; 114: 1441–8

100. Wilson N, Sloper K, Silverman M. Effect of continuous treatment with topical corticosteroid on episodic viral wheeze in preschool children. Arch Dis Child 1995; 72: 317–20

101. Doull IJ, Lampe FC, Smith S, et al. Effect of inhaled corticosteroids on episodes of wheezing associated with viral infection in school age children: randomized double blind placebo controlled trial. BMJ 1997; 315: 858–62

Lessons from human experimental rhinovirus infection in combination with allergen exposure

Robert F Lemanske Jr and William W Busse

INTRODUCTION

Viral respiratory tract infections have been epidemiologically associated with asthma in at least two major ways (Figure 15.1). First, during infancy, certain viruses have been implicated as potentially being responsible for the inception of the asthmatic phenotype. Second, in patients with established asthma, particularly children, viral upper respiratory tract infections play a significant role in producing acute exacerbations of airway obstruction that may result in frequent outpatient visits or in hospitalizations. The increased propensity for viral infections to produce lower airway symptoms in asthmatic individuals may be related, at least in part, to interactions among allergic sensitization, allergen exposure and viral infections that act as co-factors in the induction of acute episodes of airflow obstruction, and more prolonged physiological effects in the form of increased airway responsiveness that may change the airway threshold response to various environmental irritants or stimuli (e.g. exercise). This chapter highlights the latter associations by describing experiments performed in humans that have evaluated the interactions between the most common virus documented to induce asthma exacerbations, rhinovirus (RV), and aeroallergen exposure to ragweed in individuals sensitized to this pollen.[1]

BACKGROUND

Prior to the performance of the initial experiments evaluating the interactions between virus and allergen challenge on airway function, it had been demonstrated by some,[2–5] but not all investigators,[6,7] that viral upper respiratory tract infections in both normal and asthmatic individuals could enhance airway responsiveness to challenge with such chemical irritants as histamine or methacholine. However, the magnitude and duration of any observed change in responsiveness appeared to be influenced by a number of factors including the type and/or strain of virus, the severity of infection and the age of the patient.

Allergen inhalation challenge in previously sensitized individuals was also known to be followed by increases in airway responsiveness, particularly in individuals who developed biphasic alterations in airflow following allergen exposure (Figure 15.2).[8] These biphasic reactions consisted of an immediate (minutes) bronchospastic reaction, a return of airflow nearly back to baseline values, and then a second wave of airway obstruction that developed hours after the initial exposure. This latter limitation in airflow was termed a late-phase reaction, or late asthmatic response.[9] The late asthmatic response could persist for hours and, in contrast

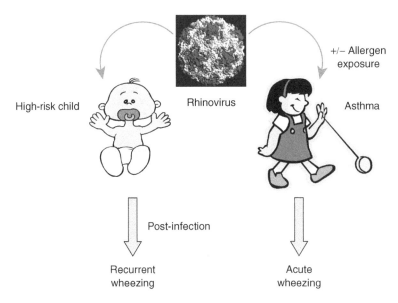

Figure 15.1 The role of rhinovirus in asthma

to an isolated immediate response, was characterized by an increase in airway responsiveness that could last for days and sometimes weeks following challenge.[10] The late asthmatic response was also demonstrated to be associated with an influx of inflammatory cells into the airway. Thus, both the physiological and inflammatory changes that ensued in association with the late asthmatic response highlighted it as a useful model for gaining improved insights into the pathophysiological mechanisms underlying chronic asthma, and for insight into how co-factors, such as viral infections, may interact with these allergen-driven responses to cause a more severe asthmatic reaction.

Indeed, both viral infections and allergen exposure were events commonly known to be associated with loss of symptom control in asthmatic patients that may be severe enough to lead to exacerbations requiring hospitalization. This loss of control was considered to be related to alterations in airway responsiveness acutely and/or chronically, thereby decreasing the threshold to the development of airflow limitation following exposure to a range of stimuli. Since airway hyperresponsiveness following allergen challenge appeared to be enhanced following a late asthmatic response (which occurred in about one-half of all subjects appropriately challenged), the relationships among viral infections, allergen exposure, the pattern of airway obstruction following these exposures and the potential for altering airway responsiveness were considered highly relevant for additional investigation.[1]

EXPERIMENTAL RHINOVIRUS INFECTION AND ALLERGEN EXPOSURE

At the time these experiments were conducted, it had already been established that RV infections were commonly involved in exacerbations of asthma. Thus, to maximize safety in these initial experiments, the individuals recruited for study ($n=10$) were subjects with allergic rhinitis, not asthma. There were eight males and two females (mean age 30.6 ± 2.2 years). All subjects had a positive immediate

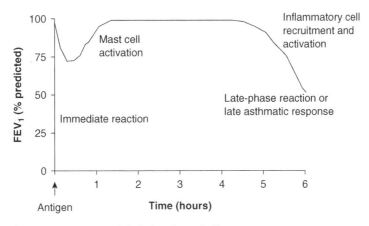

Figure 15.2 The airway response to an inhaled antigen challenge

skin test reaction to ragweed antigen, released leukocyte histamine after an *in vitro* incubation with ragweed antigen E and lacked neutralized antibody in their sera to rhinovirus 16 (RV16). None of the subjects smoked, and they were studied out of ragweed season. All subjects gave informed consent prior to enrollment.

The subjects were studied on three separate occasions, each 28 days apart, as indicated by the schematic protocol depicted in Figure 15.3: baseline, acute upper respiratory infection (URI) and recovery. At each study period, the subjects were evaluated on three consecutive days. Evaluations consisted of first, spirometry (forced expiratory volume in one second (FEV_1), forced vital capacity (FVC) and forced mid-expiratory flow ($FEF_{25–75\%}$)), which was performed during initiating bronchoprovocation studies; and second, airway responsiveness, which was measured by bronchoprovocation on separate days to aerosols of histamine (pre-antigen), ragweed antigen and histamine again (post-antigen). Airway responsiveness to histamine and ragweed antigen was determined by techniques considered to be standard at the time of the study.[11] Both histamine and antigen were administered in increasing doses until the FEV_1 fell at least 20% (PD_{20}) and was maintained at this level for at least 10 minutes. After antigen challenge,

pulmonary function evaluation was repeated at 0.5, 1, 2, 3, 4, 5 and 6 hours to determine whether a late asthmatic reaction had occurred (>15% decrease in FEV_1 from baseline values). Immediately after histamine-induced bronchoconstriction, increasing doses of isoproterenol were administered in order to evaluate maximum bronchodilatation and the concentration of isoproterenol that gave 50% maximum bronchodilatation.

The technique for RV inoculation followed previously described methodology.[12,13] Rhinoviral colds were induced in the subjects by instilling, on two consecutive days, suspensions of the virus (320–3200 $TCID_{50}$) in each nostril by pipette and then spraying approximately the same amount in each nostril with an atomizer powered by a compressor. Colds were evaluated by a questionnaire that was completed by the participant hourly during waking hours.[14] Using nasal lavage, virus shedding was evaluated using *in vitro* tissue culture methodology.[12] RV16 infection was confirmed as the etiology of the illness by obtaining at least one identified isolate and/or by a four-fold or greater increase in neutralizing antibody in the convalescent serum specimens.

Based on the definition above, all ten subjects studied were considered to have a RV infection

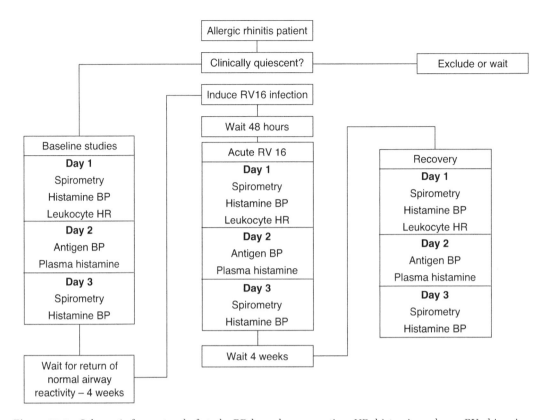

Figure 15.3 Schematic for protocol of study. BP, bronchoprovocation; HR, histamine release; RV, rhinovirus

at the time of study. Baseline spirometric values were similar at each of the three study periods: pre-infection, acute infection and post-infection, and were ≥95% of the predicted normal values for each subject. During the acute RV infection, airway responsiveness to histamine was significantly enhanced from baseline values (Figure 15.4). Only one of the subjects failed to show a fall in their histamine PD_{20} value during the acute RV infection. Airway responsiveness to ragweed antigen was also significantly enhanced over pre-infection values during the acute viral respiratory illness. When airway responsiveness to histamine was determined 24 hours after ragweed antigen challenge, a significant enhancement in airway responsiveness was noted at both baseline and during the RV infection. During the acute RV infection, airway responsiveness to

histamine, after ragweed antigen inhalation challenge, was also significantly enhanced when compared with its baseline counterpart. The relative enhancement of airway responsiveness to histamine after antigen challenge during the respiratory infection was similar to the changes in histamine responsiveness measured before viral infection.

Seven of the subjects were available for evaluation of airway responsiveness 4 weeks after virus infection (recovery period) (Figure 15.5). At this time point, airway responsiveness to histamine (pre-antigen) showed a return towards baseline values but was still significantly different from pre-infection determinants. The PD_{20} value for antigen at recovery was lower than baseline (indicating increased airway responsiveness), but differences were not significant.

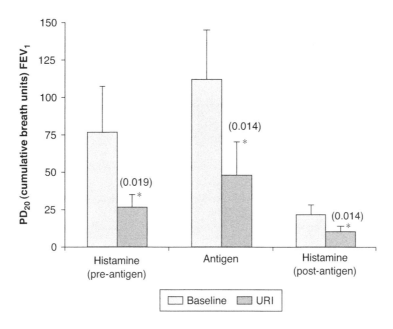

Figure 15.4 The effect of an acute rhinovirus respiratory infection on airway reactivity to histamine and ragweed antigen ($n = 10$, mean ± SEM). One inhalation unit equals one breath of a solution with 1 mg of histamine/ml or one breath of antigen extract with 1000 PNU/ml. URI, upper respiratory infection. *p value compare to baseline

In contrast, airway responsiveness to histamine post-challenge remained unchanged from values during the acute URI.

After bronchoprovocation with ragweed antigen, all subjects were evaluated for the development of late asthmatic reactions (LARs). At baseline evaluation (pre-infection), only one of the ten subjects had a LAR. When the same evaluation was performed during the acute RV infection, eight of the ten subjects had LARs (Figure 15.6). If the relationship between the development of a LAR was compared with indices of airway responsiveness, no correlations were found between the LAR and PD_{20} values for histamine or antigen, or between changes in those values from baseline measurements. This indicated that the development of a LAR was independent of enhanced airway responsiveness noted during the RV cold. Furthermore, although there was a trend towards a larger per cent fall in FEV_1 to inhaled antigen during the URI

compared to baseline, there was no significant positive correlation between the fall in FEV_1 to antigen at baseline or during the URI with the development of a LARs. Thus, this indicates that the development of a LAR was also independent of the intensity of the immediate response to antigen. Finally, during the recovery period, four of the seven subjects continued to demonstrate LARs and one additional subject developed a LAR after allergen challenge.

These latter findings indicate, in the allergic non-asthmatic individual, that viral infections have the propensity to alter the pattern of the lower airway response following antigen exposure, thereby favoring the development of late as opposed to isolated immediate responses. Since the late asthmatic response is associated with increases in airway inflammation and hyperresponsiveness, patients with allergic rhinitis could become transiently 'asthmatic' if they developed a rhinovirus infection, i.e. the

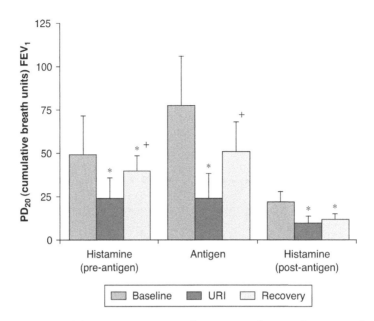

Figure 15.5 A comparison of the airway response to histamine and ragweed antigen at baseline, during an acute rhinovirus respiratory illness and 4 weeks later at recovery ($n=7$, mean ± SEM). URI, upper respiratory infection. *$p<0.05$ compared to baseline; +$p<0.05$ compared to URI

'common cold', and were simultaneously exposed to aeroallergens to which they had been previously sensitized. While the data reviewed previously indicate that these alterations would not be permanent, they would be expected to last for at least a number of weeks following the initial illness.

Based on this first experiment involving ten subjects, it was hypothesized that one mechanism by which the observed effects occurred could have been through augmented or altered mediator release by mast cells and/or basophils to favor the development of the LAR (Figure 15.7). Therefore, eight additional subjects with allergic rhinitis were studied before and during an experimentally induced RV16 infection.[15] Levels of plasma histamine and tryptase were determined, and the associated patterns of airway obstruction that developed following inhaled antigen challenge were observed. Bronchial responsiveness to histamine, methacholine and antigen were all significantly

increased during the RV16 illness. Further, reproducing the previous observations, the incidence of LAR was significantly higher (five of eight) during the infection than before. In addition, in those patients whose pattern of response following antigen challenge converted from an immediate response only before infection to a dual response (immediate plus late phase) during infection, plasma histamine concentrations after challenge were significantly greater than in those whose pattern of response did not change. It was concluded that one mechanism by which RV16 infection increases the likelihood of LAR could include enhanced mediator release from pulmonary mast cells or from circulating or recruited basophils.

These initial experiments involving whole-lung antigen challenge led to more mechanistic evaluations using the technique of segmental bronchial challenge (Figure 15.8) and lavage to evaluate cellular influx and mediator release within the airway.[16] It was hypothesized that

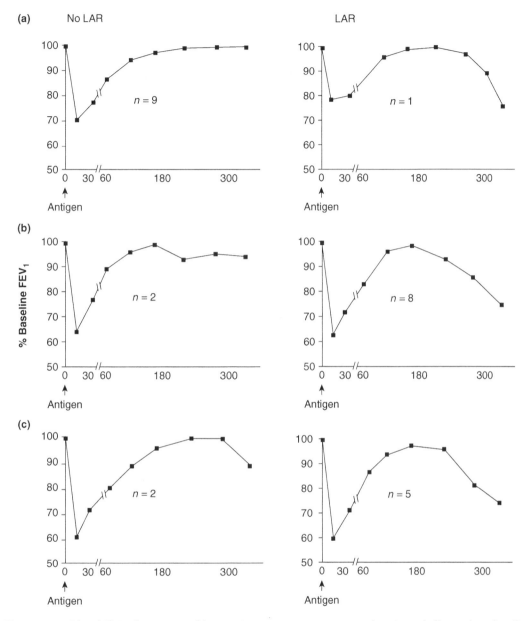

Figure 15.6 The shift in the pattern of lower airway responses to ragweed antigen challenge from baseline (a) to those seen during a viral upper respiratory infection (b) and 4–6 weeks later during the recovery period (c) The incidence of developing a late asthmatic response (LAR) was increased during the acute experimentally induced rhinovirus infection

RV colds might increase asthma by augmenting airway allergic responses (histamine release and eosinophil influx) after antigen challenge.

Seven allergic rhinitis subjects and five normal volunteers were infected with RV16 and evaluated by segmental bronchoprovocation and

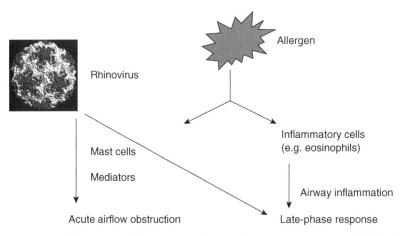

Figure 15.7   Interaction of rhinovirus and antigen to enhance the airway response to inhaled allergen

bronchoalveolar lavage (BAL). Segmental challenge with saline (right or left lung segment) and antigen (segment from contralateral lung) was performed 1 month before infection, during the acute infection and 1 month after infection during convalescence. Lavage was performed immediately and 48 hours after antigen challenge. All subjects inoculated with RV16 developed an acute respiratory infection. BAL fluid obtained from allergic rhinitis subjects during the acute viral infection, and 1 month after infection, showed the following significant RV16-associated changes after antigen challenge: (1) an enhanced release of histamine immediately after local antigen challenge; (2) persistent histamine leak 48 hours afterwards; and (3) a greater recruitment of eosinophils to the airway 48 hours after challenge. These changes were not seen in the five non-allergic volunteers when infected with RV16 and challenged with antigen, nor in the seven allergic volunteers repetitively challenged with antigen when not infected with RV16, nor in the RV16-infected allergic volunteers sham challenged with saline. Based on these results, it was concluded that RV respiratory infections significantly augment immediate and late allergic responses in the airways of allergic individuals after local

antigen challenge. These data suggest that one mechanism of increased asthma during a cold is an accentuation of allergic responses (consistent with the increased propensity of developing late asthmatic responses following whole lung antigen challenge) in the airway, which may then contribute to bronchial inflammation.

The above-described studies suggest an important interaction between existing allergic airway inflammation and the response to RV infection. In these studies, however, the variable was the RV inoculation. To determine whether the intensity of underlying allergic inflammation can affect the response to a virus inoculation, Avila and co-workers at the University of California – San Francisco[17] compared the severity of a RV infection in subjects with underlying allergic rhinitis and in similar subjects who had been actively and repetitively challenged with antigen prior to inoculation. The investigators were able to demonstrate that subjects pretreated with nasal allergen challenges had a reduction and delay in onset of cold symptoms. Furthermore, there was also a delay in the appearance of the total nasal cellular infiltrate and relative percentage of neutrophils. In addition, the appearance of cytokines interleukin (IL)-6 and IL-8 were delayed in their appearance following the cold.

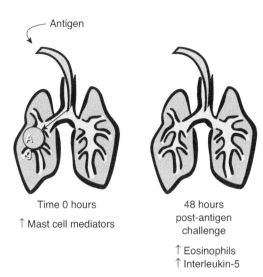

Time 0 hours

↑ Mast cell mediators

48 hours
post-antigen
challenge

↑ Eosinophils
↑ Interleukin-5

Figure 15.8 Patterns of the airway response to antigen immediately and 48 hours after antigen challenge

In analyzing their data, the investigators found an inverse correlation between nasal eosinophilia and the cold symptom score. This association suggests the possibility that, under some conditions, eosinophils, or their products, may modify the response to this respiratory infection. Alternatively, the presence of eosinophils following allergen challenge may be a marker of the co-production of other mediators (e.g. IL-10) that may confer protection from virus infection. Thus, complexities exist between allergic inflammation and responses to an infection. While evidence suggests that respiratory viruses may promote the allergic response to antigen, the reverse may not be the case.

The effects of repetitive antigen exposure in the lower airway on experimental RV16 infection-induced airway dysfunction have also been evaluated.[18] In these experiments, 36 house dust mite-allergic patients with mild-to-moderate asthma participated in a three-arm, parallel, placebo-controlled, double-blind study. Patients inhaled a low dose of house dust mite allergen for 10 subsequent working days (days 1–5 and 8–12) and/or were subsequently infected with RV16 (days 15 and 16). Allergen exposure resulted in a

significant fall in FEV_1, the provocative concentration of histamine causing a 20% fall in FEV_1, an increase in exhaled nitric oxide and an increase in the percentage of sputum eosinophils. RV16 infection led to a fall in FEV_1 and increases in the percentage of sputum neutrophils, sputum IL-8 and neutrophil elastase. Successive allergen exposure and RV16 infection had no synergistic or additive effect on any of the clinical or inflammatory outcomes. In these experiments, repeated low-dose allergen exposure and RV16 infection induced distinct inflammatory profiles within the airways in asthmatic subjects without apparent interaction between these two environmental triggers. This suggests that preceding allergen exposure, at the doses and the duration of exposure utilized, is not a determinant of the severity of RV-induced exacerbations in patients with mild-to-moderate asthma.

Recent findings by Green *et al.*,[19] in a non-experimental inoculation setting, contrast with these two previous reports. These investigators used a case–control study design to evaluate the importance of sensitization and exposure to allergens and viral infection in precipitating acute asthma in adults resulting in admission to a large district general hospital. Sixty patients aged 17–50 years who, over a year, were admitted to the hospital with acute asthma, were matched with two controls: patients with stable asthma who were recruited from the outpatient department, and patients admitted to the hospital with non-respiratory conditions (inpatient controls). The main outcome measures evaluated included atopic status (skin testing and total and specific IgE), presence of common respiratory viruses and atypical bacteria (polymerase chain reaction), dust samples from homes and exposure to allergens (enzyme-linked immunosorbent assay; ELISA: Der p 1, Fel d 1, Can f 1 and Bla g 2). Viruses were detected in 31 of 177 patients. The difference in the frequency of viruses detected between the groups was significant (admitted with asthma 26%, stable asthma 18%, inpatient controls 9%). A significantly higher proportion of patients admitted with asthma (66%) were sensitized and exposed to either mite, cat or dog allergen than patients with stable asthma (37%) and inpatient controls (15%). Being sensitized and exposed to allergens was an independent associate of the group admitted to hospital (odds ratio 2.3). Importantly, however, was the finding that the combination of sensitization, high exposure to one or more allergens and viral detection considerably increased the risk of being admitted with asthma (odds ratio 8.4). These results indicate that, in non-experimental settings, allergens and viruses have a much greater likelihood of acting as co-factors to exacerbate asthma.

SUMMARY

RV infections can enhance the airway inflammatory response to allergen in allergic subjects. These increased inflammatory responses are manifested by a greater likelihood of having a late asthmatic response to antigen, greater mast cell release of mediators and enhanced recruitment of eosinophils. The mechanisms underlying these alterations are not fully defined. Because allergic subjects appear to be more susceptible to the asthma-provoking effects of a RV infection, efforts to discover these mechanisms are of primary interest and importance. Differences in results in experimental models of infection and allergen exposure also suggest that the order and/or timing of exposure may be important in dictating the relative propensity of individual asthmatic subjects to suffer acute exacerbations.

REFERENCES

1. Lemanske RF Jr, Dick EC, Swenson CA, et al. Rhinovirus upper respiratory infection increases airway hyperreactivity and late asthmatic reactions. J Clin Invest 1989; 83: 1–10

2. Empey DW, Laitinen LA, Jacobs L, et al. Mechanisms of bronchial hyperreactivity in normal subjects after upper respiratory tract infection. Am Rev Respir Dis 1976; 113: 131–9

3. Bush RK, Busse W, Flaherty D, et al. Effects of experimental rhinovirus 16 infection on airways and leukocyte function in normal subjects. J Allergy Clin Immunol 1978; 61: 80–7

4. Hall WJ, Hall CB, Speers DM. Respiratory syncytial virus infection in adults: clinical, virologic, and serial pulmonary function studies. Ann Intern Med 1978; 88: 203–5

5. Halperin SA, Eggleston PA, Beasley P, et al. Exacerbations of asthma in adults during experimental rhinovirus infection. Am Rev Respir Dis 1985; 132: 976–80

6. Jenkins CR, Breslin AB. Upper respiratory tract infections and airway reactivity in normal and asthmatic subjects. Am Rev Respir Dis 1984; 130: 879–83

7. Halperin SA, Eggleston PA, Hendley JO, et al. Pathogenesis of lower respiratory tract symptoms in experimental rhinovirus infection. Am Rev Respir Dis 1983; 128: 806–10

8. Hargreave FE, Dolovich J, O'Byrne PM, et al. The origin of airway hyperresponsiveness. J Allergy Clin Immunol 1986; 78: 825–32

9. Lemanske RF Jr. The late phase response: clinical implications. Adv Intern Med 1991; 36: 171–93

10. Hargreave FE, Dolovich J, Robertson DG, Kerigan AT. II. The late asthmatic responses. Can Med Assoc J 1974; 110: 415–24

11. Chai H, Farr RS, Froehlich LA, et al. Standardization of bronchial inhalation challenge procedures. J Allergy Clin Immunol 1975; 56: 323–7

12. D'Alessio DJ, Peterson JA, Dick CR, Dick EC. Transmission of experimental rhinovirus colds in volunteer married couples. J Infect Dis 1976; 133: 28–36

13. D'Alessio DJ, Meschievitz CK, Peterson JA, et al. Short-duration exposure and the transmission of rhinoviral colds. J Infect Dis 1984; 15: 189–94

14. Jackson GG, Dowling HF, Spiesman IG, Boand AV. Transmission of the common cold to volunteers under controlled conditions. I. The common cold as a clinical entity. Arch Intern Med 1958; 101: 267–78

15. Calhoun WJ, Swenson CA, Dick EC, et al. Experimental rhinovirus 16 infection potentiates histamine release after antigen bronchoprovocation in allergic subjects. Am Rev Respir Dis 1991; 144: 1267–73

16. Calhoun WJ, Dick EC, Schwartz LB, Busse WW. A common cold virus, rhinovirus 16, potentiates airway inflammation after segmental antigen bronchoprovocation in allergic subjects. J Clin Invest 1994; 94: 2200–8

17. Avila PC, Abisheganaden JA, Wong H, et al. Effects of allergic inflammation of the nasal mucosa on the severity of rhinovirus 16 cold. J Allergy Clin Immunol 2000; 105: 923–32

18. De Kluijver J, Evertse CE, Sont JK, et al. Are rhinovirus-induced airway responses in asthma aggravated by chronic allergen exposure? Am J Respir Crit Care Med 2003; 168: 1174–80

19. Green RM, Custovic A, Sanderson G, et al. Synergism between allergens and viruses and risk of hospital admission with asthma: case–control study. BMJ 2002; 324: 763

PART V

Treatment and prevention of asthma exacerbations

CHAPTER 16

Role of leukotriene antagonists in the treatment and prevention of acute asthma exacerbations

William W Storms and Jeffrey M Drazen

INTRODUCTION

Many lines of evidence indicate that cysteinyl leukotrienes (LTs) are mediators of airway changes in asthma. The leukotrienes LTC_4, D_4 and E_4 are released during an allergic asthmatic reaction by many different cells in the airway, including mast cells during the early-phase reaction and other inflammatory cells during the late-phase reaction. About 15% of endogenously produced cysteinyl LTs can be recovered in the urine as LTE_4. The production of cysteinyl LTs can be measured indirectly with urinary LTE_4 levels; these levels are increased during the acute asthmatic response as compared to controls and as compared to asthmatics who are not acutely ill. Another line of evidence indicating that LTs participate in the asthmatic response is that LT receptor antagonists (LTRAs) are effective treatments of this condition in adults and children. There have been numerous studies which have evaluated the safety and efficacy of LTRAs in these population groups.[1–5] These studies, which were done primarily for registration of these drugs as asthma controller treatments, have resulted in the chronic use of LTRAs for patients with asthma. In this chapter we review the published data on another use of these drugs, i.e. the use of LT antagonists in the treatment and prevention of acute asthma exacerbations.

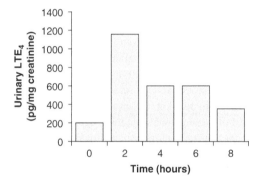

Figure 16.1 Urinary leukotriene levels in ten atopic asthmatics following allergen challenge at time 0. Adapted from reference 6

LEUKOTRIENES IN ACUTE ASTHMA

The recovery of LTs from biological fluids of patients with acute asthma is well established. Sladek *et al.*[6] evaluated ten atopic asthmatics undergoing allergen inhalation challenge and measured urinary LTE_4 levels at 2-hour intervals. They showed a large increase in urine LTE_4 within 2 hours after allergen challenge, with a drop in LTE_4 levels over the subsequent 6 hours (Figure 16.1). The increase in levels was higher in those who showed a later asthmatic response after allergen challenge as compared to those who had only an early asthmatic response.

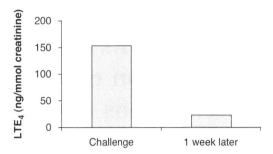

Figure 16.2 Urinary leukotriene LTE$_4$ in 3-hour urine samples from atopic subjects challenged with inhaled antigen and 1 week later during normal lung function. Adapted from reference 7

Taylor et al.[7] measured urinary LTE$_4$ excretion in patients with allergic asthma and allergic rhinitis. Urine was collected after allergen inhalation challenge from eight patients, both immediately after the challenge and 1 week later. The authors studied 29 non-asthmatic volunteers, 14 female and 15 male, aged 19–60 years, with no history of asthma or airway disease. Eight of these were atopic men, aged 22–44 years with a history of atopy, but no history of asthma. They had positive allergy skin testing to either grass pollen or dust mite. They also studied another group, an acute asthmatic group of 20 patients including seven males and 13 females, who were admitted to the hospital through the emergency department with acute exacerbations of asthma. Urine collection for LTs was obtained within 1–5 hours of hospital admission.

Antigen challenge was performed in the non-asthmatic rhinitis patients with the appropriate allergen to which they were sensitive; the antigen challenge was continued until a 20% fall in forced expiratory volume (FEV$_1$) or a maximum dose of 10^5 units/ml was reached. Urine was collected for 3 hours after the final dose of allergen challenge and also a week later (Figure 16.2). The urinary LTE$_4$ was elevated post-challenge; it had returned to normal a week later.

In the component of the study in which patients with acute asthma were admitted to the emergency department, the mean LTE$_4$

level in the urine was 78.3 ng/mmol creatinine, much higher than the control subjects' levels of 23.8 ng/mmol creatinine. The highest level of urinary LTE$_4$ was seen in one patient who required mechanical ventilation on admission. Urinary LTE$_4$ was significantly higher after the antigen challenge in the asthmatics (153 ng/mmol creatinine) as compared to the controls (23 ng/mmol creatinine). After 1 week of treatment the elevated levels of the asthmatic patients had returned to normal.

Drazen et al.[8] demonstrated an increased level of LTE$_4$ in the urine of subjects presenting for emergency treatment of acute airway obstruction. They studied 72 patients who came to the emergency department with signs and symptoms of asthma. They were treated in the usual manner with nebulized albuterol, given at 20-minute intervals. The authors noted that 22 of the 72 had a marked increase (doubling) of their peak flow rates after albuterol, whereas 19 of the 72 failed to raise their peak flows more than 25% after treatment. These groups were designated as 'responders' and 'non-responders'. Of the 22 responders, 16 had urinary LTE$_4$ measurements, as did 12 of the 19 non-responders and 13 normal subjects. They found that the responders had a much higher urinary LTE$_4$ excretion than the control subjects ($p < 0.0001$), but the responders did not have a significant increase of urinary LTE$_4$ over the non-responders ($p = 0.071$). This was due to the fact that four of the 12 non-responders had very low urinary LTE$_4$ levels. The remainder had quite high levels. The authors concluded that patients with acute asthma have enhanced recovery of LTE$_4$ from their urine, which suggests a bronchoconstrictor role for the cysteinyl LTs in spontaneous acute asthma.

Sampson et al.[9] carried out a similar study in children. These authors measured urinary LTs in ten asthmatic children aged 5–10 years who were being evaluated for acute exacerbations of asthma. These were children with a history of asthma who were admitted to the emergency department with acute shortness of breath and

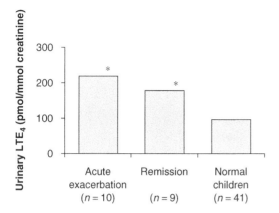

Figure 16.3 Urinary LTE_4 in asthmatic children during acute exacerbations and remission, and in normal children ($*p < 0.003$ compared to normal children). Adapted from reference 9

Table 16.1 Levels of urinary LTE_4 (pg/mg creatinine) measured before inhalation of the diluent or the sensitizing agent, between 2 and 3 hours and between 6 and 7 hours after inhalation. A significant increase* in urinary LTE_4 ($p = 0.041$) occured after the early asthmatic response. Adapted from reference 10

	0 hours	2–3 hours	6–7 hours
Diluent	0	0	0
Sensitizing agent	150	1816*	300

wheezing, and peak expiratory flow readings of less than 65% predicted. Nine out of ten of the children had readings less than 40% predicted. All of the children had taken inhaled β-agonists, but only one was taking inhaled steroids. Nine of the ten subjects were available for urine samples at least 1 month after the acute episode. The control subjects were children with a negative personal and family history of atopy, who had no history of any respiratory problems and who were taking no medication. The authors followed their patients with a 1-month follow-up visit. LTE_4 was much higher in the asthmatic children (210 pmol/mmol creatinine) as compared to the normal children (98 pmol/mmol creatinine). At follow-up the asthmatics' levels had dropped to 179 pmol/mmol creatinine. The authors noted this increase in LTE_4 acutely and pointed out that it continued to be high 1 month after the asthmatic episode. They suggested that this was related to continuing LT production in the chronic inflammation of asthma as well as the acute inflammation (Figure 16.3).

Manning *et al.*[10] evaluated LT production in an allergen challenge model. The authors studied 18 subjects with isolated early asthmatic responses, isolated late asthmatic responses or dual early and late asthmatic responses.

Patients were studied on 2 days. On the first day an inhalation challenge with allergen was performed and the response was measured. The 18 subjects for this study were chosen because they had known asthmatic responses after inhaling either allergens or occupational sensitizers. Fifteen of the subjects were atopic as indicated by positive skin prick tests to a battery of 15 common allergens. This study was performed at a time when the patient's asthma was mild or controlled by bronchodilators alone; no other medications were taken. The allergen inhalation testing was performed with the allergen to which they were sensitive and continued until there was at least a 10% drop in FEV_1. The inhalation test with occupational sensitizers was performed with sensitizing agents in powder form (guar gum, flour, western red cedar). Challenges with agents in vapor or liquid form were performed in a challenge room (toluene diisocyanate (TDI), hexamethylene diisocyanate (HDI) and tertiary amine). On the second day an inhalation challenge without the offending allergen was performed. The authors found a significant increase in urinary LTE_4 levels in the early asthmatic responders, with a change from 150 pg/mg of creatinine at baseline to 1816 pg/mg of creatinine after the early response ($p = 0.041$) (Table 16.1). The degree of maximal bronchoconstriction during the early asthmatic response correlated with levels of LTE_4. The authors suggested that LTs are important bronchoconstrictor mediators in the early asthmatic response after allergen inhalation.

TREATMENT OF ACUTE ASTHMA WITH LEUKOTRIENE RECEPTOR ANTAGONISTS

Inhibitors of the action of LTs at the Cys LT_1 receptor (LTRAs) have been the most widely studied compounds for treatment of acute and chronic asthma; most commonly the agents are administered by the oral route. Fuller *et al.*[11] evaluated atopic asthmatic subjects by performing inhaled LTD_4 challenge on day 1, allergen challenge on day 2 and then the same studies 3 weeks later. This was a study of six male atopic subjects aged 26–38, who were not taking any medication and did not have symptoms of asthma at the time of the study. Five of the six were sensitive to dust mite and the other patient was sensitive to grass antigen based on allergy skin prick testing. Allergen challenge was performed using the appropriate allergen to which the patient was sensitive. On each study day subjects received 400 mg of LY171883, an oral LTD_4 antagonist, or placebo in a double-blind manner. The forced expiratory flow at 40% of vital capacity was used as the endpoint for the allergen challenge and, when a greater than 40% fall in this measurement was obtained, the allergen challenge was stopped. The results showed that after antigen challenge, the forced expiratory flow rate at 40% vital capacity dropped 54.7% after placebo pre-treatment and 35.8% after pre-treatment with a LTRA ($p < 0.05$).

There was also a significant reduction in the area under the curve during the early-phase response for active treatment versus placebo and the authors concluded that LY171883 is a LT antagonist and that LTs play a role in the early bronchoconstrictor receptor response to inhaled allergen.

Another study of LTRAs in allergen-induced bronchospasm was performed by Findlay *et al.*[12] In this study, 15 patients with asthma participated in a double-blind randomized placebo-controlled crossover study. Patients ranged in age from 18 to 50 and all of them had diagnostic

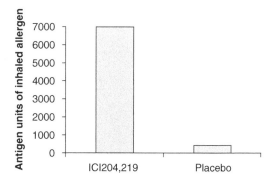

Figure 16.4 Effects of ICI204,219 (zafirlukast) or placebo given 2 hours prior to allergen inhalation challenge. Results measured as antigen units of inhaled allergen which produced a 20% drop in FEV_1. Pretreatment with study drug provided the patients a larger amount of inhaled allergen before a 20% drop in FEV_1 occurred. Adapted from reference 12

criteria for asthma and were non-smokers. None had clinical signs of airway obstruction or required medications and all had an FEV_1 of greater than 65% predicted and a positive skin test to cat antigen. Two weeks before the study, patients had a physical examination, laboratory tests and a bronchoprovocation test to cat dander. Allergen inhalation challenge was performed on two separate days and patients received either ICI204,219 (now known as zafirlukast) or placebo prior to the challenge. This study was performed to see whether acute treatment with this LTRA would prevent or attenuate the bronchospasm from allergen challenge. The LTRA was given 2 hours before allergen challenge. The endpoint was a 20% decrease in FEV_1 (PC_{20}). There was a ten-fold increase in the PC_{20} for those patients who were pretreated with ICI204,219 versus placebo (6996 AU/ml versus 460 AU/ml) (AU, antigen units of inhaled allergen). In addition, the area under the curve of the FEV_1 response was significantly less between ICI204,219 than placebo ($p < 0.05$). This study showed that pre-treatment with a LTRA is effective in acute asthma as evidenced by this laboratory evaluation of allergen-induced asthma (Figure 16.4).

Treatment

Cylly *et al.*[13] evaluated the acute response to oral montelukast. They selected 70 patients with asthma, mean age 64 years, with FEV_1 per cent predicted of 56%. A placebo group with similar characteristics was also evaluated. All patients had at least a 1-year history of asthma and a bronchodilator response to an inhaled β-agonist. At the time of the study, 11 of the 70 patients were taking no medications; nine were using only a short-acting inhaled β-agonist as needed; and 50 patients were using regular daily inhaled corticosteroids plus inhaled β-agonists as needed. All patients were seen during an acute flare of their asthma with 17 of the patients seen in the outpatient clinic and 53 patients in the emergency room. All patients were hospitalized for at least 24 hours for follow-up, regardless of asthma severity. They studied the acute effects of oral montelukast on the peak expiratory flow rate after 24 hours of treatment. The study was performed in a single-blind manner with the following study groups: 10 mg oral montelukast plus intravenous prednisolone, intravenous prednisolone alone or placebo. After randomization into one of the three treatment groups all of the patients immediately received aerosolized terbutaline sulfate, a total of 100 µg in three separate doses over 1 hour; patients were followed for 24 hours. Montelukast plus prednisolone and prednisolone alone showed a 42% improvement and 39.9% improvement, respectively, from baseline in peak expiratory flow rate. Placebo patients had a 10% improvement. The steroid plus montelukast patients had a statistically greater improvement in peak flow than the placebo patients ($p < 0.05$). The montelukast plus prednisolone group tended to have higher peak flows than the prednisolone alone, but the differences were not statistically significant. The montelukast plus prednisolone group tended to require less short-acting prednisolone β-agonists than the other two groups. The authors concluded that adding montelukast

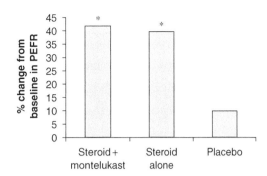

Figure 16.5 Acute treatment response to oral montelukast plus intravenous prednisolone, or the steroid alone or placebo. Results expressed as improvement in FEV_1 after 24 hours of treatment. PEFR, peak expiratory flow rate; $*p < 0.05$. Adapted from reference 13

to a steroid in acute asthma may give additive improvement in lung function (Figure 16.5).

INTRAVENOUS MONTELUKAST FOR ACUTE ASTHMA

The original studies on LTRAs in asthma were performed with oral formulations of montelukast, zafirlukast or pranlukast. Recent studies have been performed using an intravenous formulation of montelukast. Dockhorn *et al.*[14] evaluated 51 asthmatic patients in a double-blind single-dose crossover study. The patients included 22 women and 29 men, ages 15–56 with a duration of asthma of 2–50 years. For enrollment in the study patients were required to have an FEV_1 of 40–80% predicted with an improvement of 15% after inhalation of albuterol. No current smokers were enrolled. No patients had received oral, intravenous or intramuscular corticosteroids during the month prior to the study; 25% of the patients were receiving treatment with inhaled corticosteroids at a stable dose. Long-acting antihistamines were discontinued 2 weeks before the study, oral or long-acting inhaled β-agonists, cromolyn sodium or nedocromil or inhaled corticosteroids 1 week before the study. This was a

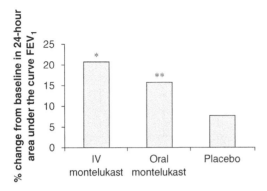

Figure 16.6 Crossover study of three treatments in patients with chronic ashthma. Results expressed as the area under the curve of FEV_1 for 24 hours after a single dose of each treatment. *IV montelukast vs. placebo, $p=0.001$; **oral montelukast vs. placebo, $p=0.02$). Adapted from reference 14

multicenter, double-blind, randomized placebo-controlled three-period crossover study. The three treatment periods were: intravenous montelukast, 7 mg; oral montelukast, 10 mg; or placebo. Each treatment period was separated by at least 4 but not more than 14 days; study medication was administered at the same time in the morning on each treatment day and patients were observed at least 24 hours for FEV_1 changes. Spirometry was performed repeatedly for 24 hours following the intervention, with analysis of the area under the curve of FEV_1 over 24 hours. The mean FEV_1 at baseline was 63% of predicted (range 42–80% predicted). There was a significant increase in FEV_1, as per cent change from baseline with intravenous montelukast as compared to placebo ($20.70\pm6.27\%$ vs. $7.75\pm6\%$, $p\leq0.001$). Following treatment with intravenous montelukast there was greater change in FEV_1 than following oral montelukast ($20.70\pm6.27\%$ vs. $15.72\pm7.13\%$, $p=0.067$). Both treatments were significantly ($p\leq0.001$ and $p=0.020$, respectively) better than placebo (Figure 16.6).

The authors concluded that both oral and intravenous montelukast improved lung function in patients with asthma and that intravenous montelukast had a faster onset than oral montelukast. They pointed out that there was a trend towards a greater improvement in FEV_1 with intravenous rather than oral montelukast and suggested that further studies should be done to look at intravenous montelukast for acute asthma treatment.

Camargo et al. [15] reported a multi-clinic study, primarily in emergency departments. They studied 194 patients who presented for medical care for acute asthma. The study was a randomized, placebo-controlled, double-blind trial comparing acute treatment of asthma in the emergency room with and without intravenous montelukast (at one of two doses) or placebo. During the screening for their acute asthma exacerbations, treatment was allowed with inhaled albuterol by nebulizer and oxygen supplementation. Spirometry was performed pre- and post-albuterol therapy and subjects who did not have a 20 percentage point improvement were excluded from the study. At this point patients were given either 7 mg or 14 mg of intravenous montelukast or placebo. Spirometry was carried out after treatment. The results showed that the two montelukast dosing groups gave the same improvement in FEV_1 and then the data were pooled. Montelukast improved the FEV_1 within 20 minutes by 14.8% versus 3.6% for the placebo group. This improvement was noted continually throughout the entire 2-hour treatment period. Those patients who were treated with montelukast had tended to receive less β-agonist treatment and tended to have fewer treatment failures than the patients receiving placebo. There were no adverse events noted in the montelukast group different from the placebo group. The authors concluded that intravenous montelukast can be used in addition to standard therapy, that it has a rapid benefit and that there were few acute side-effects. This study design is important, because it evaluated patients after they had responded to a β-agonist and showed that adding a LTRA gives benefit over and above the bronchodilatation seen with the β-agonist.

USE OF LEUKOTRIENE ANTAGONISTS IN THE PREVENTION OF ASTHMA

In the studies that were performed for registration for leukotriene antagonists for use in chronic daily asthma, the authors often gathered data on asthma exacerbations during the clinical trials. Although the number of asthma exacerbations was not the primary endpoint, the data were still collected and often reported. LTRAs resulted in a significant reduction in asthma exacerbations in these studies.[1–5] Although these trials had somewhat different definitions of asthma exacerbations, for the most part they were clinical exacerbations which were identified by either increased symptoms, requirement for extra asthma medication, a drop in pulmonary function or an emergency room visit or hospitalization. These data support the concept that LTRAs are effective therapy for the prevention of asthma exacerbations.

Barnes and Miller[16] published an integrated analysis of the risk of asthma exacerbations from published clinical trials with zafirlukast. Five double-blind multicenter randomized placebo-controlled 13-week trials comparing zafirlukast 20 mg twice daily were evaluated in a patient population of mild-to-moderate asthma. Asthma exacerbation information was prospectively collected during the studies; the pooled data were used to assess the relative risk of asthma exacerbations using three criteria: worsening of asthma leading to withdrawal from the study; requirement for additional anti-asthmatic therapy; and use of oral corticosteroid rescue therapy. The risk of an asthma exacerbation requiring withdrawal zafirlukast treatment was half that of placebo ($p=0.003$). Patients treated with zafirlukast also required less asthma medication for control ($p=0.001$) and less oral corticosteroid rescue ($p=0.01$) than the patients treated with placebo. The authors point out that, in these patients with mild-to-moderate asthma, zafirlukast 20 mg twice a day reduced the risk of exacerbations and the need for additional anti-asthmatic therapy.

Another study[17] was caried out to evaluate whether montelukast would prevent virus-induced asthma exacerbations in children aged 2–5. This was a 1-year double-blind parallel group study of patients with asthma exacerbations associated with respiratory infections and minimal symptoms between exacerbations. All children had a clinical history of intermittent asthma resulting from upper respiratory infections. No children were entered who had symptoms on a regular basis. Subjects were treated with either montelukast 4 mg daily prophylactically or placebo for 1 year. The primary efficacy variable was the number of asthma exacerbations (three consecutive days with daytime symptoms with at least two treatments of inhaled β-agonists daily, or rescue use of inhaled/oral steroids or a hospitalization due to asthma). Over 12 months of therapy, montelukast significantly reduced the rate of asthma exacerbations by 31.9% compared to placebo (relative exacerbation rate for montelukast vs. placebo, 0.68; 95% CI 0.56–0.83). The average rate of exacerbations per patient was 1.60 per year on montelukast versus 2.34 on placebo. The median time to first exacerbation was delayed by 2 months for montelukast-treated patients compared to placebo ($p=0.024$). The authors concluded that montelukast decreased the rate of asthma exacerbations and increased the time to exacerbation in 2–5-year-old asthmatic patients whose symptoms were intermittent.

SUMMARY

Multiple lines of evidence implicate the cysteinyl LTs as one of the mediators of airway constriction in patients with asthma. There are substantial clinical data that treatment of patients with acute airway obstruction in the setting of an asthmatic exacerbation with LTRAs results in physiological benefit. Studies in children with virus-induced asthma show an attenuation of the episodes in montelukast-treated children. Patients presenting in emergency settings for asthma treatment have often received repeated treatments with inhaled β-agonists but may not have received LTRA treatment. Although definitive appropriately powered randomized controlled trials have not been completed, it does not seem unreasonable to add LTRAs to the regimen provided for the patient who is otherwise not responding to the treatment of an asthma exacerbation.

REFERENCES

1. Reiss TF, Chervinsky P, Dockhorn RJ, et al. Montelukast, a one-daily leukotriene receptor antagonist, in treatment of chronic asthma. Arch Intern Med 1998; 158: 1213–20

2. Baumgartner RA, Martinez G, Edelman JM, et al. Distribution of therapeutic response in asthma control between oral montelukast and inhaled beclomethasone. Eur Respir J 2003; 21: 123–8

3. Knorr B, Matz J, Bernstein JA, et al. Montelukast for chronic asthma in 6 to 14-year-old children. J Am Med Assoc 1998; 279: 1181–6

4. Israel E, Chervinsky PS, Friedman B, et al. Effects of montelukast and beclomethasone on airway function and asthma control. J Allergy Clin Immunol 2002; 110: 847–54

5. Laviolette M, Malmstrom K, Lu S, et al. Montelukast added to inhaled beclomethasone in treatment of asthma. Am J Respir Crit Care Med 1999; 160: 1862–8

6. Sladek K, Dworski R, Fitzgerald GA, et al. Allergen-stimulated release of thromboxane A2 and leukotriene E4 in humans. Am Rev Respir Dis 1990; 141: 1441–5

7. Taylor GW, Taylor I, Black P, et al. Urinary leukotriene E4 after antigen challenge and in acute asthma and allergic rhinitis. Lancet 1989; 1: 584–8

8. Drazen JM, O'Brien J, Sparrow D, et al. Recovery of leukotriene E4 from the urine of patients with airway obstruction. Am Rev Respir Dis 1992; 146: 104–8

9. Sampson AP, Castling DP, Green CP, Price JF. Persistent increase in plasma and urinary leukotrienes after acute asthma. Arch Dis Child 1995; 73: 221–5

10. Manning PJ, Rokach J, Malo J, et al. Urinary leukotriene E4 levels during early and late asthmatic responses. J Allergy Clin Immunol 1990; 86: 211–20

11. Fuller RW, Black PN, Dollery CT. Effect of the oral leukotriene D4 antagonist LY171883 on inhaled and intradermal challenge with antigen and leukotriene D4 in atopic subjects. J Allergy Clin Immunol 1989; 83: 939–44

12. Findlay SR, Barden JM, Easley CB, Glass M. Effect of the oral leukotriene antagonist, ICI 204,219, on antigen-induced bronchoconstriction in subjects with asthma. J Allergy Clin Immunol 1992; 89: 1040–5

13. Cylly A, Kara A, Ozdemir T, et al. Effects of oral montelukast on airway function in acute asthma. Respir Med 2003; 97: 533–6

14. Dockhorn RJ, Baumgartner RA, Leff JA, et al. Comparison of the effects of intravenous and oral montelukast on airway function: a double-blind, placebo controlled, three period, crossover study in asthmatic patients. Thorax 2000; 55: 260–5

15. Camargo CA Jr, Smithline HA, Malice M, et al. A randomized controlled trial of intravenous montelukast in acute asthma. Am J Respir Crit Care Med 2003; 167: 528–33

16. Barnes NC, Miller CJ. Effective leukotriene receptor antagonist therapy on the risk of asthma exacerbations in patients with mild to moderate asthma: an integrated analysis of zafirlukast trials. Thorax 2000; 55: 478–83

17. Bisgaard H, Zielen S, Garcia-Garcia ML, et al. Montelukast reduces asthma exacerbations in 2 to 5-year-old children with intermittent asthma. Am J Respir Crit Care Med 2005; 171: 315–22

Treatment and prevention of asthma exacerbations: how good are inhaled corticosteroids alone at preventing asthma exacerbations?

Sara J Uekert, Robert F Lemanske Jr and William W Busse

INTRODUCTION

Viral infections are the major cause for asthma exacerbations in both children and adults. Current therapy for virus-induced wheezing generally includes the additional use of bronchodilators, increasing doses of inhaled corticosteroids (ICS) and, if symptoms persist or worsen, the administration of systemic corticosteroids. With the development of higher-potency topical corticosteroids, recent trials have also investigated the efficacy of high-dose ICS given either prophylactically or as an acute intervention in the management of these wheezing episodes. The efficacy of various ICS therapeutic interventions for the acute symptoms of wheezing, tachypnea and hypoxemia that may occur as a result of viral upper respiratory tract infections (URTIs) has been controversial due to differences in study design, the inability to rapidly and conveniently measure pulmonary physiological variables and the choice of outcome measures evaluated. Furthermore, it has been difficult to extrapolate these recommendations to infants and young children who wheeze in the presence of viral

infections, yet in whom the diagnosis of asthma has not yet been fully established. In these children, recurrent episodic wheezing secondary to viral respiratory infections may represent a unique illness that is distinct from persistent allergic asthma. It is the goal of this chapter to review recent pediatric and adult experiences as they pertain to the use of high-dose ICS in preventing or attenuating asthma exacerbations due both to naturally occurring viral respiratory illnesses and to experimental colds.

EXPERIENCES WITH INHALED CORTICOSTEROIDS IN CHILDREN

Episodic wheezing provoked by respiratory infections

Current National Heart, Lung and Blood Institute (NHLBI) Guidelines for the Diagnosis and Management of Asthma recommend the addition of oral corticosteroids for moderate to severe asthma exacerbations that are unresponsive to bronchodilators. The Guidelines also suggest doubling the maintenance dose of ICS for mild episodes unresponsive to bronchodilators.[1] The efficacy of this recommendation for ICS intervention has been evaluated in children by at least six different research groups (Table 17.1). First, Wilson and Silverman[2] examined the administration of beclomethasone dipropionate (750 μg three times daily for 5 days administered via metered dose inhaler (MDI)) at the first sign of an asthma episode in children 1–5 years of age with a respiratory infection. Although failing to alter the need for additional therapy, ICS therapy was associated with improvement in asthma symptoms during the first week of the episode. Second, Daugbjerg et al.[3] conducted a double-blind, placebo-controlled trial to compare the effects of an inhaled bronchodilator alone or its use in combination with either high-dose ICS (budesonide nebulization, 0.5 mg every 4 hours until discharge) or systemic corticosteroid (prednisolone) in children below 18 months of age when admitted to a hospital with acute wheezing. They found an earlier time of discharge from hospital in both the inhaled and systemic corticosteroid-treated groups, as well as a significantly accelerated rate of clinical improvement in the budesonide-treated group compared to the groups with and without oral corticosteroids.

In a third trial, Connett and Lenney[4] compared the efficacy of two doses of budesonide (800 μg or 1600 μg twice daily via MDI and a spacer device) that was initiated at the onset of upper respiratory tract symptoms in preschool-aged children with a history of recurrent wheezing with URTIs. Therapy was continued for up to 7 days or until patients were asymptomatic for 24 hours. Budesonide therapy was associated with a decrease in symptom scores during the first week of infection. Fourth, a double-blind, placebo-controlled, crossover study conducted by Svedmyr et al.[5] evaluated the administration of budesonide (200 μg qid for 3 days, tid for 3 days, bid for 3 days via MDI and spacer) or placebo to children 3–10 years of age with a history of URTI-associated deterioration

of asthma. While this approach had no significant influence on symptom scores, budesonide therapy was associated with significantly higher peak expiratory flow (PEF) rates. In a follow-up study by the same group,[6] a higher dose of budesonide (400 μg qid for 3 days, 400 μg bid for 7 days via spacer with a facemask) was compared with placebo in the management of asthma exacerbations due to URTIs in children 1–3 years of age. While the higher-dose ICS significantly improved symptom scores, it did not affect rates of hospitalization or need for oral corticosteroids.

In a recent emergency department (ED)-based study, Volovitz et al. compared the effects of inhaled budesonide and oral prednisolone in children 6–16 years of age experiencing an acute asthma exacerbation.[7] Patients received either budesonide 1600 μg by turbohaler or 2 mg/kg of oral prednisolone in the ED followed by a tapered dose of medication over the next 6 days. Both treatment groups had similar rates of improvement in the ED in terms of symptom scores and PEF. However, over the next week, the budesonide-treated group had a more rapid improvement in asthma symptoms. Children in the prednisolone group demonstrated both significantly decreased serum cortisol levels and reduced adrenocorticotropic hormone (ACTH) response by the end of the first week of therapy compared to the budesonide group; however, these values returned to the normal range 2 weeks later. This study suggests that high-dose therapy with a potent ICS may be as effective as oral prednisolone and may avoid hypothalamic–pituitary axis suppression.

Finally, a recent study evaluated the effects of high-dose ICS and oral corticosteroids in children seen in an ED for an acute severe asthma exacerbation (mean $FEV_1 < 40\%$ predicted upon presentation) and found oral corticosteroids to be superior in terms of improvement in lung function and frequency of hospitalization.[8] However, these patients were clearly in the midst of severe exacerbations, and ICS had not been utilized early in the course of the illness.

Table 17.1 Experience with inhaled corticosteroids (ICS) in children with episodic wheezing

Research group (publication date)	Study population	Intervention	Outcome
Wilson and Silverman (1990)[2]	Preschool children	DBPC Beclomethasone 750 µg tid ×5d	Significantly improved symptom score in 1st week Failed to alter need for additional treatment
Daugbjerg et al. (1993)[3]	1.5–18 months	DBPC Comparing efficacy of OCS to ICS+SABA, SABA alone or placebo	Earlier hospital discharge in both steroid groups vs. placebo Significantly improved symptom score in budesonide treated group
Connett and Lenney (1993)[4]	Preschool children	DBPC Budesonide 800–1600 µg bid ×7d	Significantly improved symptom score in treatment group
Wilson et al. (1995)[10]	0.7–6 years	DBPC Budesonide 400 µg/day ×3 months	No difference in number, severity or duration of episodes vs. placebo
Svedmyr et al. (1995)[5]	3–10 years	DBPC crossover Budesonide 0.2 mg qid ×3d, tid ×3d, bid ×3d	No difference in symptom score Improved PEF in treatment group
Doull et al. (1997)[11]	7–9 years	DBPC Beclomethasone 200 µg bid ×6 months	Significant increases in mean FEV_1 and PC_{20} in treatment group No difference in frequency, severity or duration of episodes vs. placebo
Garrett et al. (1998)[39]	6–14 years	DBPC Doubled-dose of ICS ×3d vs. maintenance dose	No difference in PEF or symptom score vs. maintenance dose
Volovitz et al. (1998)[7]	6–16 years	Double-blind ICS (budesonide) vs. OCS for discharge management from ED	Earlier symptomatic improvement and lower serum cortisol levels in budesonide treated children vs. OCS Similar improvements in PEF
Svedmyr et al. (1999)[6]	1–3 years	DBPC Budesonide 400 µg qid ×3d, then bid ×7d	Significantly improved symptom scores in treatment group No difference in need for hospitalization, ER visit or OCS

DBPC, double-blind placebo-controlled trial; OCS, oral corticosteroids; SABA, short-acting β_2-agonist; PEF, peak expiratory flow; ED, emergency department

In summary, evidence supports an approach to initiate high-dose ICS at the onset of symptoms with URTIs in order to improve symptom control. In a recent meta-analysis by McKean and Ducharme, the intermittent use of high-dose ICS was shown to attenuate the severity of asthma-like symptoms associated with viral URTIs in children and to decrease the need for oral corticosteroids by roughly one-third, particularly if given during the first week.[9] Caution should be applied in interpreting these results, however, as the intermittent use of high-dose ICS has not consistently been shown to affect other outcome measures such as need for hospitalization or ED treatment.

If intermittent high-dose ICS can modify the severity of asthma exacerbations due to viral respiratory infections in children, the next obvious question would be whether a maintenance use of low-dose ICS could further improve symptom control during an intercurrent respiratory infection. Two studies in children with episodic virus-induced wheezing have addressed this issue. First, Wilson et al. evaluated the effectiveness of regular ICS (400 μg per day of budesonide) versus placebo on episodic viral wheeze in preschool children. No differences were found in the number, duration or severity of such episodes.[10] Second, in a randomized, double-blind, placebo-controlled trial in children 7–9 years of age, Doull et al. compared the effects of twice daily administration of inhaled beclomethasone dipropionate (200 μg via Diskhaler®) versus placebo over a 6-month period on FEV_1, bronchial responsiveness to methacholine (PD_{20}) and asthma symptoms associated with URTIs.[11] Although increases in mean FEV_1 and PD_{20} values were found in the treatment group, there were no significant differences in the frequency, severity or duration of virus-induced symptoms between the two groups during the treatment period.

Known diagnosis of asthma

When looking at children who wheeze outside of respiratory infections, several studies have

identified the importance of regular inhaled corticosteroid use on the maintenance of asthma control and reduction in symptoms associated with acute exacerbations. In a large, prospective clinical trial, the investigators of the Childhood Asthma Management Program Research Group[12] found a reduction in both hospitalization and urgent care visits among children with mild-to-moderate asthma treated with 200 μg of budesonide twice daily over a period of 4–6 years. In a more recent study, by Johnston et al., children regularly treated with ICS experienced fewer asthma exacerbations during the 'September epidemic'.[13] In this study, the authors examined rates of viral detection, allergic sensitization and controller medication use in children aged 5–15 years presenting to the emergency department for asthma exacerbations after returning to school in September. When compared with age-matched controls, children requiring ED treatment demonstrated higher rates of viral recovery from nasal secretions and lower rates of prescriptions for controller medications, including inhaled corticosteroids. The authors also reported a significant decline in the number of inhaled corticosteroid prescription reimbursements during the month of August. This decrease in controller medication use combined with re-exposure to allergens in the school environment was felt to contribute to an increased vulnerability to viral respiratory pathogens. Furthermore, those children on regular ICS appeared to be protected from this seasonal epidemic.

In another recent study, findings by Murray et al. support the association of decreased ICS use and increased rates of hospitalization for acute asthma exacerbation among children aged 3–17 years.[14] In this study, children hospitalized with an acute asthma exacerbation were compared with two control groups: stable asthmatics and children hospitalized with non-respiratory conditions. Although children in the case group were more likely to be virus infected and to be both sensitized and exposed to allergens, it was only the combination of virus detection and sensitization with exposure that substantially increased the risk of hospitalization. In these children, the regular use of ICS significantly decreased this risk, leading the authors to conclude that the maintenance use of ICS in children with allergic asthma may help attenuate the synergism noted between natural viral infections and real-life allergen exposures.

Based on the above observations, high-dose inhaled corticosteroids have been shown to be at least partially effective in the acute management of exacerbations secondary to episodic viral infections in children, particularly when given during the first week. Although current evidence does not favor the initiation of maintenance low-dose ICS for the prevention of respiratory symptoms in children with episodic virus-induced wheezing, there is substantial support for the use of inhaled steroids in the pediatric asthma population as a whole for providing significant protection from other triggers of asthma exacerbations and/or those that synergize with concomitant viral respiratory infections.

EXPERIENCE WITH INHALED CORTICOSTEROIDS IN ADULTS

Treatment and prevention of acute exacerbations

In adults, several studies have evaluated the effectiveness of ICS as a replacement for oral glucocorticoids in the treatment of acute asthma exacerbations presumably arising from viral URTIs (Table 17.2). In an initial study by Levy et al.,[15] the efficacy of high-dose inhaled fluticasone (1000 µg bid) was compared with oral prednisolone (40 mg qd initially, then decreasing by 5 mg every other day) for the treatment of acute asthma exacerbations in adults presenting to their primary care physicians. Patients were eligible for enrollment if the initial PEF value was ≥60% of their personal best or predicted, but not ≥90% best/predicted (defined as entry

PEF). Treatment failures were defined as a PEF of ≤60% baseline PEF (entry value) on two or more consecutive occasions, a symptom score of ≥3 on three consecutive days, or withdrawal from the study secondary to an adverse event or uncontrolled asthma symptoms. Treatment effectiveness was considered as an increase in PEF by 10% over the course of the treatment period No significant differences were noted between treatment groups in median dose of ICS on entry, mean per cent predicted entry PEF, median symptom score during treatment period or the percentage of treatment failures. Although the authors indicated that the study was underpowered secondary to difficulties in recruitment, they felt that the negligible differences between treatment groups were sufficient to conclude that high-dose ICS may be used as an alternative treatment to oral prednisolone in the management of mild asthma exacerbations in adults with respiratory infection. It should be noted, however, that approximately one-half of patients in each treatment group were on low-dose ICS or no ICS at the time of enrollment and that the clinical response to high-dose ICS may not be noted in patients already receiving higher doses of maintenance inhaled steroids.

In a double-blind, placebo-controlled study by Foresi et al.,[16] patients with moderately severe asthma were randomized to treatment either with standard doses of budesonide plus placebo for exacerbations (400 µg bid + placebo), low-dose budesonide plus supplemental budesonide during exacerbations (100 µg bid + 200 µg qid for 7 days) or low-dose budesonide plus placebo for exacerbations (100 µg bid + placebo). Asthma control was assessed by daily symptom diaries and by monthly spirometry values over a 6-month period. Although no significant differences were noted between groups in terms of lung function or daily symptoms, the low-dose budesonide plus placebo-treated group had significantly more exacerbations and more symptomatic asthma days during exacerbations when compared to the other two study groups. The authors concluded that low-dose budesonide was effective in maintaining asthma

Table 17.2 Experience with inhaled corticosteroids (ICS) in adults

Research group (publication date)	Study population	Intervention	Outcome
Treatment of acute exacerbations			
Levy et al. (1996)[15]	Adults with moderate asthma presenting to primary MD with acute exacerbation	Double-blind, double dummy 2 mg fluticasone vs. oral prednisone taper	High-dose ICS as effective as short course of OCS
Foresi et al. (2000)[16]	Adults with moderate asthma	Double-blind Bud 400 µg bid + placebo qid × 7 days vs. Bud 100 µg bid + placebo qid × 7 days or Bud 100 µg bid + Bud 200 µg qid × 7 days	Low-dose ICS as effective as standard dose once control achieved For exacerbations, standard dose and low dose + Bud both superior to low dose alone
FitzGerald et al. (2000)[17]	15–70 years ER presentation for acute asthma	Double-blind, double dummy Bud 600 µg qid vs. OCS × 7–10 days	Bud as effective as OCS in preventing relapse hospital admission No difference in FEV_1, PEF, symptoms or quality of life score
Harrison et al. (2004)[18]	16+ years Mild, stable asthma	Double-blind Active (doubled corticosteroid dose) vs. placebo inhaler added to daily regimen with fall in PEF or symptom control	No difference in duration, severity, PEF or need for OCS between groups No evidence to support 'doubled dose' recommendations
FitzGerald et al. (2004)[19]	Adults with moderate asthma	Double-blind Maintenance dose ICS + placebo vs. Maintenance dose ICS + maintenance dose for acute exacerbations	No difference between groups No evidence to support 'doubled dose' recommendations
Prevention of acute exacerbations			
Pauwels et al. (1997)[20]	18–70 years Mild-to-moderate asthma	Double-blind, parallel-group Bud 100 µg bid + placebo bid Bud 100 µg bid + formoterol bid Bud 400 µg bid + placebo bid Bud 400 µg bid + formoterol bid	When looking at ICS arms only: decreased rates of exacerbations in high-dose Bud group vs. low-dose
Bateman et al. (2004)[21]	12–79 years Mild-to-moderate asthma	Double-blind, randomized, stratified Parallel-group Stepwise increases in salmeterol/fluticasone vs. fluticasone alone until control achieved	Decreased rates of exacerbations as dose of ICS increased

OCS, oral corticosteroids; Bud, budesonide; PEF, peak expiratory flow; ER, emergency room control and that the addition of supplemental ICS during exacerbations had a beneficial clinical effect when compared with placebo. In an ED-based study, FitzGerald et al.[17] randomized patients 15–70 years of age who were admitted for acute asthma exacerbations to either 2400 µg inhaled budesonide per day (600 µg qid via turbohaler) or 40 mg oral prednisone per day for a duration of 7–10 days. Relapse rates requiring emergency department visits were considered as the primary outcome measure with assessments in FEV_1, asthma symptoms, PEF and quality of life as secondary endpoints. Treatment groups were noted to have similar relapse rates and no statistical differences in secondary outcome measures. This led the authors to conclude that, in stabilized patients, high-dose budesonide could provide an alternative to oral glucocorticoids for discharge management from the ED in cases of acute asthma exacerbation. As patients with a recent course of oral corticosteroids (<1 month) were excluded from this study, these results cannot be extrapolated to those patients presenting with a second exacerbation within a short period of time. Furthermore, the majority of these patients were not receiving maintenance ICS at the time of enrollment, and their favorable responses to high-dose ICS may differ from those of patients receiving regular doses of inhaled corticosteroids prior to exacerbations.

In a more recent study, Harrison and colleagues[18] evaluated the current NHLBI Guidelines' recommendation to double the daily maintenance dose of ICS during acute asthma exacerbations by comparing the addition of active ICS inhaler (effectively doubling the dose) versus placebo inhaler. Patients were instructed to add the study inhaler twice daily to their maintenance medication for a period of 14 days when peak flow values or control of asthma symptoms began to deteriorate. The primary outcome (number of individuals requiring oral prednisolone) did not differ between treatment groups. Criteria for initiating prednisolone treatment were a 40% decrease in

peak flow, advice from a general practitioner or a subjective deterioration in asthma control.

In a similar study, by FitzGerald et al.,[19] patients with well-characterized asthma were randomly assigned to receive a MDI containing either a placebo or ICS (resulting in a doubled dose of their maintenance ICS) which was to be added twice daily to their maintenance ICS during acute asthma exacerbations. The primary outcome in this study was the proportion of patients failing to regain control after developing symptoms of an impending asthma exacerbation, defined by the investigators as need for oral corticosteroids or an unscheduled physician visit after 14 days of initiating treatment. Treatment failure was equivalent in both study groups, as were secondary outcome measures such as number, duration and severity of exacerbations. A subgroup analysis examining baseline ICS dosage revealed that subjects in the higher dose range (≥400 µg/day) at enrollment were more likely to develop treatment failure in both the intervention and placebo groups when compared with subjects using ≤400 µg/day at enrollment, suggesting that it may be the dose of maintenance ICS rather than the supplemental ICS that determines the outcome of acute asthma exacerbations. These studies conclude that, although it is often endorsed as a treatment approach, recommendations to double the dose of maintenance ICS during exacerbations are not supported by clinical studies and do not appear to be sufficiently effective in managing acute asthma exacerbations secondary to URTIs in adults.

Despite the disappointing results of supplemental ICS use during asthma exacerbations, there is substantial support for the regular use of low-dose inhaled steroids for the prevention of exacerbations and reduction in asthma-related mortality. In a large double-blind, parallel group trial, Pauwels and colleagues[20] randomized patients aged 18–70 to one of four treatment arms: low-dose (100 µg) budesonide plus placebo or formoterol, or high-dose (400 µg) budesonide plus placebo or formoterol, administered twice daily over 1 year.

Rates of exacerbations, symptoms and lung functions were analyzed. Although combination therapy was shown to be superior over ICS alone, the authors noted that rates of severe and mild exacerbations were decreased by 49% and 37%, respectively, in the high-dose budesonide group. Similarly, Bateman et al.[21] compared the use of fluticasone to fluticasone/salmeterol in a group of mild-to-moderate asthmatics 12–80 years of age. Prior to randomization, patients were stratified on the basis of corticosteroid use (stratum 1, 2 and 3: previously corticosteroid-free, low- and moderate-dose corticosteroid users, respectively). Treatment was stepped up until either total control or a maximum dose of 500 µg bid of corticosteroid was reached. Definition of control was based on PEF, rescue medication use, symptoms, night-time awakenings, exacerbations, emergency visits and adverse events. Among patients receiving ICS alone, total control was achieved in 31% in stratum 1, 20% in stratum 2 and 8% in stratum 3 during the first phase of the study in which corticosteroid dosing was escalated. During phase two, patients were maintained at either the dose providing total control or the maximum corticosteroid dose allowed (500 µg fluticasone bid). Rates of exacerbations continued to decline in all groups with total control being achieved in 40%, 28% and 16%, in strata 1–3, respectively. These and other studies continue to support the role of using maintenance ICS as a means of obtaining optimal asthma control and preventing or reducing symptoms associated with acute exacerbations. However, although maintenance ICS can reduce asthma exacerbations, it is important to emphasize that this therapy does not totally ameliorate them.

In addition to providing improved daily control of asthma symptoms, ICS have also been shown to reduce asthma-related mortality. Several studies have examined the relationship between patterns of ICS use and rates of severe asthma exacerbations resulting in significant morbidity and/or mortality. In an early study by Ernst et al.,[22] patients receiving one or more MDI of beclomethasone per month had a significant reduction in fatal and near-fatal asthma exacerbations. These findings were confirmed in a larger analysis by the same group[23] in which the authors demonstrated that the risk of death from asthma was markedly reduced in those patients using low-dose inhaled corticosteroids and that the risk of death continued to decline as compliance increased. Using national health statistics and pharmaceutical sales data, two additional studies have found an inverse relationship between decreasing rates of asthma mortality and increasing sales of inhaled corticosteroids, further confirming the protective effect of this class of anti-inflammatory medications.[24,25] When looking at rates of hospitalization, Donahue et al.[26] found a 50% reduction in the relative risk for hospitalization among patients receiving ICS. These observations reflect the importance of suppressing low-grade inflammation that exists between flares and that probably places the patient at increased risk for future severe exacerbations.

Although maintenance ICS therapy is the preferred treatment for patients with mild persistent asthma, recent data generated by the Asthma Clinical Research Network suggest that this approach may not be necessary in patients with long-standing histories of asthma who currently have very mild symptoms based on guideline criteria.[27] In this trial, patients were randomized to receive either budesonide 200 µg twice daily, zafirlukast 20 mg twice daily or matching placebos for an entire year. All three groups initiated a symptom-based action plan (budesonide 800 µg twice daily for 10 days or prednisone 0.5 mg/kg for 5 days) for worsening symptoms. Treatment with only a symptom-based action plan (and not daily controller therapy) was sufficient to maintain control of peak flow, asthma exacerbations and quality of life, and did not increase loss of lung function during the 1 year of treatment. However, monotherapy with ICS in this trial significantly improved pre-bronchodilator FEV_1, bronchial reactivity, biomarkers of airway inflammation (exhaled nitric oxide and sputum eosinophils) and symptom-free days. Based on these provocative and novel findings, the authors suggested that the patient and their health-care provider may want to consider the relative merits of this increase in symptom-free days (26 per year) in the context of whether it is worth the cost of treatment, both fiscal and with respect to long-term side-effects.

EXPERIENCE WITH EXPERIMENTAL RESPIRATORY INFECTIONS

As many of the above *in vivo* studies have shown, inhaled glucocorticoids appear to provide some level of benefit in modulating the effects of acute asthma exacerbations. Since viral infections are a common cause of exacerbations in both children and adults, the mechanisms by which glucocorticoids modify asthmatic host response to these infections have been evaluated in a number of different experimental paradigms. In studies that utilize experimental infections, an understanding of the pathogenesis of virus-induced exacerbations has been gained, particularly in the role of both rhinovirus (RV) infections and intercellular adhesion molecule-1 (ICAM-1). ICAM-1, a ligand for integrin receptors on leukocytes, is expressed on respiratory epithelial cells and functions both to recruit inflammatory cells to the airways during viral infections and as a cellular receptor for the majority of RVs.[28] Several research groups have evaluated the role of inhaled corticosteroids in modulating the effects of lower respiratory tract inflammatory changes that occur with RV infections. Papi *et al.*[29] investigated the effects of systemic and topical corticosteroids on the development of RV-induced ICAM-1 expression. As they had shown previously, ICAM-1 surface expression on human bronchial and pulmonary epithelial cells is increased during RV infection.[30] Cultured primary bronchial or transformed (A549) respiratory epithelial cells

were pretreated with corticosteroids, infected with RV16 and evaluated for ICAM-1 surface expression via flow cytometry. The investigators found that, while both topical and systemic corticosteroids had no direct effect on RV infectivity or replication in cultured cells, the pretreatment with corticosteroids resulted in a significant decrease in RV-induced ICAM-1 upregulation in respiratory epithelial cells in these *in vitro* conditions.

In a similar study, by Suzuki *et al.*,[31] human tracheal epithelial cells were incubated with dexamethasone or vehicle for 3 days prior to culture with RV2 or RV14. Analysis of supernatants and cell lysates revealed significantly lower RV14 titers in cells pretreated with dexamethasone. Inhibition of RV14 replication correlated in a dose-dependent fashion with maximal benefit noted at $1\,\mu mol/l$ of dexamethasone. Incubation with dexamethasone also decreased the susceptibility of these cells to RV14 infection as demonstrated by a ten-fold increase in the minimum dose of virus necessary to cause infection. ICAM-1 expression, assayed both by flow cytometry and by Northern blot, was increased two-fold by day 3 in RV14-infected cells compared to sham-exposed cells. An increase in ICAM-1 was significantly reduced by pretreatment with dexamethasone ($1\,\mu mol/l$). The ability of dexamethasone to modulate infection with RV14, but not RV2, a member of the minor group of RVs that does not use ICAM-1 as its receptor,[32] supports the conclusion that dexamethasone probably induces inhibition of RV14 infection via reduction of cell-surface ICAM-1 expression.

While the above *in vitro* reports evaluated the role of systemic and topical corticosteroids on RV infection and ICAM-1 expression, the following studies examined the efficacy of ICS on the prevention of RV-associated asthma exacerbations *in vivo*. In a double-blind, parallel study by Grünberg *et al.*,[33] 25 corticosteroid-naive, non-smoking atopic adult subjects with mild asthma were randomized to receive

2 weeks of pretreatment with either budesonide (800 µg bid) or placebo prior to an experimental inoculation with RV16. Confirmation of infection was documented by a greater than four-fold increase in virus-specific neutralizing serum antibody titer and/or by recovery of virus from nasal washes. Treatment was continued for a total duration of 4 weeks with bronchoscopy performed 2 days prior to and 6 days after RV16 intranasal inoculation. A third group of asthmatic subjects, with the same inclusion criteria, underwent bronchial biopsies at 8-day intervals without intervention or treatment and served as a control group. When ICAM-1 expression was evaluated, no difference was found between groups in the baseline bronchial biopsies. There was, however, a significant increase in ICAM-1 expression over baseline with RV16 infection in the placebo group, and a trend towards increased expression in the budesonide group; the difference between the groups, however, was non-significant and indicates that pretreatment with budesonide did not prevent the RV16-associated increase in ICAM-1 expression. An evaluation of epithelial intactness also did not vary between groups and was not affected by either RV16 infection, or bronchoscopy alone. This study confirms the observation that an experimental RV16 infection can upregulate ICAM-1 expression on bronchial epithelium in asthma *in vivo*, and led the authors to conclude that pretreatment with ICS neither affects baseline ICAM-1 expression, nor has a protective effect against RV16-associated upregulation.

In a follow-up publication from the same study group, Grünberg and colleagues[34] evaluated the effects of budesonide pretreatment on airway hyperresponsiveness and inflammatory cell recruitment associated with an RV16 infection. In these analyses, bronchial biopsy specimens were evaluated for the presence of inflammatory cells in both the lamina propria and the respiratory epithelium. After RV16 infection, an accumulation of CD3+ cells was noted in both groups, irrespective

of pretreatment, indicating that ICS did not significantly influence the inflammatory airway response associated with RV infection. The authors also found that budesonide pretreatment was associated with improved PC_{20} during the pretreatment phase and with reduced eosinophilic airway inflammation when compared to the placebo group. It should be noted, however, that while the PC_{20} did improve during the pretreatment phase with budesonide, as would be expected, there was no change in PC_{20} in either group following RV16 inoculation. This contrasts with previous studies that have found significant increases in airway hyperresponsiveness with RV infection.[35,36] Although 21 of the 25 patients demonstrated an active infection with RV16, the lower symptom scores led the authors to speculate that a mild rhinovirus infection may result in airway inflammation without evidence for clinical worsening of asthma symptoms and that only severe respiratory infections may lead to a significant decrease in PC_{20}. Therefore, the complex interactions between the use of inhaled corticosteroids, respiratory viral infections and underlying allergic airway inflammation may provide an additional explanation and suggests that other factors might be involved during spontaneous virus-induced exacerbations vs. experimental colds in asthmatic patients.

SUMMARY

Viral respiratory infections frequently result in a transient, yet significant, worsening of symptoms in patients with asthma and represent the origin for the majority of acute exacerbations found in adults.[37,38] For this reason, further insights into the mechanisms by which respiratory infections provoke asthma are essential in providing improved directions for control, and possibly prevention, of this common cause of asthma exacerbation. While the effectiveness of the anti-inflammatory properties of inhaled corticosteroids on establishing asthma control and reducing asthma-related mortality are well documented, the efficacy of prophylactic high-dose inhaled corticosteroids for the prevention of virus-induced worsening of lower airway inflammation has been less than satisfactory. As both Harrison *et al.*[18] and FitzGerald *et al.*[19] have shown, simply doubling the dose of inhaled steroids in adults does not provide significant benefit, and further studies investigating greater increments in dose adjustment may be worthwhile. In children, the intervention of high-dose ICS at the onset of viral URTIs appears more promising, yet the majority of exacerbations continue to occur. These data suggest that the mechanisms of asthma deterioration during exacerbations may not be fully regulated by corticosteroids, and other approaches need to be considered.

REFERENCES

1. Murphy S, Bleecker ER, Boushey H, et al. Guidelines for the Diagnosis and Management of Asthma. National Asthma Education and Prevention Program. Bethesda, MD: National Institutes of Health, 1997: 1–150

2. Wilson NM, Silverman M. Treatment of acute, episodic asthma in preschool children using intermittent high dose inhaled steroids at home. Arch Dis Child 1990; 65: 407–10

3. Daugbjerg P, Brenoe E, Forchhammer H, et al. A comparison between nebulized terbutaline, nebulized corticosteroid and systemic corticosteroid for acute wheezing in children up to 18 months of age. Acta Paediatr 1993; 82: 547–51

4. Connett G, Lenney W. Prevention of viral induced asthma attacks using inhaled budesonide. Arch Dis Child 1993; 68: 85–7

5. Svedmyr J, Nyberg E, Asbrink-Nilsson E, Hedlin G. Intermittent treatment with inhaled steroids for deterioration of asthma due to upper respiratory tract infections. Acta Paediatr 1995; 84: 884–8

6. Svedmyr J, Nyberg E, Thunqvist P, et al. Prophylactic intermittent treatment with inhaled corticosteroids of asthma exacerbations due to airway infections in toddlers. Acta Paediatr 1999; 88: 42–7

7. Volovitz B, Bentur L, Finkelstein Y, et al. Effectiveness and safety of inhaled corticosteroids in controlling acute asthma attacks in children who were treated in the emergency department: a controlled comparative study with oral prednisolone. J Allergy Clin Immunol 1998; 102: 605–9

8. Schuh S, Reisman J, Alshehri M, et al. A comparison of inhaled fluticasone and oral prednisone for children with severe acute asthma. N Engl J Med 2000; 343: 689–94

9. McKean M, Ducharme F. Inhaled steroids for episodic viral wheeze of childhood. Cochrane Database Syst Rev 2000; 2: CD001107

10. Wilson N, Sloper K, Silverman M. Effect of continuous treatment with topical corticosteroid on episodic viral wheeze in preschool children. Arch Dis Child 1995; 72: 317–20

11. Doull IJ, Lampe FC, Smith S, et al. Effect of inhaled corticosteroids on episodes of wheezing associated with viral infection in school age children: randomised double blind placebo controlled trial. BMJ 1997; 315: 858–62

12. Childhood Asthma Management Program (CAMP) Research Group. Long-term effects of budesonide or nedocromil in children with asthma. N Engl J Med 2000; 343: 1054–63

13. Johnston NW, Johnston SL, Duncan JM, et al. The September epidemic of asthma exacerbations in children: a search for etiology. J Allergy Clin Immunol 2005; 115: 132–8

14. Murray C, Poletti G, Kebadze T, et al. A study of modifiable risk factors for asthma exacerbations: virus infection and allergen exposure synergistically increase risk of asthma hospitalization in children. Thorax 2006; 61: 376–82

15. Levy ML, Stevenson C, Maslen T. Comparison of short courses of oral prednisolone and fluticasone propionate in the treatment of adults with acute exacerbations of asthma in primary care. Thorax 1996; 51: 1087–92

16. Foresi A, Morelli MC, Catena E; on behalf of the Italian Study Group. Low-dose budesonide with the addition of an increased dose during exacerbations is effective in long-term asthma control. Chest 2000; 117: 440–6

17. FitzGerald JM, Shragge D, Haddon J, et al. A randomized, controlled trial of high dose, inhaled budesonide versus oral prednisone in patients discharged from the emergency department following an acute asthma exacerbation. Can Respir J 2000; 7: 61–7

18. Harrison TW, Oborne J, Newton S, Tattersfield AE. Doubling the dose of inhaled corticosteroid to prevent asthma exacerbations: randomised controlled trial. Lancet 2004; 363: 271–5

19. FitzGerald JM, Becker A, Sears MR, et al. Doubling the dose of budesonide versus maintenance treatment in asthma exacerbations. Thorax 2004; 59: 550–6

20. Pauwels RA, Löfdahl CG, Postma DS, et al. Effect of inhaled formoterol and budesonide on exacerbations of asthma. N Engl J Med 1997; 337: 1405–11

21. Bateman ED, Boushey HA, Bousquet J, et al. Can guideline-defined asthma control be achieved? The

Gaining Optimal Asthma ControL study. Am J Respir Crit Care Med 2004; 170: 836–44

22. Ernst P, Spitzer WO, Suissa S, et al. Risk of fatal and near-fatal asthma in relation to inhaled corticosteroid use. J Am Med Assoc 1992; 268: 3462–4

23. Suissa S, Ernst P, Benayoun S, et al. Low-dose inhaled corticosteroids and the prevention of death from asthma. N Engl J Med 2000; 343: 332–6

24. Goldman M, Rachmiel M, Gendler L, Katz Y. Decrease in asthma mortality rate in Israel from 1991–1995: is it related to increased use of inhaled corticosteroids? J Allergy Clin Immunol 2000; 105: 71–4

25. Sly RM, Sly RM. Changing asthma mortality and sales of inhaled bronchodilators and anti-asthmatic drugs. [Review] [16 refs]. Ann Allergy 1994; 73: 439–43

26. Donahue JG, Weiss ST, Livingston JM, et al. Inhaled steroids and the risk of hospitalization for asthma. J Am Med Assoc 1997; 277: 887–91

27. Boushey HA, Sorkness CA, King TS, et al. Daily versus as-needed corticosteroids for mild persistent asthma. N Engl J Med 2005; 352: 1519–28

28. Greve JM, Davis G, Meyer AM, et al. The major human rhinovirus receptor is ICAM-1. Cell 1989; 56: 839–47

29. Papi A, Papadopoulos NG, Degitz K, et al. Corticosteroids inhibit rhinovirus-induced intercellular adhesion molecule-1 up-regulation and promoter activation on respiratory epithelial cells. J Allergy Clin Immunol 2000; 105: 318–26

30. Papi A, Johnston SL. Rhinovirus infection induces expression of its own receptor intercellular adhesion molecule 1 (ICAM-1) via increased NF-kappaB-mediated transcription. J Biol Chem 1999; 274: 9707–20

31. Suzuki T, Yamaya M, Sekizawa K, et al. Effects of dexamethasone on rhinovirus infection in cultured human tracheal epithelial cells. Am J Physiol 2000; 278: L560–L571

32. Hofer F, Gruenberger M, Kowalski H, et al. Members of the low density lipoprotein receptor family mediate cell entry of a minor-group common cold virus. Proc Natl Acad Sci USA 1994; 91: 1839–42

33. Grunberg K, Sharon RF, Hiltermann TJ, et al. Experimental rhinovirus 16 infection increases intercellular adhesion molecule-1 expression in bronchial epithelium of asthmatics regardless of inhaled steroid treatment. Clin Exp Allergy 2000; 30: 1015–23

34. Grunberg K, Sharon RF, Sont JK, et al. Rhinovirus-induced airway inflammation in asthma: effect of treatment with inhaled corticosteroids before and during experimental infection. Am J Respir Crit Care Med 2001; 164: 1816–22

35. Grunberg K, Timmers MC, Smits HH, et al. Effect of experimental rhinovirus 16 colds on airway hyperresponsiveness to histamine and interleukin-8 in nasal lavage in asthmatic subjects in vivo. Clin Exp Allergy 1997; 27: 36–45

36. Lemanske RF Jr, Dick EC, Swenson CA, et al. Rhinovirus upper respiratory infection increases airway hyperreactivity and late asthmatic reactions. J Clin Invest 1989; 83: 1–10

37. Nicholson KG, Kent JK, Ireland DC. Respiratory viruses and exacerbations of asthma in adults. BMJ 1993; 307: 982–6

38. Johnston SL, Pattemore PK, Sanderson G, et al. Community study of role of viral infections in exacerbations of asthma in 9–11 year old children. BMJ 1995; 310: 1225–8

39. Garrett J, Williams S, Wong C, et al. Treatment of acute asthmatic exacerbations with an increased dose of inhaled steroid. Arch Dis Child 1998; 79: 12–17

Efficacy of inhaled corticosteroids/long-acting β₂-agonist combinations in preventing asthma exacerbations

Paul M O'Byrne

INTRODUCTION

Preventing asthma exacerbations has been identified as an important outcome in establishing ideal asthma control by all asthma treatment guidelines (for example, see references 1 and 2). Indeed, it may be considered the most important outcome, because asthma exacerbations are not only the occasion of greatest risk to asthma patients, but also a great cause of anxiety to patients and their families, the greatest stress on health-care providers and greatest cost to the health-care system in asthma management. Despite the importance of preventing exacerbations with asthma therapy, it has not, until relatively recently, been a major outcome variable in studies of the efficacy of drug treatment in asthma.

Severe asthma exacerbations are a common clinical manifestation of patients with severe, poorly controlled asthma and, partly as a result of this, little attention has been paid to the importance of exacerbations in patients thought to have mild asthma. This view has been challenged by the results of a number of studies in patients believed by their managing physician to have mild, stable asthma. Robertson *et al.*[3] made the important observation that 33% of 51 children who died of acute severe asthma exacerbations, over a 3-year period in the State of Victoria, Australia, were thought to have mild or trivial

asthma before their final attack. Also, in a study of patients considered by their primary care physician to have such mild asthma that they would not derive any clinical benefit from inhaled corticosteroids (ICS), up to 70% of the patients were experiencing nocturnal or early morning symptoms in the month before entering the study, and 30% of the patients receiving placebo therapy had a severe asthma exacerbation during the 4 months of the study.[4] A much larger study, the OPTIMA trial,[5] also evaluated mild patients not using ICS, and demonstrated that 33% had a severe asthma exacerbation during treatment with placebo. Similarly, in the CAMP study of children with mild-to-moderate asthma,[6] >60% of the patients receiving placebo treatment had a severe asthma exacerbation during the first year. These studies indicate that the prevalence of severe asthma exacerbations is much higher in patients with mild asthma than was previously believed.

In a study of the development and resolution of severe exacerbations, Tattersfield *et al.*[7] showed that, in a group of patients with moderate-to-severe asthma, exacerbations developed on average over 5–7 days before being recognized and treated. Once treatment with oral corticosteroids was started, the exacerbation resolved over 5–7 days. However, in occasional patients, severe life-threatening exacerbations can develop over minutes to hours.

EFFICACY OF INHALED CORTICOSTEROIDS ALONE IN PREVENTING ASTHMA EXACERBATIONS

The efficacy of ICS alone in preventing asthma exacerbations is the topic of Chapter 17, and for that reason it will not be covered in any detail here. Briefly, however, ICS have been shown consistently to be remarkably effective in preventing asthma exacerbations[8,9] and asthma fatalities.[10] These important benefits are achieved with even low doses of ICS.

EFFICACY OF β_2-AGONISTS IN PREVENTING ASTHMA EXACERBATIONS

In striking contrast to the benefits of even low doses of ICS, the overuse of short-acting inhaled β_2-agonists is associated with increased risks of asthma exacerbations[11] and asthma fatalities.[12] This issue began by the identification, in 1968, of an association between the use of a more potent formulation of isoproterenol and increases in asthma mortality in the early and mid-1960s in the UK, Australia and New Zealand (reviewed in reference 11). The increases in asthma mortality did not occur in those countries in which this formulation was not available. This controversy was rekindled by a second dramatic increase in asthma mortality in New Zealand in the late 1970s, with a less dramatic increase in many other countries. In New Zealand, the increase was temporally associated with the introduction of a β_2-agonist, fenoterol,[12] in a metered dose inhaler which delivered 200 µg per activation – twice the amount of salbutamol, even though their potencies were similar. Once again, the issue of the causality of the association between the use of fenoterol and increases in asthma mortality were vigorously debated. A subsequent analysis of the association between β_2-agonist use and asthma mortality came from a Canadian study, which showed a markedly increased odds

ratio for the risk of dying from severe asthma with the overuse of fenoterol and, to a lesser extent, salbutamol.[13] This analysis related the number of filled prescriptions for the β_2-agonists to the number of life-threatening asthma exacerbations and asthma deaths. The investigators demonstrated a dose-dependent increase in both severe exacerbations and asthma deaths.

Each of these studies was a case–control analysis and, as such, cannot impute causality to the associations between the increased use of inhaled β_2-agonists and asthma mortality. There is the possibility that the overuse of β_2-agonists to treat frequent symptoms is a marker of severe, uncontrolled asthma. Patients with severe asthma are at much greater risk of exacerbations, or of dying from asthma, than milder asthmatics; thus, the overuse of β_2-agonists may be a reflection of this severity.

One double-blind, randomized crossover trial addressed the question of the potential risks of regular use of inhaled fenoterol, compared with its intermittent use (as needed), on a number of indices of asthma morbidity. Markers of asthma control included daytime and nocturnal asthma symptoms, morning and evening measurements of peak expired flow rates, rescue use of β_2-agonists during the day and night, and asthma exacerbations.[14] The study demonstrated that overall asthma control was not as good in patients who were receiving fenoterol on a regular basis. The effect was not obviated by the use of inhaled corticosteroids. Also, the regular use of inhaled fenoterol was associated with significantly more asthma exacerbations.

The results of these studies with the short-acting inhaled β_2-agonists gave great concern when the long-acting inhaled β_2-agonist (LABA) salmeterol was initially introduced. Subsequently, these concerns were, in part, borne out in studies which have evaluated salmeterol as monotherapy in patients with moderate asthma. For example, a study that compared salmeterol monotherapy to low doses of ICS or placebo demonstrated that the salmeterol-only treatment arm had more treatment failures and more asthma exacerbations.[15] In addition, a very large prospective study to assess the safety of salmeterol was initiated in 1996, in association with the US Food and Drug Administration (FDA), called the SMART study. This was a 28-week evaluation in almost 26 000 patients where salmeterol was compared to placebo. The primary endpoint of the study was the combined number of respiratory related deaths and life-threatening asthma exacerbations. Other endpoints included asthma-related events including deaths. Fortunately, despite its very large size, the number of events were few; however, a higher though not statistically significant number of asthma-related life-threatening experiences, including deaths, occurred in the patients treated with salmeterol. There was, however, a statistically significantly greater number of asthma-related events, including deaths, in African–American patients (17% of the study population) taking salmeterol. These results, taken together, have reinforced the view that asthmatic patients with persistent symptoms should not be treated with either short- or LABA as monotherapy.

EFFICACY OF COMBINATION THERAPY WITH INHALED CORTICOSTEROIDS AND LONG-ACTING INHALED β₂-AGONISTS

The use of combination therapy with LABA and ICS has been demonstrated to reduce the doses of ICS required to maintain ideal asthma control.[16] However, because of the issues mentioned above, this treatment alternative raised concerns that patients achieving short-term benefit from this combination would be put at risk, over the longer term, of increased exacerbations. This concern existed because of the potential detrimental effect of reducing doses of ICS on the progression of airway inflammation. Indeed, in studies discussed above, where ICS were discontinued, and patients treated with LABAs alone, asthma exacerbations were shown to increase.[15]

The first study to address the question of whether adding the LABA to a low dose of ICS would increase the risks of asthma exacerbations was the FACET study.[17] In this study the LABA formoterol was added to a low dose (200 μg) or four-fold higher dose (800 μg) of inhaled budesonide and compared to those doses plus placebo. This study evaluated patients with moderate-to-severe asthma, who had moderate airflow obstruction, while on an average daily dose of ICS of close to 800 μg. The primary outcome variable in the trial was the rate of severe asthma exacerbations over 1 year of treatment. Indeed, this study was the first large prospective clinical trial to use asthma exacerbations as a primary variable and to power the study accordingly. Asthma exacerbations were defined as a decline in peak expired flows (PEF) of > 30% from baseline for two consecutive days, or a hospitalization or emergency room visit because of acute severe asthma, or an asthma exacerbation as determined by the study investigator (indeed, >70% of the exacerbations were determined in this way). The study demonstrated that a four-fold increase in ICS dose or a combination of inhaled budesonide and formoterol both improved asthma control, and also significantly reduced, rather than increased, the rate of both mild and severe asthma exacerbations over and above that achieved by either low or high doses of budesonide alone (Figure 18.1). Furthermore, another study has demonstrated that even the 'as needed' use of inhaled formoterol, when combined with ICS, reduced asthma exacerbations when compared to the 'as needed' use of a short-acting inhaled β₂-agonist terbutaline.[18] In addition, the effect of the combination of low doses of inhaled budesonide plus formoterol compared to high doses of budesonide alone on airway inflammation in asthma has also been evaluated.[19] This study confirmed that eosinophilic airway inflammation did not worsen in patients taking the combination therapy, when compared to the higher dose of budesonide alone.

Studies in patients with less severe asthma have shown somewhat different results, which

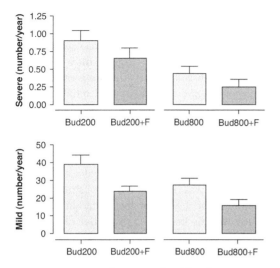

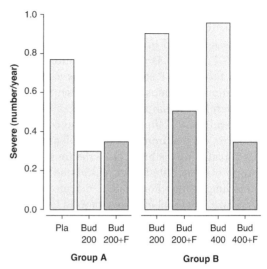

Figure 18.1 Rate of severe and mild asthma exacerbations, expressed as number/patient per year measured in the FACET study during 1 year of treatment with either budesonide 200 µg/day (Bud200) with and without formoterol (F) 12 µg twice daily, or budesonide 800 µg/day (Bud800) with and without formoterol 12 µg twice daily. A four-fold increase in the dose of budesonide reduced the rate of exacerbations by almost 50% ($p<0.001$), with an additional benefit demonstrated with the addition of formoterol ($p=0.01$)

Figure 18.2 Rate of severe asthma exacerbations, expressed as number/patient per year, measured in the patients in the OPTIMA study during 1 year of treatment. Group A consisted of patients with mild asthma not taking inhaled corticosteroids (ICS), treated with either placebo (Pla) or budesonide (Bud) 200 µg/day, with or without formoterol (F) 6 µg twice daily. Budesonide alone reduced exacerbations (RR=0.40, 95% CI 0.27–0.59), with no additional benefit from the combination of budesonide and formoterol. Group B consisted of patients not ideally controlled on low doses of ICS. Doubling the daily dose of budesonide did not significantly reduce exacerbations (RR=0.89, 95% CI 0.65–1.01) while the combination of budesonide and formoterol did (RR=0.57, 95% CI 0.46–0.72). Reprinted with permission from reference 5

seem to depend on the severity of asthma in the population studied. The OPTIMA study[5] evaluated two different populations of patients with milder asthma. These were patients with mild persisting asthma, who had not previously been treated with ICS, and a second group of patients who had mild persisting symptoms while taking a low dose of ICS (<400 µg/day budesonide). The results differed in the two groups of patients. In those patients who were steroid naive, low doses of budesonide alone had a marked effect in reducing asthma exacerbations when compared to placebo, but the combination of the LABA, formoterol and budesonide had no additional benefit when compared to budesonide alone (Figure 18.2). By contrast, in those patients already taking a low dose of ICS, but with mild persisting symptoms, the combination had a

marked effect in reducing both mild and severe asthma exacerbations (Figure 18.2).

Similar results have been reported with the combination of the LABA salmeterol and the ICS fluticasone. A meta-analysis of the studies which have compared treatment with the combination of inhaled fluticasone and salmeterol showed a 2.4% reduction in moderate or severe asthma exacerbations.[20] An even greater effect was subsequently reported in the GOAL study,[16] which evaluated the ability of

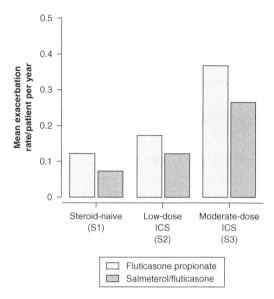

Figure 18.3 Mean rate of exacerbations requiring either oral steroids or hospitalization/emergency visit per patient per year over 1 year in the GOAL study, among patients treated with salmeterol/fluticasone or fluticasone propionate, according to use of inhaled corticosteroids (ICS) in the previous 6 months (stratum 1–stratum 3) (S1–S3). The combination of salmeterol/fluticasone significantly reduced severe exacerbations ($p \leq 0.009$ in all strata). Reproduced with permission from reference 16

increasing doses of the combination inhaler Serotide®, containing salmeterol and fluticasone, to obtain ideal asthma control in a range of patients with mild-to-severe asthma. Although the study compared the effects of treatment with Serotide to historical controls in these patients, the reduction in risk of an asthma exacerbation was approximately 25% for the entire group, but was most effective in the milder, steroid-naive population (Figure 18.3).

The combination inhaler Symbicort® contains both budesonide and formoterol, and has also been shown to improve overall asthma control as well as reduce the risk of asthma exacerbations. Zetterström and colleagues[21] have compared the use of the combination inhaler to the mono-components budesonide and formoterol given separately, and to budesonide alone. This study demonstrated that the combination inhaler was at least as effective as the mono-components given separately and significantly better than budesonide alone in reducing the risk of asthma exacerbations.

It has been possible to study a newer management approach to reduce asthma exacerbations using Symbicort. This is because the LABA component of Symbicort has an onset of action that is similar to that of the short-acting inhaled β₂-agonists salbutamol[22] or terbutaline, and is shorter than salmeterol.[23] This means that formoterol, although having a long duration of action, has been approved for rescue use in many countries. This led to the hypothesis that Symbicort, if used as rescue treatment added to a low-maintenance dose of the combination, may reduce the risk of exacerbations occurring. This is based on the fact that most severe asthma exacerbations develop over several days, with progressively worsening symptoms and reductions in flow rates.[7] Thus, if Symbicort were to be used as rescue treatment during this period of deterioration, the risk of the exacerbation developing may be reduced.

This hypothesis has been tested in the STAY study.[24] In this study, Symbicort as rescue treatment added to a low-maintenance dose of Symbicort was compared to the short-acting inhaled β₂-agonist terbutaline added to the same maintenance dose of Symbicort, or to a four-fold higher dose of budesonide. The study demonstrated a 45% lower severe asthma exacerbation risk when Symbicort was used as rescue when compared to terbutaline (Figure 18.4), and the time to second and third asthma exacerbations was also significantly prolonged. The magnitude of the benefits achieved in the current study with Symbicort for maintenance and relief, when compared with a four-fold higher maintenance dose of budesonide, was surprising and suggests that it is the timing of the increase in ICS dose, resulting from as-needed use of Symbicort in response to symptoms, rather than the total inhaled dose of ICS that

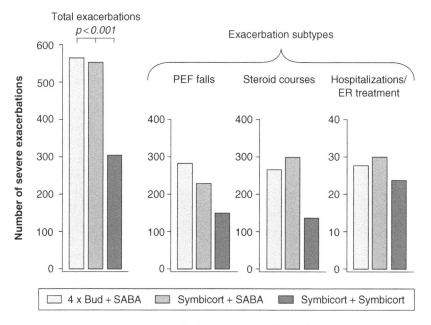

Figure 18.4 Absolute number of severe exacerbations in the STAY study during 1 year of treatment with budesonide 800 µg/day (Bud) with the short-acting inhaled β_2-agonist (SABA) terbutaline as rescue inhaler, or Symbicort 200/6 µg/day with terbutaline as rescue inhaler, or Symbicort 200/6 µg/day with Symbicort as rescue inhaler (left panel). Also shown are the number of exacerbations defined by the fall in the inhaled corticosteriod (PEF) criterion (>30% from baseline for two consecutive days), or by the number of oral corticosteroid courses decided by the managing physician, or by a hospitalization of emergency room (ER) visit. Symbicort used both as maintenance and rescue significantly reduced the number of exacerbations in all categories. Redrawn from data in reference 24

improves efficacy. Studies that simply doubled the maintenance dose of ICS well into the course of an exacerbation have generally failed to show added benefits.[25,26]

MECHANISMS OF COMBINATION THERAPY IN REDUCING ASTHMA EXACERBATIONS

The precise mechanism by which the combination of ICS and LABA reduces the risk of asthma exacerbations more effectively than ICS alone has not yet been elucidated. However, a number of recent studies have suggested a synergistic effect at a molecular level. Eickelberg and colleagues[27] were the first to identify a

ligand-independent activation of the glucocorticoid receptor by the β_2-agonists salbutamol and salmeterol. This effect was mediated by activation of the β_2-receptor. This suggested that β_2-agonists could have an anti-inflammatory effect by activating glucocorticoid response elements and steroid responsive genes. Additional effects of the combination have been shown to suppress T-cell proliferation and Th1 cytokine production in normal subjects,[28] while increasing peripheral blood T-cell apoptosis when compared with ICS alone.[29] Finally, Roth and colleagues[30] have demonstrated that the combination of formoterol and budesonide reduced airway smooth muscle proliferation better than either alone. However, whether any or all of these synergistic effects explain the benefit in reducing exacerbation risk remains to be clarified.

Another possible mechanism has been evaluated by Edwards et al.,[31] who have demonstrated a synergistic effect of salmeterol and fluticasone in respiratory epithelial cells, in their ability to reduce human rhinovirus-induced proinflammatory cytokine production. This may be an important mechanism of the combination of ICS and LABA, as human rhinoviruses are known to be an important cause of asthma exacerbations.[32]

CONCLUSIONS

Severe asthma exacerbations are common in patients with all grades of asthma severity. Most exacerbations develop over several days before being identified and treated. Even low doses of inhaled corticosteroids markedly reduce the risk of developing an asthma exacerbation. If patients are using a low dose of ICS and identify the onset of an exacerbation, a four-fold increase in inhaled corticosteroid dose may reduce the risk of the exacerbation progressing. The combination of ICS and long-acting inhaled β₂-agonists also reduces the risks of exacerbations to a greater extent than high-dose ICS alone. This has been best demonstrated with the combination of budesonide and formoterol. Other treatments including leukotriene receptor antagonists[33] and anti-IgE monoclonal antibody[34] also reduce the risks of asthma exacerbations. Their benefit, in this regard, has not yet been compared to the combination of ICS and long-acting inhaled β₂-agonists.

REFERENCES

1. National Institutes of Health. Global Strategy for Asthma Management and Prevention. NIH Publication No 02-3659, 2004

2. Lemiere C, Bai TR, Balter M, et al. Adult Asthma Consensus Guidelines Update 2003. Can Respir J 2004; 11: A9–A18

3. Robertson CF, Rubinfeld AR, Bowes G. Pediatric asthma deaths in Victoria: the mild are at risk. Pediatr Pulmonol 1992; 13: 95–100

4. O'Byrne PM, Cuddy L, Taylor DW, et al. The clinical efficacy and cost benefit of inhaled corticosteroids as therapy in patients with mild asthma in primary care practice. Can Respir J 1996; 3: 169–75

5. O'Byrne PM, Barnes PJ, Rodriguez-Roisin R, et al. Low dose inhaled budesonide and formoterol in mild persistent asthma: the OPTIMA randomized trial. Am J Respir Crit Care Med 2001; 164: 1392–7

6. Long-term effects of budesonide or nedocromil in children with asthma. The Childhood Asthma Management Program Research Group. N Engl J Med 2000; 343: 1054–63

7. Tattersfield AE, Postma DS, Barnes PJ, et al. Exacerbations of asthma: a descriptive study of 425 severe exacerbations. The FACET International Study Group. Am J Respir Crit Care Med 1999; 160: 594–9

8. Barnes PJ, Pedersen S, Busse WW. Efficacy and safety of inhaled corticosteroids: new developments. Am J Respir Crit Care Med 1998; 157: 1–53

9. Pedersen S, O'Byrne PM. A comparison of the efficacy and safety of inhaled corticosteroids in asthma. Allergy 1997; 52: 1–34

10. Suissa S, Ernst P. Inhaled corticosteroids: impact on asthma morbidity and mortality. J Allergy Clin Immunol 2001; 107: 937–44

11. Sears MR, Taylor DR. Regular beta-agonist therapy – the quality of the evidence. Eur Respir J 1992; 5: 896–7

12. Crane J, Pearce N, Flatt A, et al. Prescribed fenoterol and death from asthma in New Zealand, 1981–83: case–control study. Lancet 1989; 1: 917–22

13. Suissa S, Ernst P, Boivin JF, et al. A cohort analysis of excess mortality in asthma and the use of inhaled beta-agonists. Am J Respir Crit Care Med 1994; 149: 604–10

14. Sears MR, Taylor DR, Print CG, et al. Regular inhaled beta-agonist treatment in bronchial asthma. Lancet 1990; 336: 1391–6

15. Lazarus SC, Boushey HA, Fahy JV, et al. Long-acting beta2-agonist monotherapy vs continued therapy with inhaled corticosteroids in patients with persistent asthma: a randomized controlled trial. J Am Med Assoc 2001; 285: 2583–93

16. Bateman ED, Boushey HA, Bousquet J, et al. Can guideline-defined asthma control be achieved? The Gaining Optimal Asthma ControL study. Am J Respir Crit Care Med 2004; 170: 836–44

17. Pauwels RA, Lofdahl C-G, Postma DS, et al. Effect of inhaled formoterol and budesonide on exacerbations of asthma. N Engl J Med 1997; 337: 1405–11

18. Tattersfield AE, Lofdahl CG, Postma DS, et al. Comparison of formoterol and terbutaline for as-needed treatment of asthma: a randomised trial. Lancet 2001; 357: 257–61

19. Kips JC, O'Connor BJ, Inman MD, et al. A long-term study of the antiinflammatory effect of low-dose budesonide plus formoterol versus high-dose budesonide in asthma. Am J Respir Crit Care Med 2000; 161: 996–1001

20. Shrewsbury S, Pyke S, Britton M. Meta-analysis of increased dose of inhaled steroid or addition of salmeterol in symptomatic asthma (MIASMA). BMJ 2000; 320: 1368–73

21. Zetterstrom O, Buhl R, Mellem H, et al. Improved asthma control with budesonide/formoterol in a single inhaler, compared with budesonide alone. Eur Respir J 2001; 18: 262–8

22. Seberova E, Andersson A. Oxis (R) (formoterol given by Turbuhaler (R)) showed as rapid an onset of action as salbutamol given by a pMDI. Respir Med 2000; 94: 607–11

23. Palmqvist M, Ibsen T, Mellen A, Lotvall J. Comparison of the relative efficacy of formoterol and salmeterol in asthmatic patients. Am J Respir Crit Care Med 1999; 160: 244–9

24. O'Byrne PM, Bisgaard H, Godard PP, et al. Budesonide/formoterol combination therapy as both maintenance and reliever medication in asthma. Am J Respir Crit Care Med 2005; 171: 129–36

25. Fitzgerald JM, Becker A, Sears MR, et al. Doubling the dose of budesonide versus maintenance treatment in asthma exacerbations. Thorax 2004; 59: 550–6

26. Harrison TW, Oborne J, Newton S, Tattersfield AE. Doubling the dose of inhaled corticosteroid to prevent asthma exacerbations: randomised controlled trial. Lancet 2004; 363: 271–5

27. Eickelberg O, Roth M, Lorx R, et al. Ligand-independent activation of the glucocorticoid receptor by beta(2)-adrenergic receptor agonists in primary human lung fibroblasts and vascular smooth muscle cells. J Biol Chem 1999; 274: 1005–10

28. Goleva E, Dunlap A, Leung DYM. Differential control of T(H)1 versus T(H)2 cell responses by the combination of low-dose steroids with beta(2)-adrenergic agonists. J Allergy Clin Immunol 2004; 114: 183–91

29. Pace E, Gagliardo R, Melis M, et al. Synergistic effects of fluticasone propionate and salmeterol on in vitro T-cell activation and apoptosis in asthma. J Allergy Clin Immunol 2004; 114: 1216–23

30. Roth M, Johnson PRA, Rudiger JJ, et al. Interaction between glucocorticoids and beta(2) agonists on bronchial airway smooth muscle cells through synchronised cellular signalling. Lancet 2002; 360: 1293–9

31. Edwards MR, Laza-Stanca V, Johnson M, Johnston SL. Mechanisms of suppression of human rhinovirus induced pro-inflammatory cytokine production by combination therapy in vitro. Proc Am Thorac Soc 2005; 2: 583

32. Johnston SL, Pattemore PK, Sanderson G, et al. Community study of role of viral-infections in exacerbations of asthma in 9–11 year-old children. BMJ 1995; 310: 1225–9

33. Laviolette M, Malmstrom K, Lu S, et al. Montelukast added to inhaled beclomethasone in treatment of asthma. Am J Respir Crit Care Med 1999; 160: 1862–6

34. Busse WW. Anti-immunoglobulin E (omalizumab) therapy in allergic asthma. Am J Respir Crit Care Med 2001; 164: S12–S17

PART VI

Delivery of care

CHAPTER 19

Role of self-management in preventing asthma exacerbations

Heather Powell and Peter G Gibson

INTRODUCTION

Exacerbations are responsible for a disproportionate amount of the morbidity and mortality from asthma. Exacerbations of asthma usually occur gradually over several days to weeks, or on a background of chronic poor asthma control.[1,2] This provides an opportunity for early intervention with corticosteroids and β-agonists which act to reverse airflow obstruction and reduce the severity of the exacerbation. People with asthma can learn to recognize the symptoms of an asthma exacerbation and how to respond, to prevent further deterioration. This approach, when combined with appropriate maintenance pharmacotherapy, is an effective way to prevent severe asthma exacerbations. A written action plan facilitates the early detection and treatment of an exacerbation, and is an essential part of the self-management of exacerbations.[3]

Asthma is characterized by episodes of expiratory airflow obstruction, which occur in response to multiple stimuli. The frequency and severity of these episodes varies greatly, both between and within individuals. Since all individuals with asthma are susceptible to exacerbations of asthma, it follows that all people with diagnosed asthma need to know how to manage these episodes. This instruction in self-management can be formalized as a written action plan. For these reasons, all asthmatics are candidates for a written action plan. This contrasts with the need for inhaled anti-inflammatory therapy, which only becomes necessary when the frequency and/or severity of exacerbations is sufficiently great or asthma control is poor. At present, however, there is a paradoxical situation where the majority of people are prescribed regular inhaled corticosteroids, yet only a minority of patients either have[4,5] or use[6] a written action plan. An effective way to address this problem is to teach people with asthma how to detect and manage asthma exacerbations as early as possible. This chapter examines a variety of approaches that can be used to minimize the impact of exacerbations.

ASTHMA SELF-MANAGEMENT EDUCATION

Asthma self-management education is an effective strategy for the prevention and management of severe asthma exacerbations. Four main components of asthma education programs can be identified; these include information, self-monitoring, regular review and provision of a written action plan. Education programs can be classified in terms of these four components. Interventions that provide two or more components are termed asthma self-management education. Interventions using all four components are termed optimal self-management education.

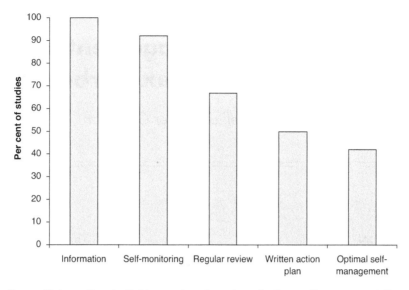

Figure 19.1   Types of intervention studied in a systematic review of asthma self-management. From reference 3

- *Information*   This is the transfer of information about asthma and its management.
- *Self-monitoring*   This involves regular assessment of either symptoms or peak expiratory flow by the person with asthma.
- *Regular medical review*   The assessment of asthma control, severity and medications by a medical practitioner forms the basis of the regular medical review component.
- *A written action plan*   This is an individualized written plan produced for the purpose of self-management of asthma exacerbations. The action plan is characterized by being individualized to the person's underlying asthma severity, treatment and individual circumstance. The action plan also informs the person with asthma when and how to modify medications and when and how to access the medical system in response to worsening asthma.

The effects of asthma self-management education on asthma outcomes have been evaluated in a systematic review of 36 randomized controlled trials involving 6090 participants.[3] The content of the asthma self-management interventions

described in the 36 studies is shown in Figure 19.1. Most programs offered information and instruction in self-monitoring, whereas 50% provided a written action plan.

Interventions using all four components are considered to provide an optimal self-management program. There were 15 studies that compared an optimal self-management program, or its components, to usual care. When these studies were examined by meta-analysis, the results showed that, with a self-management program, there was a reduction in the proportion of subjects requiring hospitalization and emergency room visits for asthma, unscheduled doctors' visits for asthma, days lost from work due to asthma and episodes of nocturnal asthma. The effects were large enough to be of both clinical and statistical significance (Figures 19.2 and 19.3). For example, the number of people who need to complete an optimal asthma self-management education program in order to prevent one severe asthma exacerbation (hospitalization number needed to treat; NNT) is 21. There was also a gradation of effect. Those interventions that included a

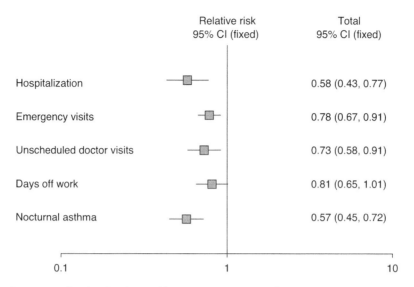

	Relative risk 95% CI (fixed)	Total 95% CI (fixed)
Hospitalization		0.58 (0.43, 0.77)
Emergency visits		0.78 (0.67, 0.91)
Unscheduled doctor visits		0.73 (0.58, 0.91)
Days off work		0.81 (0.65, 1.01)
Nocturnal asthma		0.57 (0.45, 0.72)

Figure 19.2 Outcomes of optimal asthma self-management. From reference 3

written action plan consistently showed an effect, whereas less intense interventions were not always of obvious benefit.

OPTIONS FOR SELF-MANAGEMENT

Asthma self-management complements the use of optimal pharmacotherapy. Asthma education can improve adherence[7] and thereby facilitate the use of pharmacotherapy. Guidelines recommend that asthma education be delivered together with pharmacotherapy. When this happens, as in an optimal asthma self-management program, then there is a significant improvement in asthma morbidity (Figure 19.2).

Studies have attempted to identify the improvement in asthma that can be attributed to education and separate this from that attributable to therapy.[8] In four randomized controlled trials (RCTs), there was optimization of pharmacotherapy prior to administration of an education program. In these studies, pharmacotherapy was optimized via regular medical review and was compared to regular medical review combined with an optimal

self-management program. These trials also compared two forms of adjustment of medication, usually inhaled corticosteroids, in order to achieve improved asthma control. The usual means was by regular review by a doctor. This was contrasted with self-adjustment by the patient according to written, predetermined criteria. Overall there was no difference in asthma outcomes between the two forms of asthma management. In particular, hospitalizations for asthma were not different between groups, and unscheduled doctor visits, disrupted days and lung function were not significantly different. These results indicate that regular medical review is an acceptable alternative to an asthma education program, provided that the medical review includes assessment of severity, optimization of medication and instruction on management of exacerbations.

Other variations of optimal self-management have also been compared.[8] The receipt of an optimal self-management program that did not include regular medical review led to an increase in health center visits and sickness days in comparison to those receiving a full optimal self-management program.[9] While in a program

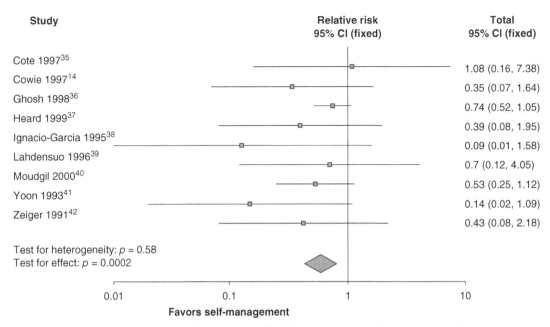

Study	Relative risk 95% CI (fixed)	Total 95% CI (fixed)
Cote 1997[35]		1.08 (0.16, 7.38)
Cowie 1997[14]		0.35 (0.07, 1.64)
Ghosh 1998[36]		0.74 (0.52, 1.05)
Heard 1999[37]		0.39 (0.08, 1.95)
Ignacio-Garcia 1995[38]		0.09 (0.01, 1.58)
Lahdensuo 1996[39]		0.7 (0.12, 4.05)
Moudgil 2000[40]		0.53 (0.25, 1.12)
Yoon 1993[41]		0.14 (0.02, 1.09)
Zeiger 1991[42]		0.43 (0.08, 2.18)

Test for heterogeneity: $p = 0.58$
Test for effect: $p = 0.0002$

Favors self-management

Figure 19.3 A comparison of the effects of optimal self-management on hospitalizations for asthma. From reference 3

where the intensity of the asthma education was reduced, there was a significant increase in the proportion of subjects requiring unscheduled doctor visits.[10] Optimal self-management programs including verbal instructions have also been compared to a written action plan with no difference reported in asthma outcomes between the two interventions.[11]

ASTHMA EDUCATION IN CHILDREN

Asthma self-management education has been evaluated in children and adolescents in a systematic review of 32 trials.[12] The included trials used a variety of educational interventions including group sessions, individual sessions or a combination of both, and ranged in intensity from one session to a majority of the trials utilizing three or more sessions. Self-management education was associated with improvements in lung function and reductions in days away from school and emergency department

visits (Figures 19.4 and 19.5). The effects were greater in the trials including children with moderate–severe asthma and those incorporating a self-management programme based on peak expiratory flow.[12]

WRITTEN ASTHMA ACTION PLANS

A written asthma action plan is a key component of an asthma education intervention. Written asthma action plans contain four essential components (Table 19.1). These are: an instruction on when to increase treatment, how to increase treatment, the duration of the treatment increase and when to cease self-management and seek medical help.[13]

Action plan: when to increase treatment

The instruction specifying when to increase treatment represents the point at which the

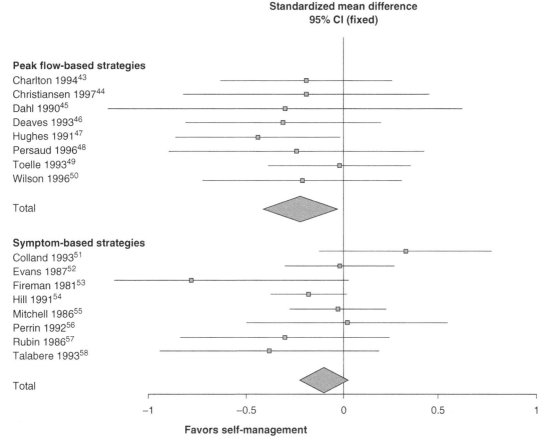

Figure 19.4 A comparison of the effects of self-management education for children on school absences. From reference 12

action plan is to be activated, i.e. the action point. This may be based on symptoms or peak expiratory flow (PEF) values. Six studies compared self-management using a written action plan based on PEF to self-management using a symptom-based written action plan. The results were similar for the proportion of subjects requiring hospitalization, and unscheduled visits to the doctor.[8] Emergency room visits were significantly reduced by PEF self-management in one study[14] but were similar to symptom self-management in four other studies. Symptom-based self-management reduced the number of subjects requiring a course of oral corticosteroids in one study.[15]

This is an important issue, since self-monitoring of PEF involves the regular measurement of PEF and recording the best of three measurements in a diary, morning and night. Medication is then adjusted according to changes in PEF levels. In contrast, adjustment of medications can be made according to the patient's symptoms such as nocturnal asthma or an increased need for reliever medication. Both PEF and symptom self-monitoring have their limitations. Compliance with PEF monitoring in the long term is poor and some patients are poor perceivers of their symptoms. In reviewing the six trials that compared PEF and symptom self-monitoring, no significant differences in health

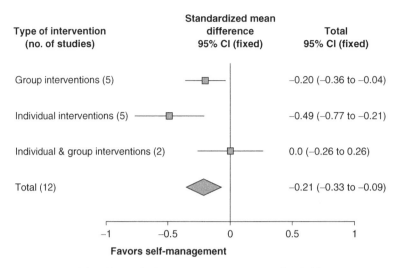

Type of intervention (no. of studies)	Standardized mean difference 95% CI (fixed)	Total 95% CI (fixed)
Group interventions (5)		−0.20 (−0.36 to −0.04)
Individual interventions (5)		−0.49 (−0.77 to −0.21)
Individual & group interventions (2)		0.0 (−0.26 to 0.26)
Total (12)		−0.21 (−0.33 to −0.09)

Favors self-management

Figure 19.5 A comparison of the effects of self-management education for children on emergency department visits. From reference 12

Table 19.1 Components of a written asthma action plan. From reference 13

1. **When to increase treatment**
    symptoms vs. peak expiratory flow (PEF)
    PEF: % predicted vs. personal best
    number of action points: 2, 3, 4
    presentation: 'traffic light'

2. **How to increase treatment**
    inhaled corticosteroid
    oral corticosteroid
    inhaled and oral corticosteroid
    inhaled corticosteroid and long-acting
    β_2-agonist

3. **For how long**
    duration of treatment increase

4. **When to call for help**

outcomes were found, suggesting that the use of either method is effective. This is a clinically important observation as self-monitoring can be tailored to patient preference, patient characteristics and the resources available.

Action points that use PEF can be based on PEF expressed as a percentage of the predicted PEF or as a percentage of the individual's best

PEF (personal best). Action points based on personal best PEF were consistently associated with improved outcomes (Figure 19.6). Therefore, action plans should use symptoms and/or personal best PEF when defining the best point to initiate therapy.

When specifying action points, these can be further subdivided as 80% or 60% of the best value (two action points), or as 90%, 70%, 60%, 40% of the best (four action points). A comparison of written action plans found those using two action points gave similar results to those using four action points (Figure 19.6). The action points can be further presented using color coding, where orange represents one action level, and red another. This approach, termed a 'traffic light' configuration, was not obviously better than the standard presentation.[13] A further modification is to base action points on the result of a statistical process control (SPC) analysis. Process control analysis requires the recording of the daily PEF over an 8–10-day period of stable medication. In its simplest form, a lower control limit is defined as 3 standard deviations below the mean PEF for that person. The probability of observing a PEF below that level is less

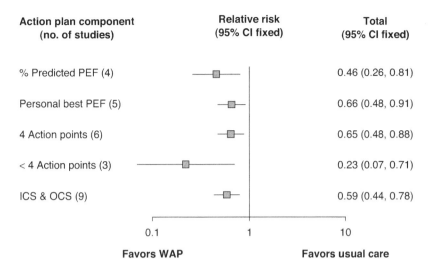

Action plan component (no. of studies)	Relative risk (95% CI fixed)	Total (95% CI fixed)
% Predicted PEF (4)		0.46 (0.26, 0.81)
Personal best PEF (5)		0.66 (0.48, 0.91)
4 Action points (6)		0.65 (0.48, 0.88)
< 4 Action points (3)		0.23 (0.07, 0.71)
ICS & OCS (9)		0.59 (0.44, 0.78)

0.1   1   10

Favors WAP   Favors usual care

Figure 19.6 A comparison of the effects of action plan components on hospitalizations for asthma. PEF, peak expiratory flow; ICS, inhaled corticosteroids; OCS, oral corticosteroids; WAP, written action plan

than one in a thousand, and so this may represent a specific but individualized action point. SPC action points appear to be more accurate, but require more data manipulation.[16,17]

Action plan: how to increase treatment

The treatment instruction is a crucial part of an asthma action plan. This instructs the person with asthma how to adjust their medication in response to deteriorating asthma. The options include inhaled corticosteroids (ICS) and oral corticosteroids (OCS), or ICS and long-acting β_2-agonists (LABA). The instructions regarding treatment showed that action plans recommending increased ICS together with the commencement of OCS were beneficial (Figure 19.6). Increased ICS alone appeared to be ineffective. Whereas one study showed a similar effect of inhaled fluticasone 1 mg to oral prednisone,[18] other work has found that doubling the dose of ICS in an asthma exacerbation may not be effective.[19,20] These recommendations for action plan use are summarized in Table 19.2.

INCREASED LONG-ACTING β-AGONIST/INHALED CORTICOSTEROID FOR EXACERBATIONS

Several studies have examined the use of LABA/ICS during exacerbations.[21–27] In these RCTs, people with asthma were treated with budesonide/formoterol in a single inhaler and instructed to increase their maintenance dose of budesonide/formoterol in response to deteriorating symptoms and/or peak flow (Tables 19.3 and 19.4).

In a multicenter trial conducted in Italy, 2358 people over the age of 6 with ICS-dependent asthma were randomized to budesonide/formoterol in a single inhaler to either a fixed dose regimen or an adjustable maintenance dose for 12 weeks (Table 19.4).[21] The adjustable maintenance group were given written instruction for their asthma management and stepped their dose up or down according to their level of asthma control. At the end of the treatment period both groups showed similar results, with a low frequency of exacerbations, improved lung function, fewer nocturnal wakings and fewer asthma symptoms. However, the adjustable

Table 19.2 Action plan variations: summary of results. From reference 13

Action plan variation	Result
Action point	
Symptoms vs. PEF triggered	Equivalent
Standard written instruction	Consistently beneficial
Traffic light configuration	Not clearly better than standard instruction
2–3 action points	Consistently beneficial
4 action points	Not clearly better than <4 points
PEF based on personal best PEF	Consistently beneficial
PEF based on % predicted PEF	Not consistently better than usual care
Treatment instruction	
Individualized WAP using ICS and OCS	Consistently beneficial
Individualized WAP using OCS only	Insufficient data to evaluate
Individualized WAP using ICS only	Insufficient data to evaluate

PEF, peak expiratory flow; WAP, written action plan; ICS, inhaled corticosteroid; OCS, oral corticosteroid

Table 19.3 Adjustable dosing: criteria for step-up or step-down. From reference 22

Initial step-down to one inhalation twice daily*
The patient felt well in his/her asthma and met both of the following in the previous 7 days:
- Reliever medication ≤2 times in previous 7 days
- No nocturnal awakening due to asthma

Step-up to four inhalations twice daily
If on two consecutive days or nights, the patient met any of the following:
- Reliever medication on three or more occasions during the day
- Nocturnal awakening due to asthma
- Morning PEF <85% of the mean baseline value

Step-down to one inhalation twice daily after a period of worsening asthma (i.e. after a step-up period)[†]
During the previous 2 days or nights, the patient met all of the following:
- No more asthma symptoms than before the worsening of asthma, as judged by the patient
- No reliever medication use for symptom relief
- No nocturnal awakenings due to asthma
- Morning PEF ≥85% of the mean baseline value

PEF peak expiratory flow
*Initial step-down criteria were assessed by the physician at visit 2 and were reassessed at visits 3 and 4. If patients did not meet the initial step-down criteria, the maintenance dose during run-in (two inhalations twice daily) was continued until patients fulfilled the initial step-down criteria
†Patients were able to step down their dose after 7 or 14 days of increased dosing (step-up period) if the criteria were met. If patients did not meet the step-up criteria after 14 days, they were instructed to contact the investigator for a decision

maintenance dose group used significantly less study medication at significantly lower costs.[21]

Stallberg *et al.* reported significantly fewer exacerbations ($p < 0.05$, NNT = 30) (Figure 19.7), a significantly lower study medication dose and lower costs over 6 months ($p < 0.001$) for the group of those with asthma randomized to an adjustable maintenance dose of budesonide/formoterol, according to their symptom control, compared to those randomized to a fixed dose regimen (Table 19.4).[22]

A 5-month RCT of fixed versus adjustable maintenance budesonide/formoterol dose was conducted in adults and adolescents (>12 years) with ICS-dependent asthma (Table 19.4).[23] Patients in both groups were provided

Table 19.4 Increased long-acting β_2-agonist/inhaled corticosteroid (ICS) for exacerbations

Reference	Participants' age (years)	n	Intervention	Dose adjustment criteria	Treatment duration	Outcome
Canonica[21]	≥6	2358	Budesonide/formoterol 'Symbicort' (160/4.5 μg or 80/4.5 μg) depending on pre-study ICS dose	FD: 2 puffs bid AMD: 2 puffs bid, step up to 4 puffs bid (max 14 days then see investigator) or step down to 1 puff bid or 2 puffs nocte according to written AP	4-week run-in on FD; 12 weeks' treatment	Exacerbations, asthma severity, FEV₁, PEF, rescue medications, symptom-free days, asthma control weeks, nocturnal waking, study medication dose, health economics, safety
Stallberg[22]	≥12	1034	Budesonide/formoterol 'Symbicort' (160/4.5 μg or 80/4.5 μg) depending on pre-study ICS dose	FD: 2 puffs bid AMD: 2 puffs bid, step up to 4 puffs bid if symptoms worsened (max 14 days then see investigator) or step down to 1 puff bid if symptoms well controlled	4-week run-in on FD; 6 months' treatment	Exacerbations, study medication dose, rescue medications, nocturnal waking, health economics, safety
Fitzgerald[23]	≥12	995	Budesonide/formoterol 'Symbicort' (160/4.5 μg or 80/4.5 μg) depending on pre-study ICS dose	FD: 2 puffs bid + AP AMD: 2 puffs bid, step up to 4 puffs bid (max 14 days then see investigator) or step down to 1 puff bid according to written AP	4-week run-in on FD; 5 months' treatment	Exacerbations, asthma severity, PEF, rescue medications, nocturnal waking, unscheduled health-care visits, days off work/school, health economics, safety
Leuppi[24]	≥12	127	Budesonide/formoterol 'Symbicort' (160/4.5 μg)	FD: 2 puffs bid + AP AMD: 2 puffs bid, step up to 4 puffs bid (14 days then see investigator) or step down to 1 puff bid or 2 puffs nocte according to written AP	4-week run-in on FD; 12 weeks' treatment	Number of treatment successes or treatment failures (predefined), FEV, PEF, nocturnal waking, rescue medications, QOL, study medication dose, safety
Aalbers[25]	≥12	658	Budesonide/formoterol 'Symbicort' (160/4.5 μg) Salmeterol/fluticasone 'Seretide' (50/250 μg)	FD: 1 budesonide/formoterol 2 puffs bid 2 salmeterol/fluticasone 2 puffs bid AMD: budesonide/formoterol 2 puffs bid, step up to 4 puffs bid (7–14 days) or step down to 1 puff bid according to predefined asthma control + written AP	2-week run-in on usual ICS, then 1 month FD; 6 months' treatment	Asthma control weeks, study medication dose, exacerbations, rescue medications, PEF, symptom score, nocturnal waking
Buhl[26]	18–50	4025	Budesonide/formoterol 'Symbicort' (160/4.5 μg)	FD: 2 puffs bid AMD: 1 puff bid if symptoms controlled, stepping up to 2 or 4 puffs bid if symptoms worsened (min 7 days prior to stepping down)	4-week run-in on FD; 12 weeks' treatment	QOL, asthma control (PEF, symptom severity score, nocturnal waking, rescue medications), study medication dose, safety
Price[27]	>18	1553	Budesonide/formoterol 'Symbicort' (160/4.5 μg or 80/4.5 μg) depending on pre-study ICS dose	FD: 2 puffs bid AMD: 1, 2 or 4 puffs bid according to a written AP (max 14 days at 4 puffs then see investigator)	4-week run-in on FD; 12 weeks' treatment	QOL, symptom-free days without SABA, health economics

FD, fixed dose; AMD, adjustable maintenance dose; AP, action plan; FEV₁, forced expiratory volume in 1 second; PEF, peak expiratory flow; QOL, quality of life; SABA, short-acting β_2-agonist with written instructions on how to use their medications and, for the adjustable dose group, criteria for stepping up or down their dose according to perceived asthma control. The authors reported significantly fewer exacerbations ($p=0.002$, NNT$=21$), lower study medication dose ($p<0.0001$) and lower total costs for the adjustable maintenance dose group compared to the fixed dose group. Asthma severity was maintained or improved in both groups.[23] Leuppi et al. conducted a RCT of 12 weeks' treatment with budesonide/formoterol adjusted according to predefined criteria compared to fixed dose in subjects with ICS-dependent asthma (Table 19.4).[24] Subjects in both groups were given a written action plan for dealing with exacerbations and deteriorating asthma. At the end of the treatment period there was no difference in lung function, treatment failure and reductions in asthma severity (significant for the adjustable maintenance group) for both treatment groups. For the adjustable maintenance dose group there was significantly less study medication used ($p<0.0001$), less rescue medication used ($p<0.0001$) and less nocturnal waking ($p=0.006$) compared to the fixed dose group.[24]

Subjects with ICS-dependent asthma randomized to an adjustable maintenance dose of budesonide/formoterol were significantly more likely to achieve an asthma control week compared to those randomized to a fixed dose of either budesonide/formoterol or salmeterol/fluticasone after 6 months' treatment in one study (OR 1.34; 95% CI 1.001, 1.78) (Table 19.4).[25] Subjects in the adjustable maintenance-dose group received oral and written instructions regarding self-management and actions for worsening asthma. For this group there was also significantly less rescue medication used compared to both fixed-dose groups ($p=0.001$, $p=0.011$) and reduced (15%) average study medication use. There was no reported difference for other clinical outcomes.[25]

In a large RCT Buhl et al. compared the effect of adjustable maintenance to fixed budesonide/formoterol dose on health-related quality of life and asthma control (Table 19.4).[26] After 12 weeks' treatment the authors reported clinically significant improvements in quality of life score, PEF and symptom severity score for both treatment groups. However, this was achieved with a significantly lower dose of study medication for the adjustable maintenance dose group compared to the fixed dose group ($p<0.001$).[26]

Similarly, quality of life improved for subjects randomized to either an adjustable maintenance dose or fixed dose regimen of budesonide/formoterol for 12 weeks in another study (Table 19.4).[27] Price et al. also reported no difference between groups in effectiveness parameters but a significantly lower mean daily cost for the adjustable dose group.[27]

These results demonstrate that ICS/OCS or ICS/LABA can be effectively used as part of an action plan to manage deteriorating asthma.

SELF-ADJUSTMENT OF THERAPY IN ASTHMA

There are several limitations to asthma self-management and written action plans. Physicians seldom provide a written action plan,[28,29] and patients may not follow their self-management instructions. For example, in adults, Turner et al.[30] found that there was between 52 and 65% adherence to the self-management plan. Furthermore, although patients like the concept of action plans, they modify their asthma plan according to their own perceptions and experience of asthma.[31] This emphasizes the need to investigate alternative approaches to the prevention and management of exacerbations. One approach uses a simplified action plan in combination with LABA–ICS therapy. In this approach, the budesonide/formoterol combination is used both as a reliever and as maintenance therapy. O'Byrne et al.[32] tested this approach in a large RCT. The study included patients who were using inhaled corticosteroid therapy but still had symptomatic asthma and significant reversibility.

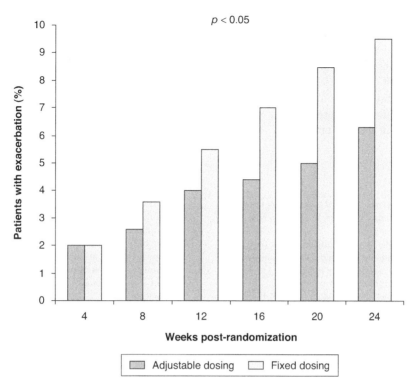

Figure 19.7 A comparison of adjustable and fixed maintenance dosing on time to first exacerbation. From reference 22

The intervention was Symbicort® (budesonide/formoterol) as maintenance and reliever therapy (SMART), and this was compared with budesonide/formoterol in a fixed dose and with high-dose budesonide. Compared with fixed-dose therapy, there was a significant reduction in exacerbations with SMART. The number of patients who needed to be treated with a SMART approach in order to prevent one severe exacerbation was 11. This suggests that SMART may be an effective way to minimize severe exacerbations of asthma.

POOR PERCEIVERS

A concern with all self-management approaches is that undertreatment of asthma could occur if patients failed to perceive deteriorating asthma. Poor perception is a recognized problem in asthma. For example, in a study of exacerbations, Tattersfield *et al.*[33] found that 18% of exacerbations were associated with a significant fall in lung function, but this was not perceived by the patient, and OCS were not used. Perception of airway narrowing is known to be impaired during a mild asthma exacerbation, and this is related to concurrent changes in airway hyperresponsiveness and resting lung function.[34] This can be dealt with by the use of objective airflow measurements and adherence to a written action plan.

CONCLUSIONS

Asthma exacerbations are responsible for a significant burden of illness in the community.

Active interventions are required to reduce this burden. Several approaches have been tested and found to be effective. These include regular medical review, asthma self-management education and LABA/ICS as maintenance and reliever therapy. The challenge for clinicians is to be skilled in the delivery of these interventions and also to implement them in practice.

REFERENCES

1. Turner M, Noertjojo K, Vedal S, et al. Risk factors for near fatal asthma. Am J Respir Crit Care Med 1998; 157: 1804–9

2. Chan-Yeung M, Chang J, Manfreda J, et al. Changes in peak flow, symptom score and the use of medications during acute exacerbations of asthma. Am J Respir Crit Care Med 1996; 154: 889–93

3. Gibson P, Powell H, Coughlin J, et al. Self-management education and regular practitioner review for adults with asthma (Cochrane Review). The Cochrane Library, Issue 4. Chichester, UK: John Wiley & Sons, 2004

4. Matheson M, Wicking J, Raven J, et al. Asthma management: how effective is it in the community? Intern Med J 2002; 32: 51–6

5. Hartert T, Windom HH, Peebles RS Jr, et al. Inadequate out-patient medical therapy for patients with asthma admitted to two urban hospitals. Am J Med 1996; 100: 386–94

6. Marks G, Burney P, Premaratne U, et al. Asthma in Greenwich UK: impact of the disease and current management practices. Eur Respir J 1997; 10: 1224–9

7. Bailey W, Richards J, Brooks C, et al. A randomised trial to improve self-management practices of adults with asthma. Arch Intern Med 1990; 150: 1664–8

8. Powell H, Gibson P. Options for self-management education for adults with asthma (Cochrane Review). The Cochrane Library, Issue 4. Chichester, UK: John Wiley & Sons, 2004

9. Kauppinen R, Sintonen H, Tukiainen H. One year economic evaluation of intensive versus conventional patient education and supervision for self-management of new asthmatic patients. Respir Med 1998; 92: 300–7

10. Cote J, Bowie D, Robichaud P, et al. Evaluation of two different educational interventions for adult patients consulting with an acute asthma exacerbation. Am J Respir Crit Care Med 2001; 163: 1415–19

11. Baldwin D, Pathak U, King R, et al. Outcome of asthmatics attending asthma clinics utilizing self-management plans in general practice. Asthma Gen Pract 1997; 5: 31–2

12. Wolf F, Guevara J, Grum C, et al. Educational interventions for asthma in children. The Cochrane Library of Systematic Reviews, Issue 4. Chichester UK: John Wiley & Sons, 2002

13. Gibson P, Powell H. Written action plans for asthma: an evidence-based review of the key components. Thorax 2004; 59: 94–9

14. Cowie R, Revitt S, Underwood M, Field S. The effect of a peak flow-based action plan in the prevention of exacerbations of asthma. Chest 1997; 112: 1534–8

15. Charlton I, Charlton G, Broomfield J, Mullee M. Evaluation of peak flow and symptoms only self-management plans for control of asthma in general practice. BMJ 1990; 301: 1355–9

16. Gibson P, Wlodarczyk J, Hensley M, et al. Using quality-control analysis of peak expiratory flow recordings to guide therapy for asthma. Ann Intern Med 1995; 123: 488–92

17. Boggs P, Hayati F, Washburne W, Wheeler D. Using statistical process control charts for the continual improvement of asthma care. Jt Comm J Qual Improv 1999; 25: 163–81

18. Levy M, Stevenson C, Maslen T. Comparison of short courses of oral prednisolone and fluticasone propionate in the treatment of adults with acute exacerbation of asthma in primary care. Thorax 1996; 51: 1087–92

19. Harrison T, Osborne J, Newton S, Tattersfield A. Doubling the dose of inhaled corticosteroid to prevent asthma exacerbations: a randomised controlled trial. Lancet 2004; 363: 271–5

20. Fitzgerald J, Becker A, Sears M, et al.; and the Canadian Asthma Exacerbation Study Group. Doubling the dose of budesonide versus maintenance treatment in asthma exacerbations. Thorax 2004; 59: 550–6

21. Canonica G, Castellini P, Cazzola M, et al. Adjustable maintenance dosing with budesonide/formoterol in a single inhaler provides effective asthma symptom control at a lower dose than fixed maintenance dosing. Pulmon Pharmacol Ther 2004; 17: 239–47

22. Stallberg B, Olsson P, Jorgensen L, et al. Budesonide/formoterol adjustable maintenance dosing reduces asthma exacerbations versus fixed dosing. Int J Clin Pract 2003; 57: 656–61

23. Fitzgerald J, Sears M, Boulet L-P, et al. Adjustable maintenance dosing with budesonide/formoterol reduces asthma exacerbations compared with traditional fixed dosing: a five month multicentre Canadian study. Can Respir J 2003; 10: 427–34

24. Leuppi J, Salzberg M, Meyer L, et al. An individualized, adjustable maintenance regimen of budesonide/formoterol provides effective asthma symptom control at a lower dose than fixed dosing. Swiss Med Weekly 2003; 133: 302–9

25. Aalbers R, Backer V, Kava T, et al. Adjustable maintenance dosing with budesonide/formoterol compared

with fixed-dose salmeterol/fluticasone in moderate to severe asthma. Curr Med Res Opin 2004; 20: 225–40

26. Buhl R, Kardos P, Richter K, et al. The effect of adjustable dosing with budesonide/formoterol on health-related quality of life and asthma control compared with fixed dosing. Curr Med Res Opin 2004; 20: 1209–20

27. Price D, Haughney J, Lloyd A, et al. An economic evaluation of adjustable and fixed dosing with budesonide/formoterol via a single inhaler in asthma patients: the ASSURE study. Curr Med Res Opin 2004; 20: 1671–79

28. Rabe K, Vermeire P, Soriano J, Maier W. Clinical management of asthma in 1999: the Asthma Insights and Reality in Europe (AIRE) study. Eur Respir J 2000; 16: 802–7

29. Wilson D, Adams R, Appleton S, et al. Prevalence of asthma action plans in South Australia: population surveys from 1990 to 2001. Med J Aust 2003; 178: 483–5

30. Turner M, Taylor D, Bennett R, Fitzgerald J. A randomized trial comparing peak expiratory flow and symptom self-management plans for patients with asthma attending a primary care clinic. Am J Respir Crit Care Med 1998; 157: 540–6

31. Douglass J, Aroni R, Goeman D, et al. A qualitative study of action plans for asthma. BMJ 2002; 324: 1003–5

32. O'Byrne P, Bisgaard H, Godard P, et al. Budesonide/formoterol combination therapy as both maintenance and reliever medication in asthma. Am J Respir Crit Care Med 2005; 171: 129–36

33. Tattersfield A, Postma D, Barnes P, et al. Exacerbations of asthma: a descriptive study of 425 severe exacerbations. The FACET International Study Group. Am J Respir Crit Care Med 1999; 160: 594–9

34. Salome C, Leuppi J, Freed R, Marks G. Perception of airway narrowing during reduction of inhaled corticosteroids and asthma exacerbation. Thorax 2003; 58: 1042–7

35. Cote J, Cartier A, Robichaud P, et al. Influence on asthma morbidity of asthma education programs based on self-management plans following treatment optimization. Am J Respir Crit Care Med 1997; 155: 1509–14

36. Ghosh C, Ravindran P, Joshi M, Stearns S. Reductions in hospital use from self management training for chronic asthmatics. Soc Sci Med 1998; 46: 1087–93

37. Heard A, Richards I, Alpers J, et al. Randomised controlled trial of general practice based asthma clinics. Med J Aust 1999; 171: 68–71

38. Ignacio-Garcia J, Gonzalez-Santos P. Asthma self-management education program by home monitoring of peak expiratory flow. Am J Respir Crit Care Med 1995; 151: 353–9

39. Lahdensuo A, Haahtela T, Herrala J, et al. Randomised comparison of guided self-management and traditional treatment of asthma over one year. BMJ 1996; 312: 748–52

40. Moudgil H, Marshall T, Honeybourne D. Asthma education and quality of life in the community: a randomised controlled study to evaluate the impact on white European and Indian subcontinent ethnic groups from socioeconomically deprived areas in Birmingham, UK. Thorax 2000; 55: 177–83

41. Yoon R, McKenzie D, Bauman A, Miles D. Controlled trial evaluation of an asthma education program for adults. Thorax 1993; 48: 1110–16

42. Zeiger R, Heller S, Mellon M, et al. Facilitated referral to asthma specialist reduces relapses in asthma emergency room visits. J Allergy Clin Immunol 1991; 87: 1160–8

43. Charlton I, Antonio A, Atkinson J, et al. Asthma at the interface: bridging the gap between general practice and a district general hospital. Arch Dis Child 1994; 70: 313–18

44. Christiansen S, Martin S, Schleicher N, et al. Evaluation of a school-based asthma education program for inner-city children. J Allergy Clin Immunol 1997; 100: 613–17

45. Dahl J, Gustafsson D, Melin L. Effects of a behavioral treatment program on children with asthma. J Asthma 1990; 27: 41–6

46. Deaves D. An assessment of the value of health education in the prevention of childhood asthma. J Adv Nurs 1993; 18: 354–63

47. Hughes D, McLeod M, Garner B, Goldbloom R. Controlled trial of a home and ambulatory program for asthmatic children. Pediatrics 1991; 87: 54–61

48. Persaud D, Barnett S, Weller S, et al. An asthma self-management program for children, including instruction in peak flow monitoring by school nurses. J Asthma 1996; 33: 37–43

49. Toelle B, Peat J, Salome C, et al. Evaluation of a community-based asthma management program in a population sample of school children. Med J Aust 1993; 158: 742–6

50. Wilson S, Latini D, Starr N, et al. Education of parents of infants and very young children with asthma: a developmental evaluation of the Wee Wheezers program. J Asthma 1996; 33: 239–54

51. Colland V. Learning to cope with asthma: a behavioral self-management program for children. Patient Educ Couns 1993; 22: 141–52

52. Evans D, Clark N, Feldman C, et al. A school health education program for children with asthma aged 8–11 years. Health Educ Q 1987; 14: 267–79

53. Fireman P, Friday G, Gira C, et al. Teaching self-management skills to asthmatic children and their parents in an ambulatory care setting. Pediatrics 1981; 68: 341–8

54. Hill R, Williams J, Britton J, Tattersfield L. Can morbidity associated with untreated asthma in primary

school children be reduced? A controlled intervention study. BMJ 1991; 303: 1169–74

55.   Mitchell E, Ferguson V, Norwood M. Asthma education by community child health nurses. Arch Dis Child 1986; 61: 1184–9

56.   Perrin J, MacLean W, Gortmaker S, Asher K. Improving the psychological status of children with asthma: a randomized controlled trial. J Dev Behav Pediatr 1992; 13: 241–7

57.   Rubin D, Leventhal J, Sadock R, et al. Educational intervention by computer in childhood asthma: a randomized clinical trial testing the use of a new teaching intervention in childhood asthma. Pediatrics 1986; 77: 1–10

58.   Talabere LR. The effects of an asthma education program on selected health behaviors of school-aged children with asthma. In Funk S, ed. Aspects of Caring for the Chronically Ill: Hospital and Home. New York: Springer Publications, 1993: 319–30

CHAPTER 20

Psychosocial factors in severe asthma in adults

Jane R Smith and Brian DW Harrison

INTRODUCTION

The role of patient-related factors in asthma and the complex relationship between psychosocial characteristics and asthma have long been recognized.[1] Despite this, improved understanding of the pathophysiology and pharmacology of asthma in the middle of the past century led to increasing neglect of psychosocial factors, as asthma became more amenable to treatment within a traditional biomedical model. In recent years, however, recognition of the significance of adherence to treatment, the importance of patients taking an active role in self-management and the need for a biopsychosocial perspective in understanding chronic illness has meant that interest in the role of psychosocial factors in asthma, and severe asthma in particular, has re-emerged.

WHAT DO WE MEAN BY PSYCHOSOCIAL FACTORS?

Here, the term psychosocial is used to encompass both psychological and social factors and processes. The two are often inextricably linked. Psychological factors include behaviors (e.g. medication adherence, trigger avoidance, attendance at health services), cognitions (e.g. knowledge, perceptions, beliefs, attitudes) and emotions (e.g. anxiety, depression). The term 'coping' is commonly used to describe complex and dynamic patterns of behaviors, cognitions and emotions in which people engage when faced with challenges: the experience of living with and managing chronic problems, including illness, or acute events.[2] 'Personality' refers to an individual's patterns of behavior, cognitions or emotions that remain more stable over time and situations.[2] Social factors of importance include sociodemographics (e.g. age, gender, ethnicity), socioeconomic characteristics, relationships and interactions with others, and culture. The biopsychosocial approach suggests that these are linked with disease primarily via psychological processes operating at the individual level.[2] It is psychological factors, and the way in which they are related to asthma and linked to broader social issues, that are the focus of this chapter.

WHAT DO WE MEAN BY SEVERE ASTHMA?

For ease of identification, patients can be defined as having severe asthma when they have had one or more hospital admissions for acute severe asthma or when they are prescribed British Thoracic Society (BTS) step 4 or 5 treatment,[3] equivalent to three or more classes of asthma drugs.[4] In practice, there are overlaps between severe, poorly controlled and 'difficult' asthma, the latter being present when, in a patient with a confirmed diagnosis of asthma, symptoms and/or lung function are poorly controlled with prescribed treatment that experience suggests would usually be effective.[5] This chapter refers to severe asthma, but many of the issues equally apply to poorly controlled and difficult asthma.

Common indicators of asthma severity include symptom control; exacerbations resulting in emergency attendances, hospital admissions, near-fatal attacks or death; medication use; pulmonary function; or some combination of these.[6] However, even at the level of defining severity, psychosocial factors play a role. Each of the above manifestations of asthma can be directly affected by psychological processes, highlighting the fact that patients with problematic asthma or problematic patients with asthma[7] may present with severe disease and be at increased risk of frequent or severe exacerbations. For example, the experience of symptoms is affected by co-existing psychiatric problems such as panic, explaining why hyperventilation is sometimes confused with acute asthma.[8] Since reports of symptoms are subjective, patients' perceptions and interpretations of symptoms also play a role, and a wide range of underlying psychosocial factors influence these.[9] Presentation with exacerbations, or delays in seeking help which may contribute to the severity of an attack on presentation, are determined by patient decision-making regarding self-care and health-care attendance which are in turn subject to a range of other psychosocial influences.[10] Furthermore, psychosocial 'triggers' can contribute to the onset of attacks.[11] Medication use is a patient behavior, subject to the psychosocial influences of any health-related behavior,[12] and even lung function and peak flow assessment may be influenced by changes in emotional status and patients' motivation to comply with testing.[13] The role of psychosocial factors in defining severity is further discussed elsewhere[14] and explored in more depth below.

OVERVIEW

The above discussion highlights the complexity and circularity inherent in considering psychosocial factors in severe asthma and makes structuring a review of the topic difficult. However, this chapter attempts:

(1) To review research highlighting associations between psychosocial factors and various forms of severe asthma;
(2) To discuss pathways by which psychosocial factors and severe asthma are likely to be linked, with reference to wider research on psychosocial factors in asthma and relevant psychological literature;
(3) To outline approaches to addressing psychosocial issues in patients with severe asthma and examine evidence on the effectiveness of psychoeducational interventions;
(4) To discuss implications for current clinical practice and future research.

Since the majority of research and the authors' expertise are in adult asthma, the focus is on psychosocial factors in adults with severe asthma. Most of the issues, and some additional psychosocial concerns (e.g. family and peer influences), are relevant to children and adolescents with severe disease and are discussed further elsewhere.[15,16]

ARE PSYCHOSOCIAL FACTORS ASSOCIATED WITH SEVERE ASTHMA?

Research on different manifestations of severe asthma, including asthma deaths, near-fatal asthma (NFA), asthma leading to hospital

Table 20.1 Adverse psychosocial and behavioral factors in fatal, near-fatal (NFA) and brittle asthma

	Fatal asthma	NFA	Brittle asthma
Depression or other psychiatric illness currently or previously	+[17–22,26,30]	+[27,28]	+
Denial	+[18–21,30]	+[27,28,31]	+
Poor compliance	+[18–22,24,26,30]	+[28,30,31]	
Personality disorder	+[22]		
Psychiatric caseness	+[30]	+[28]	+
Current or recent use of major tranquilizers or sedatives	+[23,40]	+[23]	
Deliberate self-harm	+[18]		
Learning disability or mentally retarded	+[18,26]	+[31]	
Psychiatric history in a first-degree relative	+[30]	+[28]	
Alcohol or drug abuse	+[17–20,22]	+[31]	
Recent bereavement	+[22]		
Severe domestic stress	+[18]	+[31]	
Social isolation, living alone, homeless	+[17,18]	+[31]	
Unemployment, self-employment, threatened redundancy	+[18,22,24,26]	+[31]	
Marital problems	+[17]		
Separated or single parenthood	+[18]	+[31]	
Extreme poverty	+[18]		
Childhood abuse	+[17,18]		+
Smoking or passive smoking	+[18]	+[31]	
Legal problems	+[17]		

admissions and brittle asthma, provides reliable and internationally consistent evidence on the importance of psychosocial factors.

Are psychosocial factors associated with death from asthma?

Interest in the role of psychosocial factors was revived during the 1990s as a result of studies of asthma mortality. For example, five confidential enquiries covering 222 asthma deaths in the UK[17–21] provided growing evidence for the importance of psychosocial factors.

These showed that asthma deaths are associated with disease, medical management and patient-related factors. Patients dying from asthma usually have chronically severe disease and a high frequency of previous near-fatal attacks, hospital admissions or emergency attendances and requirement for three or more classes of asthma medication. Only in a minority does the fatal attack occur suddenly against a background of mild or moderately severe asthma. With regard to medical management, there is frequently undertreatment with inhaled or oral steroids, inadequate monitoring of peak flow, lack of follow-up or specialist referral, underuse of written management plans and, in some cases, inappropriate prescription of β-blockers, non-steroidal anti-inflammatories or sedatives.

Psychological and behavioral factors associated with asthma deaths are detailed in Table 20.1. We would highlight poor compliance, including failure to attend appointments and self-discharge from hospital, depression or other psychiatric history, denial, drug or alcohol abuse and learning difficulties. Social adversities listed in Table 20.1 encompass isolation, childhood abuse and employment, income, domestic, marital or legal problems.

Confidential enquiries indicate a high prevalence of psychosocial problems amongst those dying of asthma, consistently identifying significant psychological or social problems in around three-quarters of patients. These case-series studies do not indicate the extent to which these patients differ from other groups with asthma, and thus whether these factors are likely to have played a contributory role. However, case–control studies[22–26] comparing patients dying from asthma to hospitalized and/or community-based patients provide stronger, confirmatory evidence.

The earliest of these[22] found that psychosocial problems were recorded in the notes of 44 patients dying from asthma significantly more often than in 39 matched hospitalized patients and that this was associated with a 3.5 times increase in the risk of death. In most other respects the hospitalized patients were similar to those who died, but both groups differed from 44 community controls with asthma. The largest and most recent case–control study,[26] undertaken in seven regions of Britain, compared 533 patients who died from asthma to 533 matched patients hospitalized for severe asthma at the same time as the death. It again revealed similarities between patients who died and those hospitalized, since 48% and 42% had a health behavior problem, and 85% and 86%, respectively, a psychosocial problem recorded in their notes. The following psychosocial factors were, however, associated with a significantly increased risk of death: repeated non-attendance/poor inhaler technique; psychoses; alcohol/drug abuse; financial/employment problems; and learning difficulties. Anxiety/prescription of antidepressant drugs and the mention of sexual problems in the patients' records were associated with a reduced risk of death.

Other case–control studies have tended to examine psychosocial factors in less detail, but generally support the findings that there are: (1) clear differences between patients dying from asthma and community controls;[22–25] (2) similarities between patients dying from asthma and those admitted to hospital;[24,26] and (3) some psychosocial factors (e.g. non-attendance) which may distinguish between the latter groups.[24,26]

Are psychosocial factors associated with near-fatal asthma?

Case-series studies suggest a similar prevalence of psychosocial problems amongst patients experiencing near-fatal asthma (NFA) to those dying from asthma.[27,28] Case–control studies in New Zealand,[29] Australia[30] and England,[31] comparing a total of 590 asthma deaths with 732 episodes of NFA, suggest that patients with NFA and fatal asthma come from the same population, since they share almost identical adverse psychosocial characteristics (Table 20.1). We would highlight poor compliance, depression or other psychiatric illness, denial and employment or domestic problems.

A case–control study from New Zealand examined social[32] and psychological[33] factors in 77 patients admitted to hospital with severe life-threatening asthma and 239 patients admitted with acute asthma but without NFA matched for timing of presentation. Despite similar sociodemographic characteristics and access to care, patients with NFA demonstrated deficiencies in the management of their acute attack with regard to use of medications and mode of presentation.[32] The only other difference between the NFA patients and the hospital controls was a lower incidence of previous counseling for emotional problems in the NFA group,[33] providing an interesting parallel with a lower risk of death amongst patients prescribed antidepressants in the study by Sturdy et al.[26]

Another investigation of admissions for asthma in the USA, comparing 42 intubated patients with 333 non-intubated controls, found that recorded psychosocial problems (e.g. psychiatric diagnosis, family or employment issues, poor compliance), little formal education and low socioeconomic status were associated with a significantly increased risk of NFA.[34] It is not apparent, however, that potential relationships between these and other influencing factors (e.g. severity) were accounted for using multivariate analyses. A Canadian study found that, as well as differing with respect to disease and medical management factors, 45 patients experiencing NFA were more likely to identify stress as a trigger for the acute attack than 197 patients attending the emergency department, and had significantly higher feelings of vulnerability than 303 community controls.[35]

These studies suggest that: (1) patients experiencing fatal and near-fatal attacks are largely indistinguishable with respect to their psychosocial chararacteristics;[29–31] (2) there are many similarities between patients experiencing NFA and those admitted to hospital with asthma;[32,33] and (3) some psychosocial factors (e.g. poor self-management, stress) may distinguish between individuals experiencing NFA and those experiencing less severe exacerbations.[32–35]

Are psychosocial factors associated with hospital admissions for asthma?

In one report of the New Zealand study reviewed above,[33] hospitalized patients, both those with NFA and those admitted without NFA, were compared to a random sample of 100 community controls with asthma, and striking differences were apparent. Caseness for anxiety and depression and major life events were more common in the hospitalized groups. There were particularly marked differences in the frequency with which hospitalized patients had had a close relative or friend imprisoned (14% and 16% in the NFA and hospital groups vs. 2% in the community controls) or had looked for work for more than a month (29% and 24% vs. 3%, respectively).

Other studies comparing patients hospitalized with asthma to community controls have tended to focus on clinical and environmental, rather than psychosocial, factors associated with admissions. However, cross-sectional studies, mainly conducted in the USA, suggest that patients from ethnic minority and low socio-economic groups are over-represented in asthma admission statistics.[36–38] A qualitative study of influences on admissions amongst Asian and white ethnic groups in London[39] suggested that psychological factors such as adherence,

confidence in controlling asthma, beliefs and knowledge may explain these patterns.

Several longitudinal studies have examined factors predictive of increased risk of future admissions or other asthma events in selected cohorts. Again, most have focused on identifying clinical indicators associated with excerbations, with findings consistently showing that disease severity and previous admissions or NFA, especially within the previous year, are the factors most closely associated with subsequent hospitalizations, NFA and death.[4,27,40,41] An Australian study of 293 outpatients with moderate–severe asthma followed up for a year identified that, in addition to clinical and medical management factors, use of avoidant coping and lower preference for autonomy were associated with a significantly greater risk of admission for asthma and re-admission.[42] Studies of patients attending the accident and emergency (A&E) department generally show similar findings to those of admissions,[42] but again psychosocial factors are infrequently studied.

Are adverse psychosocial factors associated with brittle asthma?

Two types of brittle asthma represent a further manifestation of severe disease. In type 1 there is a greater than 40% diurnal variation in peak expiratory flow for more than 50% of days, for at least 150 days, together with persistent symptoms despite multiple drug treatment.[43] In type 2 the asthma becomes severe within minutes or a few hours, despite little instability during the preceding days.[43]

Type 1 brittle asthma has been studied by Ayres and Miles in Birmingham, UK (Table 20.1). They identified that 80% of patients with type 1 brittle asthma admitted to having been either physically or sexually abused on a regular basis at some stage in their life.[43] A case–control study found significantly higher lifetime prevalence of psychiatric disorders amongst 20 patients with brittle asthma compared to matched control patients with less severe disease, but, perhaps due to the small numbers, other differences in psychosocial characteristics were not significant.[44] An extension of this work identified psychiatric caseness amongst 21 of 29 patients with brittle asthma, compared with only three of 29 controls.[45] Brittle asthma patients also demonstrated poorer self-management, with respect to seeking help and using medications, in response to scenarios of deteriorating asthma.[45]

Patients with type 2 brittle asthma have not been studied so systematically. They are frequently admitted with NFA[46] or die from asthma,[47] sometimes with 'empty lungs' at autopsy. Such attacks may be associated with profound emotional upsets, high concentrations of air pollutants, aeroallergens, weather changes or sensitization to foodstuffs, preservatives or aspirin.[47] There is overlap in the characteristics of patients with brittle asthma, NFA and those dying of asthma (Table 20.1).

Are psychosocial factors associated with other forms of severe asthma?

Investigations of psychosocial factors in studies that have defined severity in ways other than on the basis of experiences of acute exacerbations or respiratory functioning are limited. However, a Dutch study[48] compared psychological characteristics in 90 patients with severe asthma defined on the basis that they were taking medication equivalent to BTS step 4 or 5 treatment, and 37 patients with mild asthma. It found no differences with respect to general psychiatric caseness, anxiety caseness or personality dimensions assessed. The only significant difference was that patients with severe asthma had a lower external locus of control, suggesting that they had less trust in physicians and medication with regard to influencing asthma, than patients with milder disease.

What are the conclusions from these studies?

Although there are an increasing number of studies aimed at improving understanding of severe asthma, most continue to focus on disease and clinical factors and do not consider associations with psychosocial characteristics.[49] Those that do generally suggest high levels of social adversity, emotional and psychiatric difficulties and behavioral problems amongst patients experiencing various forms of severe asthma. However, the strength of associations may vary depending on how severity is defined, with the results of one study[48] suggesting that it is patients experiencing acute severe exacerbations or poorly controlled disease, rather than severe chronic asthma per se, in whom psychosocial problems are most apparent.

Although the current literature is lacking in longitudinal studies which would provide greater insight into the direction of relationships between psychosocial factors and severe asthma, wider asthma and psychological research provides clues as to possible mechanisms.

HOW DO PSYCHOSOCIAL FACTORS AND ASTHMA INTERACT?

Relationships of asthma morbidity with psychosocial factors are two-way. They are also likely to be operating at a number of levels, related to the experience of symptoms, changes in underlying disease processes and the development of, and presentation with, acute exacerbations (Figure 20.1). Partly due to their interaction with psychosocial factors in the ways outlined here, symptoms, disease processes and exacerbations may or may not be closely allied to each other and have differential influences on whether patients present with severe disease.

Psychosocial impacts of asthma

As with other conditions, clinical observations and qualitative studies suggest that the experience of asthma, and resulting symptoms, physical limitations and acute events, can impact on a range of domains of psychosocial well-being.[50] These include effects on emotional, cognitive,

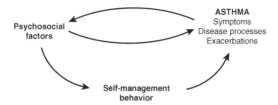

Figure 20.1 Relationships between psychosocial factors and asthma

social, sexual and occupational functioning,[51] which may go on to have socioeconomic consequences.[52] Furthermore, certain asthma medications are known to affect mood,[53] and treatment regimes and other aspects of asthma management (e.g. trigger avoidance) place additional burdens and limitations on patients which can have psychosocial consequences.[50]

Impacts of asthma on subjective well-being, including psychosocial functioning, can be assessed via an increasing array of generic, respiratory disease-specific and asthma-specific health status and health-related quality of life (HRQL) scales, reviewed elsewhere.[54,55] A review on the impact of asthma on HRQL[50] highlights that relationships of severity with HRQL are generally as would be anticipated, where worse disease is associated with greater limitations in physical and psychosocial functioning. However, findings are somewhat inconsistent and depend on the sample, measures and severity indicator used.[50] Subjective definitions of severity based on symptoms tend to be more closely associated with HRQL than pulmonary function, and composite indicators show the most marked inverse relationships between HRQL and severity.[50]

At present, most literature on asthma-specific HRQL questionnaires[51,56,57] reports on studies concerned with their development, testing and use as outcome measures in clinical trials. Few descriptive studies have examined HRQL in different asthma subgroups.[50] However, in testing the Marks Asthma Quality of Life Questionnaire (AQLQ), one study[57] showed that patients recently treated with oral steroids had

significantly higher scores on breathlessness, concerns and social dimensions, and patients hospitalized in the past year had significantly higher scores on the concerns dimension, than those with milder disease. In an emergency department setting,[58] patients classified as having more severe exacerbations on the basis of their respiratory function had significantly worse overall HRQL, and significantly greater impairments in the symptom and activity limitation domains of the Juniper AQLQ.[56] Differences in emotional functioning were of borderline significance.[58]

Studies using generic health status or HRQL scales (e.g. Short-Form health surveys (SF36, SF12)[59,60]), and questionnaires assessing specific domains of psychological functioning (e.g. Hospital Anxiety and Depression Scale (HADS);[61] General Health Questionnaires (GHQ12, GHQ28, GHQ60)),[62] provide additional data on psychosocial impacts of asthma, and severe disease. In two studies using the SF36,[59] the greatest differences between patients with mild and severe asthma were apparent in domains of physical functioning, physical role functioning, health perceptions,[63,64] emotional role functioning[63] and energy–vitality.[64] A small study[65] identified deficits in cognitive functioning amongst patients experiencing nocturnal asthma, a commonly used indicator of poorly controlled disease, compared to non-asthmatic controls. Studies reviewed above suggest that there are high levels of emotional disturbance (e.g. psychiatric caseness, anxiety, depression) amongst patients experiencing frequent or severe exacerbations compared to those experiencing less severe exacerbations or community controls.[25,33] However, since the study reviewed above comparing asthma classified as mild or severe on the basis of medication use showed no significant differences between groups with respect to general psychiatric morbidity (GHQ) or anxiety, it may be acute events, rather than just severe disease, that have the greatest impacts on psychological functioning.[48] Impacts of acute exacerbations are beginning to be further explored with the development of an acute version of the Juniper AQLQ.[66] Given that research highlights the presence of long-term cognitive and emotional problems in patients discharged from intensive care,[67] further studies on the psychosocial impacts of NFA and other acute events are warranted.

One of the complications with studying the psychosocial effects of asthma is that impacts appear to be mediated by other psychosocial characteristics. Examining the influence of sociodemographic factors on HRQL in asthma, there are inconsistent findings with respect to age, and most studies suggest women and ethnic minorities with asthma experience poorer HRQL across all domains.[50] Higher levels of education are sometimes associated with better HRQL, but socioeconomic differences and how these might link to sociodemographic factors are yet to be fully explored.[50] Impacts on HRQL are likely to reflect higher levels of asthma morbidity amongst particular groups, which in turn might have longer-term effects on a person's ability to work or study and thus contribute to socioeconomic disparities.[52] However, socioeconomic and sociodemographic factors may also influence psychological processes related to perceiving, interpreting and coping with symptoms and impacts on functioning, thus mediating the link between disease severity and subjectively assessed HRQL.[68]

Examining the influence of social[50] and psychological factors[69,70] on HRQL in asthma reiterates the circularity inherent in this field, namely: (1) do psychosocial difficulties result from severe asthma and the impacts it has on HRQL?; (2) do psychosocial problems predispose people to the development of and presentation with severe asthma which leads to reduced HRQL?; or (3) do psychosocial characteristics mediate the link between severe asthma and its impacts on HRQL? Existing studies phrase their research questions in different ways, but since they are mostly cross-sectional, they do little more than provide evidence of associations between severity, HRQL and psychosocial factors. They

also frequently fail to consider that different pathways may be operating simultaneously or at different times in the natural history of the disease and a patient's life, potentially contributing to a downward spiral of disability.

What can be concluded is that the combination of severe asthma and co-existing psychosocial problems (whether related or unrelated to, and preceding or resulting from, asthma) is associated with significantly poorer HRQL.[28,70] Our own unpublished data demonstrate that patients with severe asthma who had high levels of co-existing psychosocial problems (e.g. poor compliance, social problems, psychiatric morbidity) had worse health status across all SF36[59] domains, and poorer asthma-specific HRQL assessed using Hyland's Living with Asthma Questionnaire,[51] than patients with severe asthma alone, and clinical[63,71,72] or general population samples[73] studied elsewhere (Figures 20.2 and 20.3).

This highlights the opinion that potential impacts of asthma, severe asthma and acute episodes on psychosocial functioning must be considered, recognized and managed. Using brief HRQL questionnaires[57,60,74] and domain-specific scales designed for use in patients with physical health problems (e.g. HADS[61]) in clinical practice can aid in the identification and discussion of psychosocial impacts, highlight whether psychiatric or other intervention may be necessary to deal with these, and be used to monitor any changes resulting from treatment or events occurring in the course of patients' lives.[75] At present, there are difficulties with the interpretation and meaning of HRQL scores in clinical practice (e.g. clinically important differences) but research on these issues is increasing.[76]

The fact that pharmacological treatments improve HRQL[50] emphasizes the need for effective medical management of severe disease to minimize its impacts. That psychosocial processes may affect the degree to which asthma is perceived to result in symptoms, compromise HRQL or affect specific domains of functioning

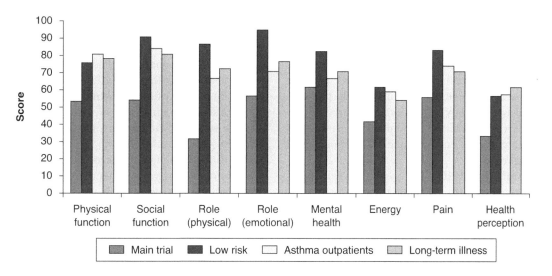

Figure 20.2 Mean SF36 subscale scores[59] (lower scores indicate poorer health status) for patients with severe asthma plus psychosocial problems and severe asthma alone compared to asthma outpatients[63] and chronic disease patients[73] in two other studies

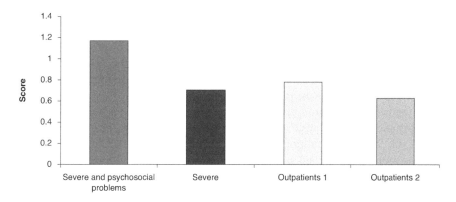

Figure 20.3 Mean asthma-specific quality of life scores[51] (higher scores indicate poorer quality of life) for patients with severe asthma plus psychosocial problems and severe asthma alone compared to asthma outpatients in two other studies[71,72]

means that impacts can also be reduced by identifying and addressing other intervention points. Since psychosocial factors influence the experience, perception, interpretation and reporting of breathlessness and other symptoms, subjectively severe asthma or disability that does not objectively reflect severe disease should be investigated. Alternative causes of symptoms

(e.g. cardiac problems, hyperventilation, panic) should be eliminated and self-monitoring of peak flow encouraged in those oversensitive or insensitive to changes in pulmonary function to ensure timely presentation with, and appropriate management of, exacerbations.[77] Inappropriate understanding of, or beliefs about, asthma may need to be addressed to aid in the interpretation and correct attribution of symptoms and impairments to asthma.[9] Furthermore, patients might be encouraged to develop more effective strategies for coping with the illness (e.g. problem-focused coping comprising self-management) and the impacts it has (e.g. emotion-focused coping to deal with anxiety).[9] Identifying underlying psychosocial influences on symptom perception and coping is also important and an area for further research.

Since the HRQL and psychosocial consequences of asthma predict future morbidity and adverse events,[78] the additional pathways by which psychosocial factors and asthma are linked must also be considered to prevent a downward spiral of morbidity and disability (Figure 20.1).

Direct effects of psychosocial factors on asthma: psychosocial triggers

There are a number of ways in which psychosocial factors can directly affect asthma disease processes. At one level, blue-collar occupations, poor housing and other socioeconomic adversity may result in increased exposure to irritants, allergens and pathogens in the workplace or home, and thus contribute directly to asthma symptoms and exacerbations.[79]

At another level, 'stress' is commonly cited as a trigger for symptoms and attacks, particularly in susceptible individuals sometimes referred to as having 'intrinsic' asthma.[80] Asthma, the impacts it has, treatment demands, life events and psychosocial problems unrelated to asthma represent challenges or stressors for patients, especially in combination. These can lead to the experience of stress, defined as occurring when perceived demands outweigh a person's perceived ability to cope, and thus representing an interaction between person and situation or stressor and response.[2]

Epidemiological and experimental studies in asthma, along with research mapping neuroendocrinological and neuroimmunological changes

associated with the stress response, highlight ways in which stress and emotions might trigger symptoms or excerbations via various pathophysiological mechanisms implicated in both allergic and non-allergic asthma.[11,80] Although there are some contradictory findings with regard to effects of acute stress, it is increasingly accepted that, at least in some individuals, inappropriate coping with an acute stressor, or exposure to chronic stress, can lead to more prolonged physiological, behavioral, cognitive and emotional changes that may be particularly detrimental to physical and mental health.[81] Chronic stress alters immune functioning, increasing susceptibility to pathogens and potentially intensifying inflammatory and autoimmune processes which may be of importance in asthma.[80] Long-term effects of stress, and impacts of episodes of acute stress imposed upon a background of chronic stress, are complex and still poorly understood.[81] However, patients dealing with severe chronic illness or frequent acute exacerbations, especially in combination with other ongoing psychosocial problems, may be at particular risk from the effects of stress on asthma and other physical or mental health problems which can further affect the disease and its management.

Biopsychosocial factors, including personality characteristics and social support, influence perceptions of demands and a person's coping and can thus mediate the psychological and physiological effects of stress.[2] This implies the need for supportive programs incorporating training in relaxation or other techniques to help patients, especially those with high levels of anxiety or identifying psychosocial triggers, cope with stress and manage emotions. This is important since, as well as affecting asthma directly as highlighted, stress can indirectly affect asthma via behavioral pathways (Figure 20.1).

Indirect effects of psychosocial factors on asthma: self-care behavior

Psychosocial factors affect asthma indirectly via their influence on patient behaviors which can increase or reduce susceptibility to symptoms or exacerbations. Interest in psychosocial influences on asthma has indeed been revived in recent years with the emphasis placed on self-management.[3,6]

Adherence to medication is a key behavior in self-management and a vast literature covering its defintion, assessment, effects and influences in asthma and other conditions is comprehensively reviewed elsewhere.[82–85] Non-adherence, particularly to preventive medication, and other indicators of poor compliance (e.g. self-discharge from hospital, failure to attend scheduled appointments or follow advice regarding self-monitoring) have frequently been associated with a range of adverse asthma outcomes.[18,21,26,28,31] Some commentaries suggest that adherence is lowest amongst patients with mild and severe disease,[84] but empirical findings are inconsistent with regard to whether patients previously hospitalized with asthma are more or less adherent.[86,87] Despite its importance, surprisingly little is known about optimal levels of adherence for different patient groups and there is a lack of evidence on the relative importance of different aspects of compliance and other dimensions of self-care.[83] That other behaviors are important, however, is demonstrated in a study of allergy which compared 28 patients with severe disease to 26 patients with mild asthma.[88] This found that a significantly higher proportion of patients with severe asthma were sensitized and exposed to the common allergens of house dust mites, dogs and cats, illustrating not only that allergy is important in severe asthma, but also that patients with severe disease were behaving inappropriately by keeping pets to which they were allergic.

Performance of any behavior central to effective self-care, including taking and adjusting medications, monitoring asthma, avoiding triggers, seeking medical attention when needed, attending regular appointments and communicating problems, is affected by internal psychosocial characteristics and external psychosocial influences in the same way as other health-related behaviors.[12,89] For example, in a study of 138 patients admitted to hospital with asthma, management errors were mainly related to inadequate self-care behavior, which was predicted by social, economic and psychological characteristics.[10] In addition to associated disease, treatment and health-professional/consultation factors, research has identified that there is a complex relationship between psychosocial factors and adherence.[82–85]

Research has failed to identify consistent relationships between sociodemographic, socioeconomic or enduring personality characteristics and adherence;[82] however, social factors may influence access to services[90] and resources[91] to support effective self-care. Recent empirical and theoretical developments in health psychology have begun to highlight dynamic, and potentially mutable, psychological factors underpinning medication adherence,[82] although work on other self-care behaviors is more limited.[89] Beliefs about the illness and medication seem to be key in predicting whether patients adhere to preventive therapies.[92] Models of health-related behavior change suggest how these beliefs are translated into behavior and influenced by underlying stable characteristics.[2,12,82] For example, the Theory of Planned Behavior suggests that behavior is immediately determined by a person's intentions to perform the behavior and perceptions of control over the behavior.[82] The latter is similar to the concept of self-efficacy, shown to be a key predictor of a range of health-related behaviors[12,82] and which has been studied to some extent in asthma.[83] Underpinning intentions and perceived control are beliefs about, and valuations of, the costs and benefits of performing the behavior, beliefs about others' views and a patients' motivation to comply with these views, plus beliefs about internal and external factors influencing perceived ability to perform the behavior.[82] The Health Belief Model also suggests that beliefs about susceptibility to, and the severity of, an illness or outcome (e.g. exacerbations), are important.[12,82–84]

These theories highlight factors to be assessed and targeted in order to improve adherence and other self-care behaviors. They suggest the need to elicit patients' beliefs about their illness, treatment, aspects of management and the views of significant others; address any misconceptions inherent in these (e.g. in relation to side-effects of treatment); agree management goals in partnership with patients to balance costs and benefits of treatment (i.e. promote concordance); and enhance patients' skills and confidence in their ability to perform behaviors central to effective self-care.[12,82,84] Further theories, for example the Stages of Change Model,[2,12,82] recognize that since behavior change is a process rather than an event, interventions may need to be targeted according to individuals' stage of readiness to change. It provides a framework within which common psychotherapeutic principles for facilitating change, including cognitive and behavioral techniques that are increasingly used in medical settings,[12] can be used in a timely fashion to influence the above psychological factors unpinning behavior.

The potential utility of psychological theories and psychotherapeutic approaches to intervention are increasingly discussed in the adherence and asthma literature.[12,82] Although there is a growth of empirical research into their application to management of chronic diseases, research on using these approaches to understand and influence self-management behavior in asthma, and particularly severe asthma, is limited. A point to note is that being largely 'cognitive' in nature, these models tend to assume rational decision-making and negate emotional influences on behavior[82,92] which have, for example, been shown to be important in adherence.[84] Amongst people with high levels of anxiety or depression, including a significant proportion of those with severe asthma,[18,21,27,28] emotions may first need to be addressed before patients will be motivated to undertake the problem-focused coping that self-management requires.[9] Other theories (e.g. the Self-Regulatory Model) aimed at understanding patients'

responses to illness and their behavior in terms of their dynamic appraisal of, and coping with, the challenges it presents, take account of this but are less widely researched and may be more difficult to translate into interventions.[82,92] The development of measures to assess self-care behavior and its psychological correlates in order to test the utility and applicability of psychological models to asthma self-management, especially in complex patients, is an important area for future research.[82,89] In the meantime, the above findings emphasize the need for a holistic approach to management that considers each of the pathways by which psychosocial factors and asthma interact, and attempts to intervene at relevant, often multiple points, according to individual needs (Figure 20.4).

WHAT DOES THIS TELL US ABOUT IDENTIFICATION OF PATIENTS AT RISK OF ADVERSE OUTCOMES?

In the absence of more detailed research on the interactions of psychosocial factors with severe asthma, the main conclusion that can be drawn to date is that, where one or more of the adverse psychological or social characteristics discussed are coupled with severe asthma, the risk of patients experiencing frequent or severe (e.g. fatal, near-fatal) exacerbations is increased (Table 20.2). For example, a Dutch study showed that patients with severe asthma *plus* psychiatric caseness were at increased risk of frequent general practitioner and A&E visits, exacerbations and hospitalizations compared to those with severe asthma but no psychiatric problems.[93]

Since poor compliance with medical or self-care recommendations appears to be a key mechanism by which underlying psychosocial characteristics influence asthma outcomes,[18,85] we conducted a study to determine whether clinician-identified poor compliance was useful in identifying, from amongst adults with severe asthma, patients with characteristics

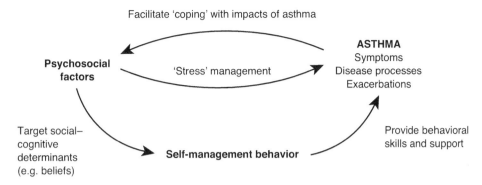

Figure 20.4 Intervention points for psychoeducational programs

Table 20.2 Patients at risk of developing near-fatal or fatal asthma or being admitted to hospital with asthma. Modified from Table 3 in reference 3

A combination of *severe asthma* recognized by one or more of:
    previous near-fatal asthma, e.g. previous ventilation or respiratory acidosis
    previous admission for asthma, especially if in the past year
    requiring BTS step 4 or 5 treatment
    brittle asthma

And *adverse behavioral or psychosocial features* recognized by one or more of:
    poor compliance with treatment or monitoring including
        failure to attend appointments
        self-discharge from hospital
    psychosis, depression, other psychiatric illness or deliberate self-harm
    current or recent major tranquilizer use
    denial
    alcohol or drug abuse
    obesity
    learning difficulties
    employment problems
    income problems
    social isolation
    childhood abuse
    severe domestic, marital or legal stress

BTS, British Thoracic Society

likely to put them at risk of experiencing adverse asthma events.[94] We also explored physical and psychosocial co-morbidities associated with patients being identified as poorly compliant. A cross-sectional study examined differences between two groups with severe asthma that differed in the extent to which they were considered compliant. We drew on common clinical experience to reflect

how poor compliance might be identified routinely, namely poor compliance indicated by patients not attending appointments, taking medication and/or monitoring asthma as agreed.

Our results suggest that, compared to compliant (C) patients with severe asthma, patients with severe asthma identified by clinicians as being poorly compliant (PC) had significantly poorer self-reported asthma control in terms of symptoms, asthma-specific quality of life, rescue and exacerbation-related medication use, absenteeism, primary care visits and A&E attendances or hospital admissions. They were also significantly more likely to be engaging in behaviors and using coping strategies indicative of poor self-management. Furthermore, PC patients shared other clinical and psychosocial characteristics with those experiencing serious adverse events (deaths, NFA) in previous studies[17-35] which were not evident amongst the C group. Co-morbid anxiety, younger age, indicators of social deprivation (being out of work, in receipt of a higher number of welfare benefits) and adverse family circumstances were shown to be psychosocial factors independently associated with patients being identified as PC. These psychosocial characteristics and adversities might be hypothesized to contribute to the poorly compliant behavior.

Our data suggest that clinicians can identify broad patterns of poor compliance in patients with severe asthma, indicated in particular by failure to attend routine appointments. This is linked to poor asthma control, co-morbidities and psychosocial difficulties, and is useful in identifying a subgroup of patients in whom a combination of poor asthma control and inadequate self-care is likely to put them at risk of future hospital admissions for asthma and near-fatal or fatal attacks.[10,26,32,33,42] These findings emphasize the complexity of the problems these patients face, the need for consideration of psychosocial issues in their routine care and the difficulty of designing and evaluating sufficiently powerful interventions to improve management of their asthma.

HOW CAN PSYCHOSOCIAL ISSUES BE ADDRESSED IN SEVERE ASTHMA?

Many psychosocial factors are potentially amenable to intervention. Programs involving education, training in self-management and/or targeting specific psychological or social issues

resulting from or impacting on asthma are increasingly being implemented alongside conventional medical treatment to address them. The emphasis on patient self-care has meant that training in self-management and asthma education in particular have become central to the overall management of asthma in recent years.[3,6]

There is increasing overlap between self-management education and other psychological and social support interventions, with recognition that there is a need for all programs to take account of psychological theories of behavior change and be tailored to address individual psychosocial and behavioral needs.[12,89] This is especially true in difficult patient groups.[84,85] An increasing number of programs also attempt to intervene at various points in the cyclical relationship between psychological factors and asthma highlighted (Figure 20.1) by incorporating, for example, education and training in self-management, relaxation and other stress management techniques and support for coping with the impact of chronic disease (Figure 20.4). For this reason, psychotherapeutic, social support, educational and self-management interventions in asthma are sometimes considered together as 'psychoeducational' programs.

ARE PSYCHOEDUCATIONAL INTERVENTIONS EFFECTIVE IN SEVERE ASTHMA?

Existing reviews suggest that some psychoeducational interventions can be effective in certain patient groups. A Cochrane review of 36 trials concluded that self-management education was effective in improving health outcomes in general adult asthma populations.[95] However, good evidence on other types of intervention addressing psychosocial issues resulting from, or impacting on, asthma is limited.[96] Furthermore, findings from most existing studies are unlikely to be generalizable to patients at risk of adverse outcomes, in whom the complex interplay of clinical and psychosocial factors

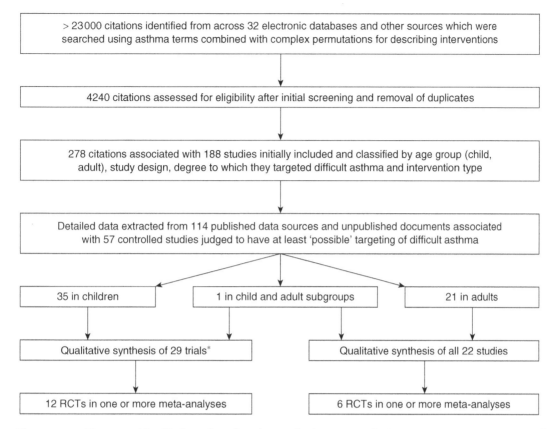

Figure 20.5 Literature identified, reviewed and contributing to conclusions in a systematic review of psychoeducational interventions for severe and difficult asthma. From reference 97. RCT, randomized controlled trial; *results from seven poor quality controlled observational studies were not considered further

frequently complicates management and who are thus often excluded from, or fail to attend, standard programs.[85] For this reason, we recently conducted a systematic review of a full range of psychoeducational interventions for severe and difficult-to-manage asthma.[97] An overview of the review process, literature identified and studies considered is presented in Figure 20.5.

Our review showed that there has been a rapid and continuing growth of research in this field, with the largest proportion of research to date conducted in the USA. Reporting of interventions and methodological quality was often poor but the majority of studies identified demonstrated some success in targeting and

following up at-risk patients. The range of outcomes assessed and variations in the ways they were measured and reported precluded quantitative synthesis for most. However, studies reporting data suitable for calculation of summary statistics were of higher quality than those that did not. These provided evidence that, compared to usual or non-psychoeducational care, psychoeducational interventions reduced admissions when data from the latest follow-ups reported were pooled across six studies targeting adult patients with severe asthma, but lacking other characteristics likely to put them at risk (RR = 0.57, 95% CI 0.34, 0.93; Figure 20.6). There was no evidence from our review of pooled

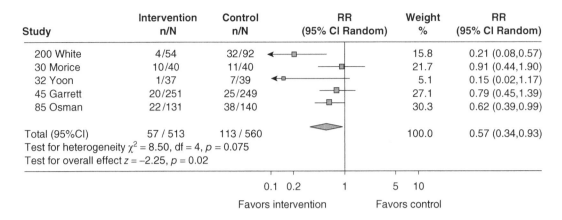

Study	Intervention n/N	Control n/N	RR (95% CI Random)	Weight %	RR (95% CI Random)
200 White	4/54	32/92		15.8	0.21 (0.08,0.57)
30 Morice	10/40	11/40		21.7	0.91 (0.44,1.90)
32 Yoon	1/37	7/39		5.1	0.15 (0.02,1.17)
45 Garrett	20/251	25/249		27.1	0.79 (0.45,1.39)
85 Osman	22/131	38/140		30.3	0.62 (0.39,0.99)
Total (95%CI)	57 / 513	113 / 560		100.0	0.57 (0.34,0.93)

Test for heterogeneity $\chi^2 = 8.50$, df = 4, $p = 0.075$
Test for overall effect $z = -2.25$, $p = 0.02$

0.1 0.2   1   5 10

Favors intervention   Favors control

Figure 20.6 Forest plot showing meta-analysis for proportions of patients admitted at latest follow-up reported by studies of psychoeducational interventions targeting adults with severe asthma but lacking other risk factors. From reference 97

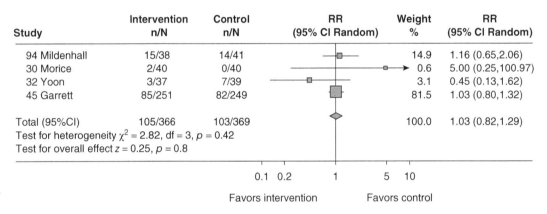

Study	Intervention n/N	Control n/N	RR (95% CI Random)	Weight %	RR (95% CI Random)
94 Mildenhall	15/38	14/41		14.9	1.16 (0.65,2.06)
30 Morice	2/40	0/40		0.6	5.00 (0.25,100.97)
32 Yoon	3/37	7/39		3.1	0.45 (0.13,1.62)
45 Garrett	85/251	82/249		81.5	1.03 (0.80,1.32)
Total (95%CI)	105/366	103/369		100.0	1.03 (0.82,1.29)

Test for heterogeneity $\chi^2 = 2.82$, df = 3, $p = 0.42$
Test for overall effect $z = 0.25$, $p = 0.8$

0.1 0.2   1   5 10

Favors intervention   Favors control

Figure 20.7 Forest plot showing meta-analysis for proportions of patients attending accident and emergency at latest follow-up reported by studies of psychoeducational interventions targeting adults with severe or difficult asthma. From reference 97

effects of psychoeducational interventions on A&E attendances from four studies in adults (RR = 1.03, 95% CI 0.82, 1.29; Figure 20.7). With respect to all other outcomes where sufficient data allowed conclusions to be drawn, studies showed mixed results or suggested limited effectiveness of psychoeducational interventions. No studies of specific psychotherapeutic or social support interventions were included in any quantitative syntheses and it was not possible to draw clear conclusions regarding the relative

effectiveness of educational, self-management and multifaceted programs. However, the delivery, setting, timing and content of interventions varied considerably, even within these broad types, suggesting that alternative ways of conceptualizing these in light of the way in which psychosocial factors and asthma interact may be necessary (Figure 20.4).

A larger evidence base on psychoeducational interventions in children with severe and difficult asthma and limited data in adults suggest

Table 20.3 Recommendations for the management of patients with severe asthma and adverse behavioral or psychosocial characteristics

Primary care
Create an at-risk register
Liaise with secondary care respiratory specialist

Secondary care
Create a special clinic with longer consultation times and input from a combination of a consultant respiratory physician, an asthma nurse and a psychological therapist

Both
Maintain contact with patients who fail to attend appointments
Always try to involve a close relative or friend in education and understanding about asthma and share the agreed management plan

that the possible benefits of psychoeducational programs indicated by our review may not extend to those most at risk.[97] For example, in our own randomized controlled trial of a 6-month home-based, nurse-led psychoeducational program for patients with severe asthma who were poorly compliant with recommended management, limited short-term changes in aspects of self-management (peak flow monitoring and use of reliever inhaler) did not translate into any changes in health outcomes in the short or long term.[98] Data also suggest that the significantly increased costs of providing the intervention were not offset by any short-term savings in use of health-care resources. Other data on costs and cost-effectiveness of psychoeducational programs for patients with severe asthma who are at particular risk of adverse outcomes are very limited in quantity and quality.

WHAT ARE THE IMPLICATIONS FOR CURRENT CARE OF PATIENTS WITH SEVERE ASTHMA?

In patients with severe asthma alone, our review suggests that provision of psychoeducational interventions (especially those incorporating formal self-management) may reduce hospital admissions but potentially at increased overall cost. There is currently a lack of evidence,

however, to warrant significant changes in clinical practice with regard to care of patients with severe asthma plus additional characteristics likely to increase their risk of experiencing adverse events.

Better identification and recognition of such patients, taking into account the different pathophysiological, clinical, compliance and psychosocial risk factors, might improve their care, enhance the value of future audit and aid in the targeting of any new interventions. There is thus a need for primary and secondary research to clarify key risk factors and develop tools for better identifying patients susceptible to adverse asthma outcomes. In the meantime, current recommendations are summarized in Table 20.3. Until further research on the effectiveness of psychoeducational interventions is available, the emphasis should be on optimization of medical care for these patients, taking account of potential complicating psychosocial factors, to ensure that the number continuing to experience poor control of symptoms and frequent exacerbations is minimized. Ideally, such patients should be managed jointly across primary and secondary care by a consultant respiratory physician and asthma nurse interested in this area. Pragmatic approaches to managing at-risk patients are summarized in Table 20.3 and our own experiences in implementing some of these are discussed below.

At-risk registers in primary care

Primary care practitioners are likely to have the most frequent contact with patients at risk of adverse asthma outcomes and be well placed to understand the complexity of the co-morbidity, psychological, social and environmental issues they face. However, despite the fact that the majority of asthma care in the UK is delivered in primary care, most interventions for these patients to date have been conducted in hospital settings.[97] Programs delivered in primary care could capitalize on opportunistic intervention and outreach to overcome many of the barriers to at-risk patients attending organized programs or accessing secondary care facilities.[85]

There are anecdotal reports (G Mohan, personal communication) for the benefit of establishing a register of patients at risk from their asthma so that they can be identified and their routine care improved. This approach was recently piloted in a local general practice.[99] Twenty-six patients with severe asthma (3% of those registered with asthma in a general practice population of 8800) plus other clinical and psychosocial characteristics consistently associated with poor outcomes were added to an at-risk register. Tags were placed in these patients' electronic and paper notes and all practice staff were provided with training to ensure recognition of the patients' at-risk status and their appropriate management. Data on service use and emergency treatments were retrospectively extracted from notes for all at-risk patients and 26 age-, sex- and treatment-matched control patients with asthma for 1 year before and 1 year after the introduction of the register. Service use was costed using published national unit cost data and the cost of introducing the register estimated on the basis of local expenditure.

In the year before introduction of the register, more at-risk than control patients were hospitalized (three vs. none), attended A&E (one vs. none) and were nebulized (four vs. none) for acute asthma. Significantly higher numbers also used out-of-hours services, attended the general practitioner, failed to attend scheduled clinics and received oral steroids for asthma (all $p < 0.025$). The year after introduction of the register, no at-risk patients were admitted or attended A&E. Although differences in the numbers receiving oral steroids remained ($p = 0.05$), other differences disappeared (all $p > 0.235$). There were notably greater reductions in overall numbers of admissions, out-of-hours attendances, general practitioner attendances, courses of steroids and total costs associated with service use amongst at-risk compared to control patients.

These preliminary data suggest that the introduction of an at-risk asthma register is a low-cost intervention (estimated at £17 per patient) that may improve appropriate use of services in a vulnerable and costly patient group. However, a formal larger-scale evaluation of this innovation is required before it can be recommended for wider implementation.

Combined clinic in secondary care

A further approach we have developed is to offer patients at risk from their asthma referral to a combined clinic run jointly by a psychiatrist and a chest physician.[100] Clearly, patients' housing, employment or relationship problems cannot be resolved at a stroke. However, we can ensure at a practical level that all appropriate benefits are being claimed and available services being accessed. Including a psychiatrist in an asthma clinic contributes a different perspective to the conventional medical one, with importance placed on the meaning given to events. We have observed that acknowledgment of issues by patients, family, doctors and nurses can be extremely helpful and lead to the exploration of strategies for coping with problems, including asthma, in a more positive and less harmful way. Some patients have been brought up in families where one or both parents see physical illness, and particularly asthma, as a weakness. In others, asthma may be the main factor keeping their parents' marriage together. Experience of death from asthma, particularly if in the same family, is bound to alter a person's approach to another relative with asthma and difficulties in relationships can complicate management.

In some patients, asthma interferes with their self-perceptions. For example, 'copers' who are often professional people, most frequently in health, other caring or teaching professions, see themselves as helping others and have difficulty adjusting to the patient role. This can lead to denial of symptoms and of the need to take necessary therapy. Sometimes there are secondary gains, since severe asthma can attract financial compensation. Especially in cases when the event initiating asthma was extremely traumatic (e.g. in the military or in an industrial accident), or when a partner has given up paid employment to look after the patient, effective management may be compromised. Several patients' asthma began during an abusive or disastrous adult relationship and triggers which bring back memories of those times can be difficult to handle, especially if they are not understood or accepted. As our psychiatrist colleagues emphasize for all patients, but especially for at-risk asthmatics, we must try to understand the meaning of their asthma and of medication to themselves and their families, and explore their beliefs about asthma, its treatment and its effects on family dynamics and social and occupational interactions.

Psychological and psychiatric interventions are often considered time consuming and the outcomes difficult to measure. Although not subject to formal evaluation, we have found that the combined clinic utilizes a psychiatrist's time in a focused manner within the context of the respiratory team with a number of benefits. Perhaps the most important is that the intervention is acceptable to patients who, when referred for separate psychiatric assessment, may not attend appointments and, indeed, may reject the suggestion, which can undermine the relationship with their physician. Understanding and

acceptance of the interactions between physical and psychosocial factors are reached more accurately and more promptly, which facilitates patient concordance with their management. The psychiatrist can access a range of psychological therapies when indicated and advise on the use of psychotropic medication and management of drug and alcohol misuse. Most of the patients we have seen have not been psychiatrically ill, meaning that many psychiatrists would not regard them as patients. It is thus important to stress that the most useful colleagues in this work are psychiatrists or psychological therapists who are interested in how people cope or manage their lives rather than whether or not they have a psychiatric diagnosis. Finally, it is important, where acceptable to the individual, to see patients with a close family member or friend. This not only aids in understanding the current situation and what might have happened in the past, but also facilitates involvement of the other person in the future support of the patient.

WHAT IS THE WAY FORWARD?

This chapter has emphasized the importance of psychosocial factors in severe asthma, brought to the fore the pathways by which psychosocial factors and asthma interact (Figure 20.1) and emphasized that psychoeducational programs targeting patients with severe asthma might be further classified and designed in terms of the pathways, or number of pathways, they target (Figure 20.4). Limited findings from our own research on severe asthma, trends in the broader evidence base and theoretical developments in psychology suggest that multidisciplinary, multifaceted interventions incorporating formal self-management and medical care, and utilizing formal psychoeducational theories or approaches in their delivery, may be the most promising approaches warranting further evaluation. Multiprofessional working is key, since an asthma nurse may be best placed to provide training in self-management skills, whilst a psychologist may be able to address the influence of psychosocial factors on self-care behaviors or provide training for nurses with respect to these aspects of care. Likewise, a respiratory clinician may understand the ways in which psychosocial factors directly impact on pathophysiological mechanisms in asthma, but may in turn need advice or input from an interested psychiatrist or clinical psychologist to find ways of addressing these and treating psychosocial difficulties resulting from living with a chronic disease. There is also a role for social care agencies and referral in dealing with more severe social consequences and determinants of poor asthma control. Recent research demonstrates that a patient's psychosocial status and beliefs may have different implications in terms of outcomes, depending on whether a patient has experienced a recent attack or not.[101] This potentially implies the need for different approaches to management for patients experiencing frequent or severe exacerbations and those experiencing chronically severe, but controlled, disease. Future programs for patients with severe asthma might be broad-based approaches addressing a range of intervention points which are adapted to individual needs for a wide spectrum of at-risk patients, or specific interventions matched to the needs of particular well-defined groups (e.g. patients with poor self-management, identifying psychosocial triggers or experiencing psychosocial difficulties resulting from asthma).

There continues to be an urgent need to educate doctors and nurses about the detection of psychological, social and behavioral problems in patients with severe asthma (Table 20.2). If we do not respond, we will be failing to meet one of the most important ongoing challenges of asthma management at the beginning of the 21st century, and countless patients will be denied effective control of their asthma. As our review of the literature indicates, there is also a need for further well-conducted research to improve our understanding of, and evaluate interventions in, this field.

REFERENCES

1. Osler W. The Principles and Practice of Medicine, 4th edn. New York: D Appleton & Co, 1901

2. Sarafino EP. Health Psychology, Biopsychosocial Interactions, 4th edn. New York: Wiley, 2001

3. British Thoracic Society, Scottish Intercollegiate Guideline Network. British guideline on the management of asthma. Thorax 2003; 58 (Suppl 1): 1i–83i

4. Crane J, Pearce N, Burgess C, et al. Markers of risk of asthma death or readmission in the 12 months following a hospital admission for asthma. Int J Epidemiol 1992; 21: 737–44

5. Harrison BDW. Difficult asthma. Thorax 2003; 58: 555–6

6. National Asthma Education and Prevention Program. Expert Panel Report 2. Guidelines for the Diagnosis and Management of Asthma. Bethesda, MD: National Heart, Lung and Blood Institute, 1997

7. Patterson R, Greenberger PA. Problem cases in asthma and problems in asthma management. Chest 1992; 101 (6 Suppl): 430–1s

8. Keeley D, Osman L. Dysfunctional breathing and asthma. BMJ 2001; 322: 1075–6

9. Salmon P. Psychology of Medicine and Surgery. Chichester: John Wiley & Sons, 2000

10. Kolbe J, Vamos M, Fergusson W, Elkind G. Determinants of management errors in acute severe asthma. Thorax 1998; 53: 14–20

11. Wright RJ, Rodriguez M, Cohen S. Review of psychosocial stress and asthma: an integrated biopsychosocial approach. Thorax 1998; 53: 1066–74

12. Kehoe WA, Katz RC. Health behaviors and pharmacotherapy. Ann Pharmacother 1998; 32: 1076–86

13. Affleck G, Apter A, Tennen H, et al. Mood states associated with transitory changes in asthma symptoms and peak expiratory flow. Psychosom Med 2000; 62: 61–8

14. Adams R, Ruffin R, Campbell D. Psychosocial factors in severe asthma. In Holgate ST, Boushey HO, Fabbri LM, eds. Difficult Asthma. London: Martin Dunitz, 1999: 413–43

15. Fregonese L, Silvestri M, Sabatini F, et al. Severe and near-fatal asthma in children and adolescents. Monaldi Arch Chest Dis 2001; 56: 423–8

16. Marshik P, Kelly HW, Murphy S. Severe asthma in childhood: special considerations. In Holgate ST, Boushey HO, Fabbri LM, eds. Difficult Asthma. London: Martin Dunitz, 1999: 225–52

17. Wareham NJ, Harrison BDW, Jenkins PF, et al. A district confidential enquiry into deaths due to asthma. Thorax 1993; 48: 1117–20

18. Mohan G, Harrison BDW, Badminton RM, et al. A confidential enquiry into deaths caused by asthma in an English health region: implications for general practice. Br J Gen Pract 1996; 46: 529–32

19. Bucknall CE, Slack R, Godley CC, et al., on behalf of SCIAD collaborators. Scottish confidential inquiry into asthma deaths (SCIAD) 1994–6. Thorax 1999; 54: 978–84

20. Burr ML, Davies BH, Hoare A, et al. A confidential inquiry into asthma deaths in Wales. Thorax 1999; 54: 985–9

21. Harrison BDW, Slack R, Berrill WT, et al. Results of a national confidential enquiry into asthma deaths. Asthma J 2000; 5: 180–6

22. Rea HH, Scragg R, Jackson R, et al. A case–control study of deaths from asthma. Thorax 1986; 41: 833–9

23. Joseph KS, Blais L, Ernst P, Suissa S. Increased morbidity and mortality related to asthma among asthmatic patients who use major tranquillisers. BMJ 1996; 312: 79–82

24. Jalaludin BB, Smith MA, Chey T, et al. Risk factors for asthma deaths: a population-based, case–control study. Aust NZ J Public Health 1999; 23: 595–600

25. Hessel PA, Mitchell I, Tough S, et al., for the Prairie Provinces Asthma Study Group. Risk factors for death from asthma. Ann Allergy Asthma Immunol 1999; 83: 362–8

26. Sturdy PM, Victor CR, Anderson HR, et al., on behalf of the Mortality and Severe Morbidity Working Group of the National Asthma Task Force. Psychological, social and health behavior risk factors for deaths certified as asthma: a national case–control study. Thorax 2002; 57: 1034–9

27. Yellowlees PM, Ruffin RE. Psychological defences and coping styles in patients following a life-threatening attack of asthma. Chest 1989; 95: 1298–303

28. Campbell DA, Yellowlees PM, McLennan G, et al. Psychiatric and medical features of near fatal asthma. Thorax 1995; 50: 254–9

29. Richards GN, Kolbe J, Fenwick J, Rea HH. Demographic characteristics of patients with severe life threatening asthma: comparison with asthma deaths. Thorax 1993; 48: 1105–9

30. Campbell DA, McLennan G, Coates JR, et al. A comparison of asthma deaths and near-fatal asthma attacks in South Australia. Eur Respir J 1994; 7: 490–7

31. Innes NJ, Reid A, Halstead J, et al. Psychosocial risk factors in near-fatal asthma and in asthma deaths. J R Coll Physicians Lond 1998; 32: 430–4

32. Kolbe J, Fergusson W, Vamos M, Garrett J. Case–control study of severe life threatening asthma (SLTA) in adults: demographics, health care, and management of the acute attack. Thorax 2000; 55: 1007–15

33. Kolbe J, Fergusson W, Vamos M, Garrett J. Case–control study of severe life threatening asthma (SLTA) in adults: psychological factors. Thorax 2002; 57: 317–22

34. LeSon S, Gershwin ME. Risk factors for intubation of adult asthma patients. J Asthma 1995; 32: 97–104

35. Mitchell I, Tough SC, Semple LK, et al. Near-fatal asthma: a population-based study of risk factors. Chest 2002; 121: 1407–13

36. Gottlieb DJ, Beiser AS, O'Connor GT. Poverty, race, and medication use are correlates of asthma hospitalization rates: a small areas analysis in Boston. Chest 1995; 108: 28–35

37. Fox Ray N, Thamer Mae, Fadillioglu B, Gergen PJ. Race, income, urbanicity, and asthma hospitalization in California: a small areas analysis. Chest 1998; 113: 1277–84

38. Gilthorpe MA, Lay-Yee R, Wilson RC, et al. Variations in hospitalization rates for asthma among black and minority ethnic communities. Respir Med 1998; 92: 642–8

39. Griffiths C, Kaur G, Gantley M, et al. Influences on hospital admission for asthma in south Asian and white adults: qualitative interview study. BMJ 2001; 323: 962

40. Ryan G, Stock H, Musk AW, et al. Risk factors for death in patients admitted to hospital with asthma: a follow-up study. Aust NZ J Med 1991; 21: 681–5

41. Ruffin RE, Latimer KM, Schembri DA. Longitudinal study of near fatal asthma. Chest 1991; 99: 77–83

42. Adams RJ, Smith BJ, Ruffin RE. Factors associated with hospital admissions and repeat emergency department visits for adults with asthma. Thorax 2000; 55: 566–73

43. Ayres J, Miles JF. Brittle asthma. In Holgate ST, Boushey HO, Fabbri LM, eds. Difficult Asthma. London: Martin Dunitz; 1999: 291–305

44. Garden GMF, Ayres JG. Psychiatric and social aspects of brittle asthma. Thorax 1993; 48: 501–5

45. Miles JF, Garden GMF, Tunnicliffe WS, et al. Psychological morbidity and coping skills in patients with brittle and non-brittle asthma: a case control study. Clin Exp Allergy 1997; 27: 1151–9

46. Wasserfallen JB, Schaller MD, Feihl F, Perret CH. Sudden asphyxic asthma: a distinct entity? Am Rev Respir Dis 1990; 142: 108–11

47. Sur S, Crotty TB, Kephart GM, et al. Sudden onset fatal asthma. A distinct entity with few eosinophils and relatively more neutrophils in the airway submucosa? Am Rev Respir Dis 1993; 148: 713–19

48. ten Brinke A, Ouwerkerk ME, Bel EH, Spinhoven PH. Similar psychological characteristics in mild and severe asthma. J Psychosom Res 2001; 50: 7–10

49. ENFUMOSA Study Group. The ENFUMOSA cross-sectional European multicentre study of the clinical phenotype of chronic severe asthma. Eur Respir J 2003; 22: 470–7

50. Schmier JK, Chan KS, Leidy NK. The impact of asthma on health-related quality of life. J Asthma 1998; 35: 585–97

51. Hyland ME, Finnis S, Irvine SH. A scale for assessing quality of life in adult asthma sufferers. J Psychosom Res 1991; 35: 99–110

52. Nocon A, Booth T. The social impact of asthma: a review of the literature. Soc Work Soc Sci Rev 1989–90; 1: 177–200

53. Brown ES, Khan DA, Nejtek VA. The psychiatric side effects of corticosteroids. Ann Allergy Asthma Immunol 1999; 83: 495–504

54. Bowling A. Measuring Disease. Buckingham: Open University Press, 2001: 163–88

55. Maillé AR, Kaptein AA, de Haes JCJM, et al., WTAM. Assessing quality of life in chronic non-specific lung disease – a review of empirical studies published between 1980 and 1994. Qual Life Res 1996; 5: 287–301

56. Juniper EF, Guyatt GH, Epstein RS, et al. Evaluation of impairment of health related quality of life in asthma: development of a questionnaire for use in clinical trials. Thorax 1992; 47: 76–83

57. Marks GB, Dunn SM, Woolcock AJ. A scale for the measurement of quality of life in adults with asthma. J Clin Epidemiol 1992; 45: 461–72

58. Rowe BH, Oxman AD. Performance of an asthma quality of life questionnaire in an outpatient setting. Am Rev Respir Dis 1993; 148: 675–81

59. Ware JE Jr, Sherbourne CD. The MOS 36-item Short-form Health Survey (SF-36). Med Care 1992; 30: 473–83

60. Ware JE, Kosinski M, Keller SD. A 12-Item Short-Form Health Survey: construction of scales and preliminary tests of reliability and validity. Med Care 1996; 34: 220–33

61. Zigmond AS, Snaith RP. The Hospital Anxiety and Depression Scale. Acta Psychiatr Scand 1983; 67: 361–70

62. Goldberg DP, Williams P. A User's Guide to the General Health Questionnaire. Windsor, UK: NFER Nelson, 1988

63. Bousquet J, Knani J, Dhivert H, et al. Quality of life in asthma. I. Internal consistency and validity of the SF-36 questionnaire. Am J Respir Crit Care Med 1994; 149: 371–5

64. Viramontes JL, O'Brien B. Relationship between symptoms and health-related quality of life in chronic lung disease. J Gen Intern Med 1994; 9: 46–8

65. Fitzpatrick MF, Engleman H, Whyte KF, et al. Morbidity in nocturnal asthma: sleep quality and daytime cognitive performance. Thorax 1991; 46: 569–73

66. Juniper EF, Svensson K, Mörk A-C, Ståhl E. Measuring health-related quality of life in adults during an acute asthma exacerbation. Chest 2004; 125: 93–7

67. Skirrow P, Jones C, Griffiths RD, Kaney S. Intensive care – easing the trauma. Psychologist 2001; 14: 640–2

68. Leidy NK, Coughlin C. Psychometric performance of the Asthma Quality of Life Questionnaire in a US sample. Qual Life Res 1998; 7: 127–34

69. Adams RJ, Ruffin RE, Smith BJ, Wilson D. Impact of coping and socioeconomic factors on quality of life in adults with asthma. Respirology 2004; 9: 87–95

70. Adams RJ, Wilson DH, Taylor AW, et al. Psychological factors and asthma quality of life: a population based study. Thorax 2004; 59: 930–5

71. Rutten-van Molken MPMH, Custers F, Van Doorslaer EKA, et al. Comparison of performance of four quality of life instruments in evaluating the effects of salmeterol on asthma quality of life. Eur Respir J 1995; 8: 888–98

72. van der Molen T, Postma DS, Schreurs AJM, et al. Discriminative aspects of two generic and two asthma-specific instruments: relation with symptoms, bronchodilator use and lung function in patients with mild asthma. Qual Life Res 1997; 6: 353–61

73. Jenkinson C, Coulter A, Wright L. SF 36 health survey questionnaire normative data for adults of working age. BMJ 1993; 306: 1437–40

74. Juniper EF, Guyatt GH, Cox FM, et al. Development and validation of the Mini Asthma Quality of Life Questionnaire. Eur Respir J 1999; 14: 32–8

75. Higginson IJ, Carr AJ. The clinical utility of quality of life measures. In Carr AJ, Higginson IJ, Robinson PG, eds. Quality of Life. London: BMJ Publishing Group, 2003

76. Jones PW. Interpreting thresholds for a clinically significant change in health status in asthma and COPD. Eur Respir J 2002; 19: 398–404

77. Rees PJ. Perception of breathlessness. Asthma J 1996; December: 11–15

78. Eisner MD, Ackerson LM, Chi F, et al. Health-related quality of life and future health care utilization for asthma. Ann Allergy Asthma Immunol 2002; 89: 46–55

79. Rona RJ. Asthma and poverty. Thorax 2000; 55: 239–44

80. Mrazek DA, Klinnert M. Asthma: psychoneuroimmunologic considerations. In Ader R, Felton DL, Cohen N, eds. Psychoneuroimmunology. San Diego: Academic Press, 1991: 1013–35

81. Klinnert MD. Evaluating the effects of stress on asthma: a paradoxical challenge. Eur Respir J 2003; 22: 574–5

82. Myers LB, Midence K, eds. Adherence to Treatment in Medical Conditions. Amsterdam: Harwood Academic Publishers, 1998

83. Schmier JK, Leidy NK. The complexity of treatment adherence in adults with asthma: challenges and opportunities. J Asthma 1998; 35: 455–72

84. Bender B, Milgrom H, Rand C. Nonadherence in asthmatic patients: is there a solution to the problem? Ann Allergy Asthma Immunol 1997; 79: 177–86

85. Uldry C, Leuenberger P. Compliance, psychosocial factors and patient education in difficult or therapy-resistant asthma. Eur Respir Rev 2000; 10: 97–101

86. Chambers CV, Markson L, Diamond JJ, et al. Health beliefs and compliance with inhaled corticosteroids by asthmatic patients in primary care practices. Respir Med 1999; 93: 88–94

87. Put C, Verleden G, Van den Bergh O, Demedts M. A study of the relationship among self-reported noncompliance, symptomatology, and psychological variables in patients with asthma. J Asthma 2000; 37: 503–10

88. Tunnicliffe WS, Fletcher TJ, Hammond K, et al. Sensitivity and exposure to indoor allergens in adults with differing asthma severity. Eur Respir J 1999; 13: 654–9

89. Wilson SR. Patient and physician behavior models related to asthma care. Med Care 1993; 31: MS49–60

90. Jones AP, Bentham G. Health service accessibility and deaths from asthma in 401 local authority districs in England and Wales, 1988–1992. Thorax 1997; 52: 218–22

91. Apter AJ, Reisine ST, Affleck G, et al. Adherence with twice-daily dosing of inhaled steroids: socio-economic and health belief differences. Am J Respir Crit Care Med 1998; 157: 1810–17

92. Horne R, Weinman J. Self-regulation and self-management in asthma: exploring the role of illness perceptions and treatment beliefs in explaining non-adherence to preventer medication. Psychol Health 2002; 17: 17–32

93. ten Brinke A, Ouwerkerk ME, Zwinderman AH, et al. Psychopathology in patients with severe asthma is associated with increased health care utilization. Am J Respir Crit Care Med 2001; 163: 1093–6

94. Smith JR, Mildenhall S, Noble M, et al. Clinician-assessed poor compliance identifies adults with severe asthma who are at-risk of adverse outcomes. J Asthma 2005; 42: 437–45

95. Gibson PG, Powell H, Coughlan J, et al. Self-management education and regular practitioner review for adults with asthma. In The Cochrane Database of Systematic Reviews. Issue 1. Chichester: John Wiley & Sons, 2005

96. Fleming SL, Pagliari C, Churchill R, et al. Psychotherapeutic interventions for adults with asthma. In The Cochrane Database of Systematic Reviews. Issue 1. Chichester: John Wiley & Sons, 2005

97. Smith JR, Mugford M, Holland R, et al. A systematic review to examine the impact of psycho-educational interventions on health outcomes and costs in adults and children with difficult asthma. Health Technol Assess 2005; 9: 1–182

98. Smith JR, Mildenhall S, Noble MJ, et al. The Coping with Asthma Study: a randomised controlled trial of a home-based, nurse-led psychoeducational intervention for adults at risk of adverse asthma outcomes. Thorax 2005; 60: 1003–11

99. Noble M, Smith JR, Windley J. A controlled retrospective pilot study of an 'at risk asthma register' in primary care. Prim Care Respir J 2006; 15: 116–24

100. McAdam EK, Noble M, Harrison BDW. A combined clinic using a medical and psychological approach for the management of poorly controlled asthma. Asthma J 2000; 5: 71–9

101. Greaves CJ, Eiser C, Seamark D, Halpin DMG. Attack context: an important mediator of the relationship between psychological status and asthma outcomes. Thorax 2002; 57: 212–21

Index

T - #0323 - 101024 - C0 - 246/189/21 [23] - CB - 9781842143186 - Gloss Lamination